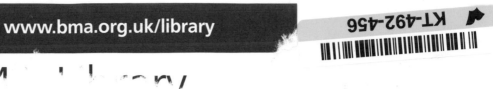
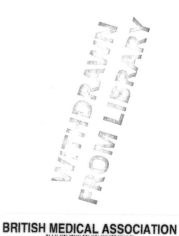

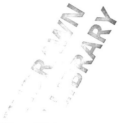

Requisites in
DERMATOLOGY
Pediatric Dermatology

For Elsevier

Commissioning Editor: Thu Nguyen
Development Editor: Claire Bonnett
Project Manager: Krishnan BalaKrishnan and Jess Thompson
Designer: Stewart Larking
Illustration Manager: Kirsteen Wright
Illustrator: Richard Prime

Requisites in DERMATOLOGY

Pediatric Dermatology

Edited by

Howard B Pride, MD

Geisinger Medical Center
Department of Pediatrics and Dermatology
Danville, PA, USA

Albert C Yan, MD

Section of Dermatology
Division of General Pediatrics
The Children's Hospital of Philadelphia,
University of Pennsylvania School of Medicine
Philadelphia, PA, USA

Andrea L Zaenglein, MD

Departments of Dermatology and Pediatrics,
Penn State University/
Milton S. Hershey Medical Center,
Hershey, PA, USA

Series editor
DIRK M ELSTON

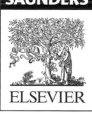

SAUNDERS

ELSEVIER

Edinburgh London New York Oxford Philadelphia St Louis Sydney Toronto 2008

SAUNDERS
ELSEVIER

An imprint of Elsevier Limited

© 2008, Elsevier Limited. All rights reserved.

First published 2008

ISBN: 978-0-7020-3022-2

British Library Cataloguing in Publication Data
A catalogue record for this book is available from the British Library

Library of Congress Cataloging in Publication Data
A catalog record for this book is available from the Library of Congress

Notice
Medical knowledge is constantly changing. Standard safety precautions must be followed, but as new research and clinical experience broaden our knowledge, changes in treatment and drug therapy may become necessary or appropriate. Readers are advised to check the most current product information provided by the manufacturer of each drug to be administered to verify the recommended dose, the method and duration of administration, and contraindications. It is the responsibility of the practitioner, relying on experience and knowledge of the patient, to determine dosages and the best treatment for each individual patient. Neither the Publisher nor the author assume any liability for any injury and/or damage to persons or property arising from this publication.

The Publisher

ELSEVIER your source for books,
journals and multimedia
in the health sciences
www.elsevierhealth.com

Working together to grow
libraries in developing countries

www.elsevier.com | www.bookaid.org | www.sabre.org

ELSEVIER   BOOK AID International   Sabre Foundation

The Publisher's policy is to use **paper manufactured from sustainable forests**

Printed in China

Last digit is the print number: 9 8 7 6 5 4 3 2 1

Contents

Contributors

Howard B Pride, MD
Geisinger Medical Center,
Department of Pediatrics and Dermatology,
Danville, PA, USA

Albert C Yan, MD
Section of Dermatology
Division of General Pediatrics
The Children's Hospital of Philadelphia
University of Pennsylvania School of Medicine
Philadelphia, PA, USA

Andrea L Zaenglein, MD
Departments of Dermatology and Pediatrics,
Penn State University/
Milton S. Hershey Medical Center,
Hershey, PA, USA

with an additional contribution by Sharon Jacob.

Series foreword

The *Requisites in Dermatology* series of textbooks is designed around the principle that learning and retention are best accomplished when the forest is clearly delineated from the trees. Topics are presented with an emphasis on the key points essential for residents and practicing clinicians. Each text is designed to stand alone as a reference or to be used as part of an integrated teaching curriculum. Many gifted physicians have contributed their time and energy to create the sort of texts we wish we had had during our own training and each of the texts in the series is accompanied by an innovative online module. Each online module is designed to complement the text, providing lecture material not possible in print format, including video and lectures with voice-over. These books have been a labor of love for all involved. We hope you enjoy them.

Dirk M Elston

Series dedication

This series of textbooks is dedicated to my wife Kathy and my children, Carly and Nate. Thank you for your love, support, and inspiration. It is also dedicated to the residents and fellows it has been my privilege to teach and to the patients who have taught me so much.

Dirk M Elston

Pediatric dermatology is a relative newcomer to the stage of medical specialties, but its growth has been explosive. In a matter of 40 years, the specialty has gone from a fledgling group of founding members to the formation of an international specialty society (the Society for Pediatric Dermatology) with highly attended meetings, the initiation of a specialty journal (*Pediatric Dermatology*), the formation of fellowship training programs and board certification, and the expectation that most dermatology training programs will have at least one pediatric dermatologist.

This text is meant to be an introduction to the exciting world of pediatric dermatology. It was designed to be a cover-to-cover read during a dermatology rotation, easily digested and covering the entities most likely to be encountered in a pediatric or general practice. The online version mirrors and enhances the text and provides a solid core lectureship for a pediatric dermatology curriculum.

This book is not intended to be exhaustive or encyclopedic. Several texts, including *Pediatric Dermatology* by Larry Schachner and Ronald Hansen, *Textbook of Pediatric Dermatology* by John Harper, Arnold Oranje and Neil Prose and the updated version of *Hurwitz Clinical Pediatric Dermatology* by Amy Paller and Anthony Mancini, are beautifully written and extremely complete texts for those who want to dive deeper into this fascinating specialty. We are also indebted to those who have preceded us in publishing elegantly written and illustrated texts, including William Weston, Alfred Lane, Joseph Morelli, Bernard Cohen, Susan Bayliss, Daniel Krowchuk and others. Once you have been energized by the study of pediatric dermatology, there will be a wealth of great reading to satisfy your appetite.

Before you dive into the text, take the time to memorize some basic dermatologic descriptions. Correctly describing a condition will enhance your communication with other practitioners and will open the door to differential diagnosis. In much the same way that a cardiologist will expect an accurate description of a heart murmur or an orthopedist a correct depiction of the X-ray findings of a fracture, dermatologists have precise language that translates the visual to the verbal.

Macule – flat discoloration, 1 cm in size or less

Patch – flat discoloration, greater than 1 cm in size

Telangiectasia (dilated blood vessel), **petechiae** (small patch of blood in the skin), and **purpura** (large patch of blood in the skin) – macules and patches have their own specific names

Papule – elevated lesion, 0.5 cm in size or less

Nodule or **tumor** (not implying malignancy) – elevated lesion, greater than 0.5 cm (nodule tends to have a deeper component)

Comedone, milium, cyst, burrow, scar, and **keloid** – all papules and nodules that imply some diagnostic assumptions and are acceptable descriptors as primary lesions

Plaque – elevated and flat-topped lesion, generally much more broad than raised

Vesicle – elevated collection of fluid, 0.5 cm in size or less

Bulla – elevated collection of fluid, greater than 0.5 cm in size

Pustule – elevated collection of pus (white blood cells)

Wheal – firm, edematous plaque resulting from fluid in the dermis

Scale, crust, ooze, erosion, ulcer, fissure, excoriation, atrophy, and lichenification are secondary lesions that can be used to modify the above descriptors.

We hope that you find this text useful and, perhaps, a first step toward a life career in this field.

References

Harper J, Oranje A, Prose N. Textbook of Pediatric Dermatology. 2nd edn. Oxford: Blackwell Science, 2006

Paller AS, Mancini AJ. Hurwitz Clinical Pediatric Dermatology, 3rd edn. Philadelphia, PA: Elsevier Saunders, 2006

Schachner LA, Hansen RC. Pediatric Dermatology, 3rd edn. Philadelphia, PA: Mosby, 2003.

Howard B Pride

Acknowledgments

I want to thank Dr. O. Fred Miller III for his leadership throughout my career in dermatology. His example and friendship have been an enormous component of my development as a dermatologist and teacher.

I would also like to acknowledge the support and encouragement of the dedicated and inquisitive dermatology residents at Geisinger Medical Center. Their thirst for knowledge, motivation, enthusiasm, and love of laughter keep me going.

Howard B Pride

Dedication

To my family, Kathy, Tianna, and Nicole, who provided support and encouragement while enduring the busy months of this book's creation.

Howard B Pride

For my patients, my mentors, and my parents who have taught me so much; and for my wife, Grace, who has helped to make all things, including this book, possible.

Albert C Yan

To Max and Trevor for all the support and always leaving the light on; and to everyone in the Penn State Department of Dermatology for their mentorship and making work fun.

Andrea L Zaenglein

Dermatitis

1

Albert C. Yan with Sharon E. Jacob

Introduction

Dermatitis is a nonspecific term that denotes an inflammatory skin rash characterized by primary changes of erythema, scaling, and exudates, as well as secondary changes of excoriation and lichenification. Various forms of dermatitis have been described, including: atopic dermatitis (AD), nummular dermatitis, seborrheic dermatitis, and contact dermatitis. The term *eczema* – derived from ancient Greek and meaning "boiling over" – is frequently used interchangeably to describe the often exudative quality of this skin disorder. However, in practical usage, many clinicians employ the term *eczema* to refer specifically to AD.

Atopic Dermatitis

Key Points

- Common, chronic inflammatory skin condition characterized by pruritus, typical morphology and distribution, periodic recurrences, and association with other atopic diseases (such as asthma, allergic rhinitis)
- Significant impact on quality of life, affecting sleep, school performance, social interactions, and self-esteem
- Influenced by immune dysregulation, but an impaired skin barrier associated with mutations in filaggrin may be a central pathogenetic factor
- The "atopic march" proposes that AD is a gateway disorder: the impaired skin barrier results in epicutaneous sensitization and can then engender other atopic diseases such as asthma and allergic rhinitis
- Atopic skin care should be the foundation of any therapeutic regimen for AD
- Topical corticosteroids represent the mainstay of treatment for acute flares of AD
- Topical calcineurin inhibitors, antihistamines, and barrier repair agents can be useful adjuncts to AD therapy

- Food allergies are uncommon triggers of AD, although parents often worry about them; when food allergies are implicated, elimination of the specific food can reduce the tendency for atopic flares
- Children with AD are especially predisposed to skin infections with bacteria and viruses, including Kaposi's varicelliform eruption

AD or atopic eczema is a chronic and relapsing, pruritic inflammatory skin condition that is frequently associated with other allergic atopic diseases such as asthma and allergic rhinitis. AD is one of the most common skin conditions encountered in childhood, and its prevalence among school-age children in industrialized nations approximates 15–20%.

Clinical presentation

Although individuals of any age can be affected, AD is principally a disease of childhood. The vast proportion of patients with AD manifest with disease during childhood and the 75–95% of those affected experience significant improvement or remission of their disease before adulthood.

Erythema, scaling, and exudates are accompanied by pruritus. The clinical findings of AD vary depending on age. In infancy, the face is commonly involved, and while the eruption can be extensive, characteristic sparing of the nose and perinasal region is observed and is referred to as the "headlight" sign or balaclava-like distribution (Figure 1-1). There is a predilection for appearance of the rash in flexural creases, including the antecubital, popliteal, wrist, ankle, and proximal posterior thigh creases (Figure 1-2). Extensor surface involvement can be seen, particularly in older infants and toddlers who may aggravate their eczema in these areas because of crawling and friction on these surfaces. At the same time, a relative sparing of intertriginous areas is generally noted. Classically, patients with AD have itchy but normal-appearing skin that will evolve into the characteristic rash of eczema with scratching ("the itch that rashes"). Chronic excoriation results in thickened, lichenified skin, often with hyperpigmentation or hypopigmentation (Figure 1-3).

The postinflammatory dyschromia that develops in AD can be distressing to patients and their families. Hypopigmentation, in particular, is often misattributed to use of topical corticosteroids (Figure 1-4). Although topical steroids can indeed cause hypopigmentation and cutaneous atrophy with chronic use (Figure 1-5), hypopigmentation is virtually always a postinflammatory response and resolves spontaneously with appropriate treatment of the underlying eczema.

Although not essential to the diagnosis of AD, certain clinical manifestations have been strongly associated with AD. Hanifin and Rajka originally described these as minor manifestations of AD, and building on these observations, the American Academy of Dermatology's 2003 Consensus Conference on Atopic Dermatitis compiled a list of associated supporting features (Box 1-1).

AD predisposes to secondary infection, particularly to *Staphylococcus aureus*, but also to herpes simplex, molluscum contagiosum, human papillomavirus, and dermatophytes.

Children with AD often later manifest other features of the so-called atopic triad: AD accompanied by asthma or allergic rhinitis. Based on data from the International Study on Asthma and Allergies in Childhood and other international studies, 10–50% of patients with AD go on to develop asthma later. Patients with AD commonly report a personal or family history of atopic disease.

The initial signs of AD are generally observed within the first 2 years of life, and by 5 years

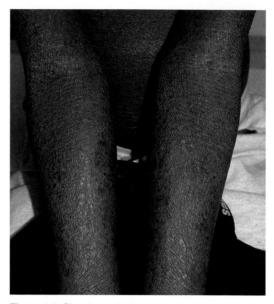

Figure 1-3 Chronic atopic dermatitis manifesting with hyperpigmented, lichenified skin

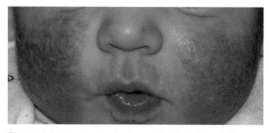

Figure 1-1 Infantile atopic dermatitis. Note the relative sparing around the nose, referred to as the "headlight" sign or "balaclava-like" distribution

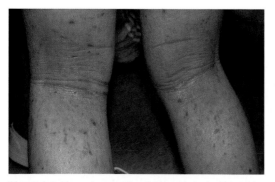

Figure 1-2 Flexural crease involvement is typical in atopic dermatitis

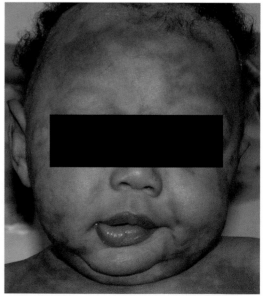

Figure 1-4 Hypopigmentation resulting from atopic dermatitis-associated inflammation. Steroids had not been previously prescribed in this patient

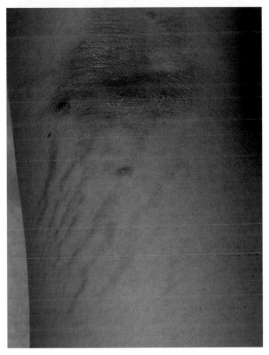

Figure 1-5 Cutaneous atrophy from chronic use of a high-potency topical corticosteroid

BOX 1-1

Features associated with atopic dermatitis: adapted from the American Academy of Dermatology's 2003 Consensus Conference on Atopic Dermatitis

Essential features

Pruritus

Eczema – typical morphology and age-specific patterns

    Infancy: face, neck, extensors

    Any age: flexural involvement

    Sparing of intertriginous zones

Chronic, relapsing history

Important features

Early age of onset

Personal or family history of atopy, immunoglobulin E reactivity

Supporting features

Atypical vascular phenomena such as facial pallor, white dermographism, delayed blanch response

Ichthyosis vulgaris

Keratosis pilaris

Ocular, periorbital, perioral, periauricular changes

Palmar hyperlinearity

Perifollicular accentuation

Prurigo and lichenification

Modified from Eichenfield LF, Hanifin JM, Luger TA, et al. Consensus conference on pediatric AD. J Am Acad Dermatol 2003;49:1088–1095.

of age, 80% of those with AD will have shown clinical signs of the disease. Approximately 60% of children will experience remission of their AD by 5 years of age, and by adolescence, some 50–90% of children will have seen remission of their disease. However, children with more severe AD have a poorer prognosis, as only about 25% of these children will remit by adolescence.

AD has a significant impact on the quality of life of patients and families. Children with AD suffer from chronic, recurrent bouts of pruritus which can interfere with sleep, school performance, and social interaction, creating anxiety and increased behavioral problems. Parents need to manage complex treatment regimens and attend frequent medical visits, leading to lost work time. It has been estimated that children with AD have 12–24 annual visits to physicians. Annual health care costs of managing AD are high and approximate or exceed those of other chronic diseases such as diabetes mellitus, inflammatory bowel disease, and respiratory syncytial virus.

Recently the implementation of multi-disciplinary and dedicated AD centers at major children's hospitals has highlighted the need to coordinate the often complex care involved in managing this disease. Children with very severe AD can receive more coordination visits with educational nursing to address skin care and adherence to treatment regimens and specialists including, but not limited to, dermatology, allergy, pulmonary medicine, and behavioral psychology.

Diagnosis

When confronted with a child who has a characteristic pruritic rash with the typical morphology and distribution, corroborated by a personal or family history of atopic disease, the diagnosis of AD can be made on clinical grounds and does not usually require laboratory testing (Box 1-1).

However, if the diagnosis is not clear from the history and physical examination, or if AD must be differentiated from other disorders, the following laboratory tests may be helpful:

- Complete blood count with differential – an elevated white blood cell count could indicate superinfection. Although not always present, the presence of a peripheral eosinophilia would be consistent with AD.
- Immunoglobulin (Ig) E levels – may be elevated and can be quite high. However, very elevated IgE levels in the appropriate context should raise the suspicion of hyperIgE syndrome.
- Radioallergosorbent test (RAST) or skin testing for food and environmental allergens – helpful in children with AD that is poorly

responsive to conventional therapy. RAST testing has good negative predictive value: i.e., if RAST testing for an allergen is negative, it is highly unlikely that the child is allergic to the allergen. However, positive RAST testing may or may not be clinically relevant. Skin testing is better at assessing clinical relevance.

- Serum zinc levels – may be decreased in patients with AD. Zinc levels may drop in the setting of inflammation as well as from increased skin turnover. If low, supplementation with zinc may improve the clinical response to topical therapy. If significantly low and associated with diarrhea, alopecia, or failure to thrive, evaluation for acquired zinc deficiency or acrodermatitis enteropathica may be indicated.
- In AD patients with signs of superinfection:
  - Bacterial culture of the skin helps to determine the identification and sensitivities of the organisms involved.
  - Direct fluorescent antibody testing, polymerase chain reaction, or viral culture can be helpful in the diagnosis of agents involved in Kaposi's varicelliform eruption.
- Skin biopsy – useful in cases where the diagnosis of AD is uncertain and other diagnoses are being considered. Findings on histology are nonspecific, but may show epidermal acanthosis, exocytosis, and eosinophils. Variable spongiosis may be present.

Differential Diagnosis

- Pityriasis alba
- Keratosis pilaris (KP)
- Seborrheic dermatitis
- Psoriasis
- Nummular dermatitis
- Lichen simplex chronicus (LSC)/prurigo
- Contact dermatitis
- Tinea capitis
- Diseases associated with chronic severe AD:
  - Hyper-IgE syndrome
  - Wiskott–Aldrich
- Diseases in which associated rashes resemble AD:
  - Acrodermatitis enteropathica and other necrolytic erythemas
  - Ataxia-telangiectasia
  - Congenital ichthyoses (such as Netherton syndrome)
  - Dermatophytosis
  - Dubowitz syndrome
  - Gluten-sensitive enteropathy
  - Immunodeficiency syndromes (selective IgA deficiency, severe combined immunodeficiency, X-linked agammaglobulinemia)
  - Langerhans cell histiocytosis

- Metabolic disorders (biotin deficiency, Hartnup's, histidinemia, phenylketonuria)
- Mucopolysaccharidoses (such as Hurler's syndrome)
- Nutritional disorders (hypervitaminosis A, kwashiorkor)
- Mycosis fungoides (cutaneous T-cell lymphoma)
- Scabies
- Syphilis, secondary

Pathogenesis

AD is an inflammatory disease that is influenced by both intrinsic and extrinsic factors. Immune dysregulation has traditionally been thought to engender cutaneous hyperreactivity and barrier disruption – the "inside-out" theory. It appears that in acute AD, a T-cell-mediated Th2 response is evident in which Th2-related cytokines such as interleukin (IL)-4, IL-5, and IL-13 predominate, while chronic AD is characterized by Th1-related responses involving IL-12 and interferon-γ. Pruritus, abnormalities in essential fatty acid metabolism, autonomic nervous system dysregulation, and increased phosphodiesterase activity have also been documented.

Recent data indicate that barrier dysfunction may play a central and primary role in its pathogenesis, suggesting an "outside-in" conception of AD. Investigators have identified mutations in filaggrin that are responsible for ichthyosis vulgaris. Many of those heterozygous for mutations in filaggrin had mild ichthyosis vulgaris and AD, while those homozygous or compound heterozygotes for mutations in filaggrin had severe ichthyosis vulgaris and all had AD. Epidemiologic studies of Irish, Scottish, and Danish patient cohorts indicate that a large percentage of those with atopic disease – asthma and AD – had a significantly

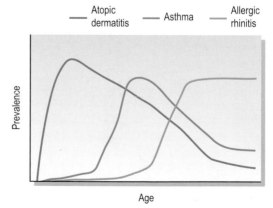

Figure 1-6 The typical evolution of atopic disease from atopic dermatitis as a "gateway disorder" with later sequential development of asthma and allergic rhinitis. (Reprinted with permission from Spergel JM, Paller AS. Atopic dermatitis and the atopic march. J Clin Allerg Immunol 2003;112:S118–S127)

greater odds ratio of having mutations in filaggrin. This increased odds ratio was not seen among those with asthma alone. This indicates that a structural skin protein – filaggrin – may play a central role in the development of not only AD, but also asthma and perhaps allergic rhinitis.

This "outside-in" conception has been characterized as the "atopic march." Many of those suffering from atopic diseases first manifest with AD and later go on to asthma and allergic rhinitis (Figure 1-6). AD may act as a gateway disorder to other atopic diseases because it engenders an impaired skin barrier that may permit environmental allergens access to regional lymph nodes and immune surveillance. Epicutaneous systemic sensitization can then occur and result in asthma and allergic rhinitis (Figure 1-7). Experimental data indicate that mice that receive skin sensitization to peanut and ovalbumin can go on to develop systemic sensitization. This theory has provided the hope that early intervention in AD to improve skin integrity could potentially decrease the incidence of other diseases in the atopic march, such as asthma or allergic rhinitis.

The predilection for infection among AD patients is well known. The impaired skin barrier aggravated by constant scratching in AD-affected skin exposes epitopes such as fibronectin that attract adherence by *Staphylococcus aureus*. Elaboration of inflammatory cytokines such as IL-4 and IL-13 may also be responsible for suppressing the production of endogenous anti-microbial peptides such as cathelicidins and defensins that normally provide the basis of normal innate immune defense in the skin. As a result, infections with bacteria (most commonly, *S. aureus*) as well as viruses (herpes simplex virus (HSV), coxsackie virus, vaccinia virus, molluscipox virus) affect patients with AD more frequently and more severely than nonatopic individuals.

Treatment

Atopic skin care (Box 1-2)

Atopic skin care should form the foundation of any AD treatment regimen. This includes the appropriate modification of bathing practices, selection of cleansers, and use of emollients. There is significant controversy regarding the frequency

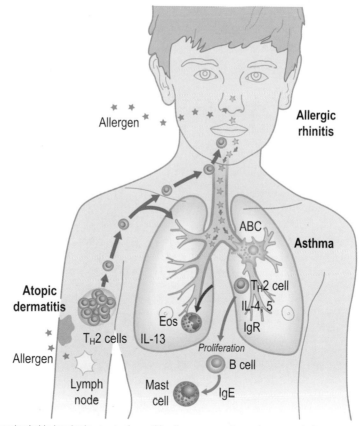

Figure 1-7 The impaired skin barrier in atopic dermatitis allows access to environmental allergens and results in skin sensitization. Allergens bind to antigen-presenting cells such as Langerhans cells and induce Th2 cells which migrate to lungs and nasal mucosa, promoting systemic sensitization. (Reprinted with permission from Spergel JM, Paller AS. Atopic dermatitis and the atopic march. J Clin Allerg Immunol 2003;112:S118–S127)

Atopic dermatitis: therapeutic options

Atopic skin care measures

- Address bathing practices
- Use of a mild soap or cleanser
- Increased use of emollients or moisturizers
- Avoidance of potential triggers

Topical corticosteroids

Topical calcineurin inhibitors

Topical barrier repair devices

Antihistamines

Antibiotics for secondary infection (antistaphylococcal, antiviral: depending on context)

Systemic agents

- Ultraviolet light phototherapy
- Systemic corticosteroids
- Systemic immunosuppressive agents (cyclosporine, methotrexate, azathioprine, mycophenolate mofetil)
- Gamma-interferon
- Biologic agents (omalizumab, efalizumab, etanercept)

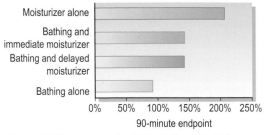

Figure 1-8 The degree of hydration in the skin at 90 min based on different bathing parameters. Cetaphil cream was used as the moisturizer in this study and a hygrometer was employed to measure skin hydration. (Based on data presented by C Chiang and Eichenfield at the Society for Investigative Dermatology Annual Meeting 2006, abstract 212)

Vehicle selection is important to optimize efficacy, safety, and compliance. Ointments are preferred in infants and younger children, due to their better tolerance since they sting less, are more occlusive, and often contain fewer potential sensitizing ingredients than their cream, gel, lotion, foam, and solution counterparts. Ointments tend to be perceived as greasy and impractical for older children, adolescents, and adults, especially on the hands, and are cosmetically less acceptable as they tend to stain clothing. In these situations, creams, gels, lotions, and foams may be selected to improve acceptability and adherence to the treatment regimen. Scalp areas are frequently involved, and medicated shampoos or oils, topical solutions, foams, and occasionally ointments (especially for thick, curly, or wiry hair) may be preferred (Table 1-1).

Topical steroids remain the mainstay of therapy for AD. Their anti-inflammatory properties typically induce a prompt and favorable clinical response. They are classified as low-potency, mid-potency, high-potency, and super-high-potency, or as within classes I–VII (I indicating most potent and VII indicating least potent). Commonly used topical steroids include: hydrocortisone acetonide 2.5% (class VII), fluticasone, fluocinolone 0.025%, and hydrocortisone valerate 0.2% (class IV), triamcinolone 0.1% (class III–IV), and desoximetasone and fluocinonide 0.05% (class II). This classification scheme is based on the vasoconstrictor assay where higher-potency ratings correlate with a greater ability to induce vasoconstriction, and this roughly correlates with greater efficacy and greater risk of adverse effects (Table 1-2). Vehicle choice also significantly influences the potency of agents and potential for adverse effects since newer topical steroids that are typically classified as potent may possess better safety profiles than older steroid formulations.

Most are indicated for once- or twice-daily application; more frequent application does not significantly improve the response and can increase the potential for adverse effects. Principal adverse effects warranting surveillance include local effects of hypopigmentation (although the underlying

of bathing, with some advocating less bathing with short, infrequent baths during the week (the so-called "dry school") to minimize excessive drying of the skin through removal of protective skin lipids and proteins, whereas others recommend more bathing with daily or even more frequent baths with longer soaks (the so-called "wet school") in an effort to hydrate the skin and minimize the risk of infection. Preliminary data indicate that less bathing does indeed provide better hydration, but more bathing also does increase hydration above baseline as long as moisturizers are also used either immediately after tubbing or within an hour afterwards. Children treated with either approach seem to improve, as long as mild cleansers or soaps are selected and emollients are applied with increased frequency, especially after bathing (Figure 1-8). Gentle soaps and cleansers that are pH-balanced include but are not limited to: Dove Sensitive skin bar, Tone, Cetaphil bar or cleanser, Aveeno, and Vanicream. More frequent use of emollients or moisturizers can reduce the reliance on topical medications. Favored moisturizers include: petrolatum, Aquaphor, Eucerin cream, Acid Mantle cream, Vanicream, and Cetaphil cream. Vegetable shortening has also been successfully used as a moisturizer in winter weather. It has the advantages of being cheap, readily available, fragrance-free, and preservative-free. While greasy ointments may be better tolerated in infants, older children and adolescents may prefer lighter emollients such as creams and lotions.

Table 1-1 Vehicle benefits and disadvantages

Vehicle	Benefits	Disadvantages
Ointment	Occlusive	Greasy
	Often fewer additives	Stains clothing
	Does not sting	
Cream	May be moisturizing	Less greasy
	Easy to spread	Causes stinging in some
Lotion	Easier to spread	Causes stinging in more
	Not greasy	Less moisturizing
Foam, hydrogel	Easiest to spread	Higher likelihood of stinging
	Not greasy	
	Increased patient preference	Less moisturizing
Solution, oil	Liquid formulation	Solution occasionally causes stinging
	Best for scalp	
		Oil can be greasy

dermatitis is much more likely to be the cause), telangiectasia formation, skin atrophy and striae, and increased ocular pressure (when used near the eye). Systemic effects such as hypothalamic–pituitary–adrenal axis suppression and growth delay due to systemic absorption can rarely be seen when used over large body surface areas and especially with more potent topical agents.

Topical calcineurin inhibitors are useful alternatives to topical steroids. These agents bind cytosolic macrolide receptors and inhibit T-cell-mediated inflammation initiated via the NF-κB pathway. Pimecrolimus is indicated for mild to moderate AD whereas tacrolimus is indicated for moderate to severe AD. Both anti-inflammatory agents can be used up to twice daily on any affected body surface area, and can be applied with reasonable safety even on periocular, facial, or intertriginous areas. They can create a burning sensation on moist skin. Unlike corticosteroids, these agents do not cause skin atrophy and are not associated with hypothalamic–pituitary–adrenal axis suppression. In January 2006, boxed warnings were issued by the US Food and Drug Administration (FDA) on both of these agents because very high doses of these agents taken orally or applied at high concentration to the skin can cause systemic immunosuppression in animal models, and systemic immunosuppression is known to increase the risk of lymphoma and skin malignancies.

Barrier repair agents represent a new category of therapeutic options for AD. These contain ingredients that may have some anti-inflammatory properties, and that seem to reduce the signs and symptoms of AD. These include topical ceramide products (CeraVe, Epiceram, Triceram), MAS063DP (Atopiclair), and palmitoylethanolamide (PEA) cream (MimyX). These agents have been evaluated and cleared for marketing through the US FDA as new medical devices. Limited data are currently available, but these agents may be useful in moderating the signs and symptoms of mild AD and in the maintenance phase of AD therapy.

Food and environmental allergies can play a role in triggering flares of AD in some patients. Strategies to improve skin barrier integrity through use of moisturizers and clothing coverage, managing dust mites, and the avoidance of triggering foods can be helpful in maintaining longer flare-free periods. However, it appears that foods play a minor role, if any, in most children with AD. Between 5 and 30% of children have relevant food allergies that trigger flares of AD, and the likelihood of food allergy triggers appears to be higher in those with more severe disease. In most cases, successful management of the AD using atopic skin care measures, topical steroids, and adjunctive agents, and avoidance of environmental allergens often assuages parental concerns of food allergies. Consultation for food allergy triggers should be considered in those children in whom a history of flares consistently occurs with exposure to specific foods, or those in whom conventional topical therapy is unsuccessful. When present, the most common food allergy triggers include: wheat, milk, eggs, soy, and nuts. Appropriate elimination of the allergenic food in these particular instances can significantly improve AD.

Antihistamines (such as diphenhydramine, hydroxyzine, cetirizine, loratadine, fexofenadine, and doxepin) are of limited benefit in relieving the itch in patients with AD. Although a subset of patients may respond, many do not. Caution should be taken when using these medications in infants since antihistamines may cause paradoxical agitation. Older children may experience sedation, especially with traditional older antihistamines such as diphenhydramine and hydroxyzine so these agents are best given at bedtime to moderate nighttime pruritus. Sedation may, in fact, account for virtually all of an antihistamine's beneficial effect. Doxepin, useful as an antipruritic, is a tricyclic agent that has antihistaminic properties and should be used with great care given its potential for toxicity.

Systemic agents may be necessary in the treatment of recalcitrant and severe AD. When considering their use, the benefits of short-term relief should be weighed against the potential long-term sequelae that may result from using these modalities. Systemic steroids have been used to

Table 1-2 Common topical corticosteroids and their associated potency rankings

Potency ranking	Vasoconstrictor class	Agent	Brand
Ultrapotent or superpotent	I	Augmented betamethasone dipropionate 0.05%	Diprolene (G, O)
		Clobetasol propionate 0.05%	Clobex (L), Cormax (C, S), Olux (F), Temovate (C, S, O)
		Diflorasone diacetate 0.05%	Psorcon (O)
		Halobetasol propionate 0.05%	Ultravate (C, O)
		Fluocinonide 0.1%	Vanos (C)
High-potency	II	Amcinonide 0.1%	Cyclocort (O)
		Augmented betamethasone dipropionate 0.05%	Diprolene AF (C)
		Betamethasone dipropionate 0.05%	Diprosone (O), Maxivate (O)
			Topicort (G, O, C)
		Desoximetasone 0.05%, 0.25%	Psorcon (C), Maxiflor (O)
		Diflorasone diacetate 0.05%	Lidex (G, S, O, C)
		Fluocinonide 0.05%	Halog (O, C)
		Halcinonide 0.1%	Elocon (O)
		Mometasone furoate 0.1%	
High-potency	III	Amcinonide 0.1%	Cyclocort (C, L)
		Betamethasone dipropionate 0.05%	Diprosone (C)
		Betamethasone valerate 0.12%, 0.1%	Luxiq (F), Valisone (O)
		Desoximetasone 0.05%	Topicort LP (C)
		Diflorasone diacetate 0.05%	Florone (C), Maxiflor (C)
		Fluocinonide 0.05%	Lidex-E (C)
		Fluticasone 0.005%	Cutivate (O)
		Triamcinolone 0.1%	Aristocort A (O)
Mid-potency	IV	Fluocinolone 0.025%	Synalar (O)
		Flurandrenolide 0.05%	Cordran (O)
		Hydrocortisone valerate 0.2%	Westcort (O)
		Mometasone 0.05%	Elocon (C)
		Triamcinolone 0.1%	Aristocort (C), Kenalog (C, O)
Mid-potency	V	Fluocinolone 0.025%	Synalar (C)
		Fluticasone 0.05%	Cutivate (C)
		Hydrocortisone butyrate 0.1%	Locoid (C), Pandel (C)
		Prednicarbate 0.1%	Dermatop (O, C)
Lower-potency	VI	Alclometasone 0.05%	Aclovate (O, C)
		Betamethasone valerate 0.1%	Valisone (L)
		Desonide 0.05%, Verdeso (F)	Desonate (H), Desowen (O, C), Tridesilon (O, C)
		Fluocinolone 0.01%	Dermasmoothe FS (S)
		Triamcinolone 0.025%	
Lower-potency	VII	Hydrocortisone 1%, 2.5%	Hytone (O, C, L)

C, cream; F, foam; G, gel; H, hydrogel; L, lotion; O, ointment; S, solution.

abate severe acute flares of AD. In general, however, systemic steroid agents should be avoided in AD patients because of their propensity for rebound flares as the steroids are tapered. Patients and their families often develop a dependence on systemic steroids due to their rapid onset of action and the significant clinical improvement seen, but patients easily become steroid-dependent. Ultraviolet light phototherapy can be helpful in providing relief from itching in severe AD patients and can be utilized as an adjunct to topical therapy. Immunosuppressive agents, including cyclosporine, methotrexate, mycophenolate mofetil, azathioprine, and interferon-γ, have demonstrated various degrees of efficacy in the management of severe AD. More recently, anecdotal reports have documented the limited efficacy of using biologic agents such as efalizumab, etanercept, and omalizumab.

Superinfection is a common complication of AD. *Staphylococcus aureus* is the most common bacterial pathogen involved in colonizing and causing superinfection. Superinfected cases of AD may become less responsive to topical anti-inflammatory therapy until the colonizing organism is treated. Indeed, it appears that the presence of staphylococcal superantigens interferes with the normal transport of steroid molecules and can induce apparent clinical steroid resistance. Limited areas of superinfection can often be successfully treated with topical mupirocin or retapamulin. More extensive involvement typically requires systemic antibiotic therapy using an antistaphylococcal agent. Beta-lactam antibiotics, such as cephalexin, dicloxacillin, or similar agents can be used initially. Clindamycin and co-trimoxazole are alternatives. Serious invasive bacterial infections or septicemia generally require parenteral antibiotics. Beta-lactam drugs still have a place in management, but those who present with spontaneous abscess and severe cellulitis, necrotizing soft-tissue infection, empyema, joint lesions, or pneumonitis should be managed with drugs effective against methicillin-resistant *S. aureus* (MRSA), including parenteral vancomycin or linezolid.

Secondary infection with viral agents such as HSV, coxsackie virus, and vaccinia virus is referred to as Kaposi's varicelliform eruption, or simply eczema herpeticum when it denotes HSV superinfection. It is for this reason that smallpox vaccination is contraindicated in patients with known AD. Affected patients typically present with acute exacerbations of AD in which vesicles and pustules appear superimposed on eczematized areas. As the blisters rupture, characteristic punched-out erosions manifest. These children feel ill, may be febrile, and often have poor oral intake with dehydration. Admission for parenteral fluids, antiviral therapy with acyclovir, and antibiotic therapy for bacterial secondary infection are indicated. Tap water soaks can assist in removing thick crust. In general, topical corticosteroids are deferred for a few days until the infection is better controlled, and then topical AD therapy can be reinstituted. Patients who have experienced eczema herpeticum should be followed for recurrences since approximately one-quarter of patients suffer from a recurrent outbreak of HSV within 6 months after an initial episode. For those with severe AD and a history of eczema herpeticum, acyclovir or related antiviral agent may be indicated as prophylaxis against recurrences.

Nummular Eczema

Key Points

- Circular patches and plaques of dermatitis
- Commonly treatment-resistant
- Treat with potent topical steroids

Clinical presentation

Individual lesions of nummular eczema present as pruritic, coin-shaped, and circular areas of erythema, scaling, and lichenification and are typically located on the torso or extremities (Figure 1-9). The margins of individual plaques are better defined than is typical of AD and lesions are circinate (round) rather than annular (ring-shaped) and can therefore be readily distinguished from tinea corporis.

Diagnosis

If scaling is prominent, a potassium hydroxide preparation or fungal culture can assist in ruling out dermatophytosis. Patch testing can be helpful in elucidating an underlying contact allergy trigger. No other laboratory testing is typically necessary. However, if the condition does not respond appropriately to therapy, a skin biopsy may be indicated.

The differential diagnosis includes AD, contact dermatitis, fixed drug eruption, psoriasis, tinea corporis, and mycosis fungoides (cutaneous T-cell lymphoma).

Pathogenesis

Although lesions of AD may be nummular in configuration, nummular dermatitis can also occur independently of AD. Nummular eczema has also been associated with nickel allergic contact dermatitis and a wide variety of other contact allergens.

Treatment

Therapeutic options for AD can also be applied to nummular dermatitis. However, lesions of nummular eczema often require more potent topical agents as they are less responsive to low-potency topical steroids. Medium-potency or short-term use of more potent topical steroids

Figure 1-9 Coin-shaped plaques of nummular eczema

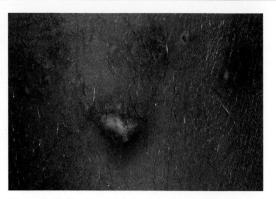

Figure 1-10 Prurigo nodularis. Note the central hypopigmentation in these keratotic nodules seen with chronic excoriation and postinflammatory hypopigmentation

is typically used either alone or under occlusion. Atopic skin care measures may help reduce the likelihood of recrudescence. For those with associated contact sensitivity, avoidance of exposure to the allergen is advised.

Lichen Simplex Chronicus and Prurigo Nodularis

Chronic scratching or friction can elicit localized areas of skin thickening, known as prurigo nodularis or the picker's papule (Figure 1-10) when picking of the skin creates lichenified papules or nodules. The expression of this phenomenon as lichenified or keratotic plaques involving larger areas is known as LSC (Figure 1-11). Lesions are most commonly observed on anatomic sites that can be easily reached, usually the arms and legs, with classic sparing of the mid-back. Prurigo and LSC are phenotypic terms that describe an endpoint resulting from chronic itching, scratching, and rubbing. These are frequent findings among chronic AD patients. Like nummular eczema, higher-potency topical steroids may be required. Occlusion will enhance penetration of the steroid and provide a barrier to further scratching.

Contact Dermatitis

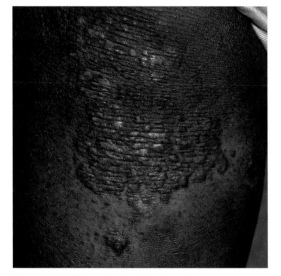

Figure 1-11 Lichen simplex chronicus

- Phytophotodermatitis is a phototoxic contact dermatitis associated with exposure to plant furocoumarins
- Patch tests can assist in identifying specific allergens

Key Points

- The principal forms of contact dermatitis can be categorized as:
  - Irritant contact dermatitis
  - Allergic contact dermatitis
  - Photocontact (phototoxic) dermatitis
  - Photoallergic contact dermatitis
- Contact dermatitis represents an "outside job" and is characterized by linearity or geometric configuration

Irritant contact dermatitis accounts for approximately 80% of all contact dermatitis cases and can appear in any location on the skin or mucosa where too *harsh* a chemical has been in contact with too *weak* an integumental surface. It can occur in anyone (i.e., naive person) and does not require previous exposure to that chemical. Irritant contact dermatitis does not represent a sensitization reaction because it is not an immunologic event. Contact with a harsh irritant can produce dermatitis, but more commonly dermatitis results from repeated exposures to weak irritants (such as soaps, urine, chlorinated diapers).

Allergic contact dermatitis has recently been recognized as an important cause of childhood dermatitis, with a prevalence rate in the range of 25–60% in children referred for epicutaneous patch testing. Recently, Jacob, Brod, and Crawford found the prevalence of clinical relevant allergens in symptomatic children significantly higher than previously reported. Furthermore, the authors found a significant number of allergens which would not have been detectable using the thin-layer rapid use epicutaneous (TRUE) test, the Hermal test, or the North American contact dermatitis standard. Their work demonstrates the importance of customized comprehensive patch testing based on the exposure experience of the individual patient. The catch is that children have small backs with little room to place allergens during testing. The art of patch testing in children is selecting the most appropriate allergens for each child. Boxes 1-3–1-8 summarize the most common allergens and factors important in the evaluation of contact allergy in children.

Phototoxic dermatitis requires light in association with a topical agent to elicit the reaction. These compounds do not require antecedent sensitization. By contrast, in allergic contact dermatitis, a small amount of the etiologic agent can elicit a delayed-type hypersensitivity reaction in a patient who has been previously sensitized. A photoallergic contact dermatitis requires light in association with a topical compound to generate the delayed-type hypersensitivity reaction. Contact urticaria, an urticarial reaction that can be either immunologically triggered (as with latex allergy) or nonimmunologically mediated, is an immediate-type hypersensitivity reaction that will not be covered in this section.

Clinical presentation

The hallmark of any contact dermatitis is its geometric or linear configuration that marks it as a so-called "outside job." Characterized by geometric or bizarre shapes that do not correspond to normal anatomic landmarks, the dermatitis is typically eczematous – there are areas of erythema and scaling; in more severe cases vesiculation, oozing, and crusting; and in chronic cases, lichenification, fissuring, and hyperpigmentation can be seen (Figure 1-12). Areas involved typically correspond to sites where contact with an irritant or allergen occurs. However, contact dermatitis that requires photoactivation will typically manifest in light-exposed areas: classically, the face (with sparing of the philtrum and chin), the ears (in those with short hair), the upper chest, and dorsal hands.

Irritant contact dermatitis is variably pruritic depending on the severity of the reaction. Allergic contact dermatitis and photoallergic contact dermatitis are often intensely itchy. Those suffering from photocontact dermatitis more commonly describe a burning sensation.

Irritant contact dermatitis among infants, children, and adolescents can occur in a variety

---

BOX 1-3

Common causes of phytophotodermatitis ("lime disease" or "harvester's dermatitis")

Fruits: citrus (limes and lemons), mangoes

Vegetables and other plants: celery, parsley, carrots, parsnips, meadow grass, giant hogweed, cocklebur, buttercups, wheat, clover, pigweed, shepherd's purse

---

BOX 1-4

Top contact allergens in children

Top allergens

Nickel

Cobalt

Thimerosal

Fragrance mix

Neomycin

Carba mix

Thiuram mix

Wool wax alcohol

Chromate

Paraphenylenediamine

Colophony

---

of contexts. Irritant diaper dermatitis arises from chronic moisture and exposure to fecal enzymes and urine. Drooling predisposes infants who are teething to perioral irritant contact dermatitis. Excessive hand washing and use of harsh soaps can trigger an irritant contact hand dermatitis.

The most important allergens involved in causing contact dermatitis in children include: *Toxicodendron* (*Rhus*) or "poison plants" (poison ivy, oak, sumac), nickel, fragrances, topical antibiotics, topical steroids, preservatives, and dyes (Figure 1-13).

Phytophotodermatitis represents a form of photocontact dermatitis. Exposure to a photosensitizing furocoumarin in common fruits and vegetables followed by exposure to sunlight results in a phototoxic skin reaction. The eruption commonly presents as either streaky areas of erythema or irregular markings corresponding to either drip marks or handprints where contact was made. Phytophotodermatitis is accompanied by a burning sensation not unlike sunburn (Figure 1-14).

The identification of the causative agent in contact dermatitis sometimes requires detailed history taking and detective work. The location and distribution of the dermatitis may provide useful clues to recognizing the possible allergens involved. Sources of irritant contact dermatitis may be obvious, as with diaper dermatitis and excessive

BOX 1-5

Investigating the exposure experience in the diagnosis of allergic contact dermatitis

Clinical index of suspicion raised due to:

New-onset dermatitis in a nonatopic distribution

Worsening of endogenous dermatoses (atopic dermatitis/psoriasis)

Clinical presentation of dishydrosis

Uncontrollable dermatitis by standard therapies

An indepth history taken based on:

Patient demographics (i.e., age, gender, atopy, etc.)

Patient's medical/medicament history

Patient's personal hygiene environment (i.e., shampoo, soap, diaper wipes, etc.)

Patient's home environment (i.e., parents' personal hygiene products to home contents)

Patient's school/daycare/caregivers' environment (i.e., school chair materials to sleep mats, to what these are cleaned with)

Patient's avocation/hobbies (i.e., baseball player, hockey player, scuba diver)

Physical examination and integrative evaluation

Geographic distribution of dermatitis

Temporal association of dermatitis location with environmental exposures

Notable negative findings

Allergen selection with consideration of:

Smaller available area for patch test placement

Higher-probability allergens selected for recurrent exposures in one or more settings[*]

Allergen placement and evaluation

The lowest number of allergens possible without compromising the ability to detect a clinically relevant allergen (this is the trick)

Allergens placed on the patient's back/arms

Allergens removed between 24[†] and 48 hours

Allergens evaluated at 48 hours and again at 72–96 hours[†]

Assignment of clinical relevance

Designation of which allergens are most likely responsible for the clinical picture

Identification of which of those allergens are found in the child's personal environment

Avoidance

[*]This is the art: for example, fragrances might be selected if the mother wears them, child has them in bubble bath. If the child eats ketchup daily, an allergen with increased probability would be cinnamic alcohol.
[†]The optimal timing of patch removal and reading is an evolving concept: Worm M, Aberer W, Agathos M, et al. Patch testing in children – recommendations of the German Contact Dermatitis Research Group (DKG). J Dtsch Dermatol Ges 2007;5:107–109.

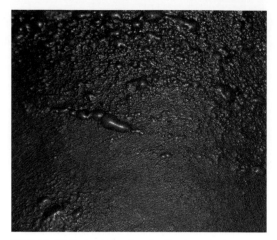

Figure 1-12 An example of acute allergic contact dermatitis secondary to poison-ivy exposure. Note the characteristic "outside job" manifesting as collections of vesicles with a linear configuration

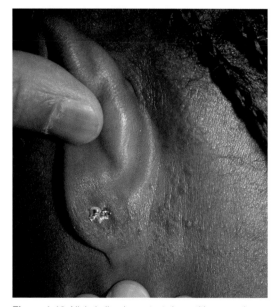

Figure 1-13 Nickel allergic contact dermatitis secondary to nickel found in earrings

handwashing dermatitis. Nail polish allergies to formaldehyde and tosylamide often manifest on eyelid, periocular areas, and other head and neck sites. Cosmetic allergies occur at sites of application and suggest the possibility of allergies to fragrances or preservatives. Nickel allergic contact dermatitis typically presents at sites of nickel contact, such as the earlobes (earrings), sides of the neck (necklaces and chains), and lower abdomen (belt buckles or pant snaps). Foot dermatitis secondary to shoe allergens suggest reactions to *para-tert*-butylphenol formaldehyde resin (PTBFR), leather and rubber allergens such as potassium dichromate, and various dyes. Reactions from bandages and electrocardiographic monitoring leads may result

BOX 1-6

Suspect allergic contact dermatitis

New-onset dermatitis in "nonatopic" areas

Worsening of endogenous dermatoses (atopy/psoriasis)

Dishydrosis presentation

Uncontrollable dermatitis by standard treatments

BOX 1-7

Differential diagnoses of eczematous diseases

Asteatotic dermatitis

Atopic dermatitis

Autosensitization reaction

Contact dermatitis

  Irritant (~80%)

  Allergic (~19%)

  Urticarial

Dishydrotic eczema

Nummular dermatitis

Psoriasis vulgaris

Seborrheic dermatitis

BOX 1-8

Steps in managing allergic contact dermatitis

Elicitation of a careful history of environmental exposures

Temporal association of dermatitis location with environmental allergen

Selection of allergens to patch test (standard screen versus individualized)

Patch test evaluation with assignment of clinical relevance to allergens

Avoidance of suspected clinically relevant allergens

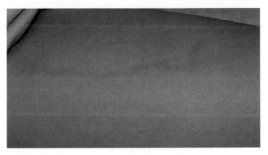

Figure 1-14 Phytophotodermatitis from lime juice presenting as a serpiginous linear eruption characterized by a burning sensation followed by postinflammatory hyperpigmentation

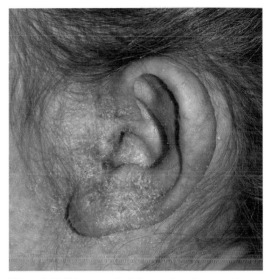

Figure 1-15 Edema, vesiculation, and oozing as part of allergic contact dermatitis secondary to the neomycin component in ear drops

from sensitization to acrylate adhesives, PTBFR, or use of concomitant topical antibiotic preparations, including bacitracin, neomycin, or polymyxin (Figure 1-15). Disperse dyes have also been more recently linked to skin reactions in children. These dyes are used in diapers and other fabrics.

Diagnosis

In most cases, a detailed history and physical examination provide the key information for identifying the etiologic allergens. Patch testing or photopatch testing where appropriate is recommended if the etiology of the contact dermatitis is not evident from history or physical examination. Patches should be custom-tailored to those allergens found in the child's environment. The standard patch test involves the placement of small epicutaneous patches containing allergen to unaffected areas of skin for 48 h. The patches are then removed and an initial reading is then performed. Typically, a repeat reading is then done at 72–96 h to identify any delayed reactions. Location of the dermatitis can assist in determining which allergens are most likely to be responsible for the contact dermatitis. Special trays of additional allergens can be used in patch testing to identify allergens if the initial set of patches does not identify a suspected contact allergen.

Although no other laboratory testing is generally needed, those suffering from severe allergic contact dermatitis may have a circulating eosinophilia. Skin biopsy is generally not needed, but often shows spongiosis, dermal edema, eosinophils, and a lymphohistiocytic infiltrate with exocytosis. Photocontact dermatitis may show frank vesiculation and neutrophils may predominate.

Treatment

Identification and avoidance of the contact agent etiologic in the contact dermatitis are the most important steps in the treatment of this condition. Once the responsible agent has been determined, patient and family education are essential since many products may contain the irritant or allergen. An especially helpful tool for those with allergic contact dermatitis is the American Contact Dermatitis Society's Contact Allergen Replacement Database (CARD), which can help create a roster of acceptable, allergen-free products that patients and their families can use to substitute for their current products.

For symptomatic relief of contact dermatitis, topical steroids of appropriate potency and, in more severe cases, oral steroids can be considered. Topical calcineurin inhibitors, particularly in sensitive areas such as the eyelids or genitals, can be helpful. In cases where the etiologic agent can be identified and exposure discontinued, treatment of the contact dermatitis typically leads to abatement of the rash within 1–4 weeks, depending on the severity and identity of the agent involved.

Seborrheic Dermatitis

Key Points

- Salmon-colored erythema with greasy scale
- Associated with colonization by *Malassezia* species
- In contrast to AD, pruritus is generally mild if present in seborrheic dermatitis
- Infantile cases of seborrheic dermatitis, referred to as "cradle cap," resolve spontaneously and often require no intervention
- The facial involvement in seborrheic dermatitis can be mistaken for lupus erythematosus
- Severe cases have been associated with underlying immunodeficiency states, including infection with human immunodeficiency virus (HIV)
- Treatment is with topical anti-inflammatory agents (topical steroids, topical calcineurin inhibitors, tar compounds) or topical antifungal medications

Clinical presentation

Seborrheic dermatitis is a chronic, inflammatory skin disorder affecting infants and adolescents, as well as adults. The condition is characterized by salmon-colored erythema and greasy scaling that classically involve the scalp, eyebrows, perinasal areas, external auditory canals, periauricular areas, and, less often, the mid-chest, axillae, and diaper or inguinal areas (Figure 1-16). In contrast to AD, pruritus is relatively minimal in seborrheic dermatitis. Although scaling and erythema may be noted on the scalp, alopecia is not typically observed. More severe involvement may be referred to as sebopsoriasis, as it is considered on a spectrum with frank psoriasis. While seborrheic dermatitis is common among infants, it tends to remit during childhood, with recrudescence seen during adolescence and adulthood.

Severe recalcitrant seborrheic dermatitis, particularly when seen in association with other systemic manifestations such as failure to thrive, diarrhea, and opportunistic infection, should raise the possibility of an underlying immunocompromised state, such as leukemia or HIV infection. Up to 40% of HIV-positive individuals and 80% of those with acquired immunodeficiency syndrome (AIDS) show clinical signs of seborrheic dermatitis.

Diagnosis

The diagnosis is made on clinical grounds. Testing for immune deficiency should be considered in the appropriate context. Biopsy is seldom needed, except when papular scalp lesions and inguinal erosions are present. In such cases, a biopsy should be done to rule out Langerhans cell histiocytosis.

Differential Diagnosis

- Facial involvement: AD, contact dermatitis, lupus erythematosus, perioral dermatitis, psoriasis, rosacea
- Scalp involvement: AD, psoriasis, sebopsoriasis, tinea capitis, Langerhans cell histiocytosis (small orange-brown papules and crusts)
- Genital or intertriginous involvement: erythrasma, intertrigo (candidal, streptococcal), Langerhans cell histiocytosis (fissuring or erosions), psoriasis, tinea cruris, zinc deficiency

Pathogenesis

The etiology of seborrheic dermatitis is unknown. However, *Malassezia* species have been associated and may aggravate the condition or might simply represent an epiphenomenon.

Treatment

Infantile seborrheic dermatitis or "cradle cap" is self-limited and resolves during infancy. Excessive scaling can be removed using baby oil and a fine-toothed comb. For those patients requiring treatment, use of either a topical anti-inflammatory agent or a topical antifungal medication can be helpful. These agents can be delivered in a variety of vehicles depending on the anatomic site(s) affected, including shampoos and solutions for hair-bearing areas, while creams, lotions, ointments, and gels are preferred for other sites. Useful topical anti-inflammatory agents include: low-potency topical corticosteroids such as hydrocortisone acetonide 2.5%, alclometasone, and desonide; topical calcineurin inhibitors such as pimecrolimus and tacrolimus; and tar-based shampoos. Topical

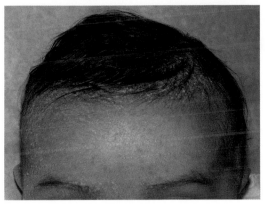

Figure 1-16 Infantile seborrheic dermatitis. Note the greasy scaling involving the scalp and eyebrow areas in particular

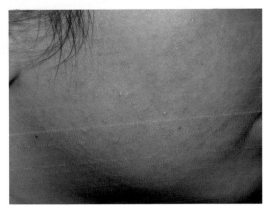

Figure 1-17 Keratosis pilaris. Follicular keratotic papules on the cheek in association with a faint telangiectatic background

antifungal medications have also been employed and include zinc pyrithione, selenium sulfide, clotrimazole, ketoconazole, and ciclopirox.

Keratosis Pilaris

Key Points

- Typically appears on the cheeks, arms, and legs
- Facial lesions tend to resolve spontaneously; lesions on the arms and legs may persist into adulthood
- Most cases require no intervention, but keratolytic moisturizers and topical retinoids can moderate the appearance of KP

Clinical presentation

KP manifests as follicular keratotic papules on the cheeks, arms, and legs (Figure 1-17). The lesions are commonly erythematous and keratin spines may be present. In extensive cases, involvement can be seen on the upper back and buttocks. These papules give the skin a sandpaper-like quality. Some cases demonstrate background telangiectatic erythema, especially on the cheeks, and are sometimes referred to as KP rubra faciei. While KP can appear during infancy, most cases manifest within the first 5 years. Involvement on the cheeks resolves spontaneously during childhood or adolescence, while findings on the arms and legs may persist into adulthood. Some of those affected report seasonal exacerbations, with most experiencing worsening during colder, winter months.

Diagnosis

KP is an easy clinical diagnosis. Histology reveals keratin plugs within hair follicles, as well as an increased granular layer accompanied by a mild superficial perivascular inflammation with hyperkeratosis, but biopsy is seldom necessary.

Differential diagnosis includes acne vulgaris, AD with perifollicular accentuation, KP atrophicans (ulyerythema ophryogenes), lichen nitidus, milia, phrynoderma (associated with vitamin A, B-complex, C, and essential fatty acid deficiency), and pityriasis rubra pilaris.

Treatment

Treatment is generally not necessary for asymptomatic cases. Keratolytic moisturizers containing ammonium lactate or urea can be useful agents to moderate the appearance of KP but the efficacy is limited. For those with pitted scarring, topical retinoids such as adapalene or tretinoin can be prescribed.

Further reading

Atopic dermatitis, nummular dermatitis, prurigo nodularis, and lichen simplex chronicus

Berger TG, Duvic M, Van Voorhees AS, et al. The use of topical calcineurin inhibitors in dermatology: safety concerns. Report of the American Academy of Dermatology Association Task Force. J Am Acad Dermatol 2006;54:818.

Charman C. Clinical evidence: atopic eczema. BMJ 1999;318:1600.

Eichenfield LF, Hanifin JM, Luger TA, et al. Consensus conference on pediatric AD. J Am Acad Dermatol 2003;49:1088–1095.

Hanifin JM, Rajka G. Diagnostic features of atopic dermatitis. Acta Derm Venereol (Stockh) 1980; 92(suppl):44–47.

Hoare C, Li Wan Po A, Williams H. Systematic review of treatments for atopic eczema. Health Technol Assess 2000;4:1.

Kang K, Polster AM, Nedorost ST, et al. Atopic dermatitis. In: Bolognia JL, Jorizzo JL, Rapini RP, et al., eds. Dermatology. New York: Mosby. 2003, 199.

Jones SM, Sampson HA. The role of allergens in atopic dermatitis. Clin Rev Allergy 1993; 11:471.

Paller AS, Lebwohl M, Fleischer AB Jr, et al. Tacrolimus ointment is more effective than pimecrolimus cream with a similar safety profile in the treatment of atopic dermatitis: results from 3 randomized, comparative studies. J Am Acad Dermatol 2005;52:810.

Rothe MJ, Grant-Kels JM. Diagnostic criteria for atopic dermatitis. Lancet 1996;348:769.

Rowland Payne CM, Wilkinson JD, McKee PH, et al. Nodular prurigo – a clinicopathological study of 46 patients. Br J Dermatol 1985;113:431–439.

Su JC, Kemp AS, Varigos GA, et al. Atopic eczema: its impact on the family and financial cost. Arch Dis Child 1997;76:159–162.

Weidinger S, Illig T, Baurecht H, et al. Loss-of-function variations within the filaggrin gene predispose for atopic dermatitis with allergic sensitizations. J Allergy Clin Immunol 2006;118:214–219.

Weidman AI, Sawicky HH. Nummular eczema; review of the literature: survey of 516 case records and follow-up of 125 patients. AMA Arch Dermatol 1956;73:58–65.

Williams HC. Clinical practice. Atopic dermatitis. N Engl J Med 2005;352:2314.

Wollenberg A, Kraft S, Oppel T, et al. Atopic dermatitis: pathogenetic mechanisms. Clin Exp Dermatol 2000;25:530.

Contact dermatitis

Atherton DJ. A review of the pathophysiology, prevention and treatment of irritant contact dermatitis. Curr Med Res Opin 2004;20:645–649.

Bruckner AL, Weston WL. Beyond poison ivy: understanding allergic contact dermatitis in children. Pediatr Ann 2001;30:203–206.

Denig NI, Hoke AW, Maibach HI. Irritant contact dermatitis. Clues to causes, clinical characteristics, and control. Postgrad Med 1998;103:199–200, 207–208, 212–213.

Kuttin B, Brehler R, Traupe H. Allergic contact dermatitis in children: strategies of prevention and risk management. Eur J Dermatol 2004;14:80–85.

Lewis VJ, Statham BN, Chowdhury MMU. Allergic contact dermatitis in 191 consecutively patch tested children. Contact Dermatitis 2004; 51:155–156.

Militello G, Jacob SE, Crawford GH. Allergic contact dermatitis in children. Curr Opin Pediatr 2006; 18:385–390.

Mortz CG, Lauritsen JM, Bindslev-Jensen C, et al. Contact allergy and allergic contact dermatitis in adolescents: prevalence measures and associations. The Odense Adolescence Cohort Study of Atopic Diseases and Dermatitis (TOACS). Acta Dermatol Venereol 2002;82:352–358.

Mozzanica N. Pathogenetic aspects of allergic and irritant contact dermatitis. Clin Dermatol 1992; 10:115–121.

Roul S, Ducombs G, Taieb A. Usefulness of the European standard series for patch testing children. A 3 year single-centre study of 337 patients. Contact Dermatitis 1999;40:232–235.

Saary J, Quereshi R, Palda V, et al. A systematic review of contact dermatitis treatment and prevention. J Am Acad Dermatol 2005;53:845.

Seidenari S, Giusti F, Pepe P, et al. Contact sensitization in 1094 children undergoing patch testing over a 7-year period. Pediatr Dermatol 2005;22:1–5.

Weston WL, Weston JA, Kinoshita J, et al. Prevalence of positive epicutaneous tests among infants, children, and adolescents. Pediatrics 1986; 78:1070–1074.

Seborrheic dermatitis

Dunic I, Vesic S, Jevtovic DJ. Oral candidiasis and seborrheic dermatitis in HIV-infected patients on highly active antiretroviral therapy. HIV Med 2004;5:50–54.

Faergemann J. *Pityrosporum* infections. J Am Acad Dermatol 1994;31:S18–S20.

Gupta AK, Madzia SE, Batra R. Etiology and management of seborrheic dermatitis. Dermatology 2004;208:89–93.

Heng MC, Henderson CL, Barker DC, et al. Correlation of *Pityrosporum ovale* density with clinical severity of seborrheic dermatitis as assessed by a simplified technique. J Am Acad Dermatol 1990;23:82–86.

Reichrath J. Antimycotics: why are they effective in the treatment of seborrheic dermatitis? Dermatology 2004;208:174–175.

Schwartz RA, Janusz CA, Janniger CK. Seborrheic dermatitis. Am Fam Physician 2006;74:125–130.

Keratosis pilaris

Lateef A, Schwartz RA. Keratosis pilaris. Cutis 1999; 63:205–207.

Poskitt L, Wilkinson JD. Natural history of keratosis pilaris. Br J Dermatol 1994;130:711–713.

Chapter 2

Papulosquamous skin eruptions

Andrea L. Zaenglein

Introduction

The papulosquamous disorders are a varied group of conditions with the shared morphology of being raised and scaly. The easiest way to visualize these disorders is to generalize: any dry and scaling, well-defined rash that resembles psoriasis in some form most often will fit into this grouping. Eczematous disorders, especially nummular dermatitis and seborrheic dermatitis, may be less well-defined plaques that are nonetheless included in the papulosquamous differential diagnosis. Lichenoid eruptions, such as lichen planus and lichen striatus, are also commonly recognized alongside papulosquamous disorders given their similar basic characteristics.

The causes of papulosquamous rashes are varied and include infectious, systemic, and primary cutaneous disorders. Therefore, it is important to consider fully the patient's history, family history, and physical examination before arriving at a diagnosis.

> ### PEARL
> Remember the axiom, "If it scales, scrape it," as tinea infection is the greatest imitator of all.

Psoriasis

Key Points

- Well-defined, symmetric pink plaques with adherent silvery scale
- Flexural and facial involvement more common in children
- *Streptococcus* is a common "trigger" in childhood

Clinical presentation

Psoriasis is a very common skin disorder that affects approximately 2–3% of the population. It can present at any age, even in early infancy, with about 10% of cases presenting before the age

of 10 and 2% under 2 years of age. The natural history of psoriasis is defined by chronic periods of flaring followed by unpredictable remission. The two most common parental questions, what caused the psoriasis? and when will it go away? are not easily answered. The etiology of psoriasis is complicated and multifactorial, and the course highly variable.

Generalized plaque psoriasis is the most common form in children and adults. Markedly well-defined pink plaques with thick silvery scaling are typical (Figure 2-1). Pruritus is variable but, if scratched, pinpoint bleeding will result due to the adherence of the scale (Auspitz sign). One of the hallmarks of psoriasis is the presence of the Koebner phenomenon (Figure 2-2). This term is used when a disorder appears at sites of trauma to the skin, whether a scratch, scrape, or sunburn. Other disorders can exhibit koebnerization but psoriasis is the classic example.

The distribution of psoriasis is generally symmetric, involving the extensor surfaces of the knees, buttocks, and elbows. The scalp is the most common site of involvement and may be solely affected in some patients. Approximately 40–60% of children will have psoriasis of the scalp.

There are several key differences in the clinical appearance of childhood psoriasis. Facial involvement (Figure 2-3) is more common, occurring in 20%, and the intertriginous areas behind the ears, axillae, and groin are frequently affected. Intertriginous involvement presents with sharply defined, moist, bright pink-red plaques with fissuring and no scale. Psoriasis should be considered in children presenting with balanitis, vulvitis, and diaper dermatitis (Figure 2-4).

Guttate psoriasis is a common childhood presentation of the disease. Drop-like pinkish-red, scaling papules and small plaques erupt suddenly on the trunk, extremities, face, and scalp (Figure 2-5). Pharyngitis with group A beta-hemolytic streptococcus can trigger

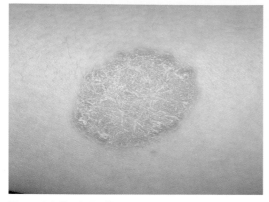

Figure 2-1 Psoriasis. Classic psoriasis plaque

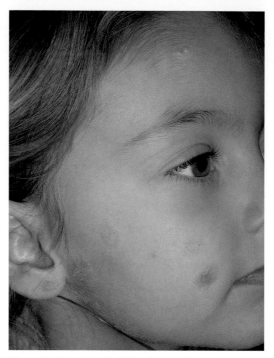

Figure 2-3 Psoriasis. Facial involvement in a 4-year-old girl

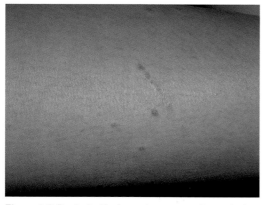

Figure 2-2 Psoriasis. Koebner phenomenon in psoriasis

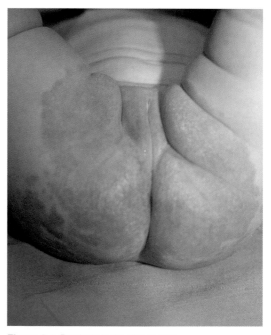

Figure 2-4 Psoriasis in the diaper area

guttate psoriasis. The patient may or may not have a known streptococcal throat infection and a culture is warranted in unclear cases. Perianal streptococcal disease should also be considered as a source and cultured in any suspected cases. Treatment of the streptococcus may or may not lead to clinical improvement of the psoriasis. Prophylactic tonsillectomy has been reported in patients with chronic streptococcal pharyngitis with variable efficacy.

Pustular forms of psoriasis, though less common in children, can occur. Annular pustular psoriasis is the most common presentation (Figure 2-6). Boys are more frequently affected than girls. The onset is typically abrupt and dramatic, accompanied by fever and malaise. Spontaneous remission can occur, but recurrences are common.

Although rare, chronic recurrent multifocal osteomyelitis, or SAPHO syndrome, has been reported in childhood. The acronym SAPHO stands for synovitis, acne, pustulosis, hyperostosis, and osteitis. Sterile pustulosis is the hallmark of this disorder affecting the joints and skin. The cutaneous manifestations include palmoplantar pustular psoriasis, generalized pustular psoriasis, or plaque psoriasis. Pyoderma gangrenosum, Sweet syndrome, and acne are associated with this systemic disorder.

Nail involvement is common, and in the absence of classic skin findings can be difficult to diagnose (Figure 2-7). The four changes found in

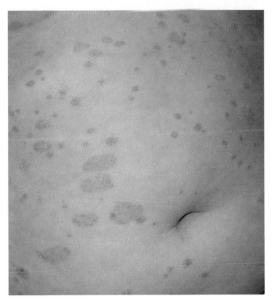

Figure 2-5 Guttate psoriasis on the abdomen

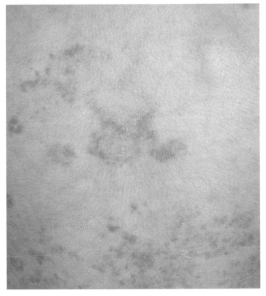

Figure 2-6 Annular pustular psoriasis

psoriatic nails are pitting, thickening, distal onycholysis (separation of the nail from the nail bed), and yellow "oil spots" (slightly translucent areas on the nail surface). Pitting alone can be the first sign of psoriasis, warranting close follow-up in patients with this clinical clue.

Palmoplantar involvement may occur in conjunction with classic plaque psoriasis or as the sole manifestation of psoriasis. The affected areas maintain their sharp borders. As the skin thickens, painful fissuring often results. Pustular palmoplantar psoriasis can also occur.

Mucosal involvement is found in over 5% of cases. The extent and presentations vary, but include geographic tongue and shallow oral aphthae. The genital mucosa may exhibit pain and fissuring.

Psoriatic arthritis can accompany any form of psoriasis. Cutaneous involvement most often precedes the onset of arthritis. Symptoms are similar to those of juvenile rheumatoid arthritis, and, without skin involvement, the two can be difficult to distinguish. A negative rheumatoid factor and absence of systemic rheumatoid symptoms favor a psoriatic diagnosis. A positive family history of psoriasis, presence of dactylitis, or nail pitting and onycholysis are highly suggestive of psoriatic arthritis. The various joint presentations include oligoarthritis involving the proximal and distal interphalangeal joints of the feet, proximal interphalangeal joints of the hands, knees, and ankles. As the disease progresses polyarthritis results, involving the elbow, wrist, and metacarpophalangeal and metatarsophalangeal joints. Blue discoloration overlying affected joints may be seen. Spinal involvement, uveitis, iridocyclitis, pericarditis, and

inflammatory bowel disease are also seen more commonly with psoriatic disease.

Diagnosis

The diagnosis of psoriasis is most often made based on a classic clinical presentation. A biopsy showing hyperkeratosis, parakeratosis, and epidermal acanthosis with loss of the granular layer is diagnostic. The dermal infiltrate is mixed with neutrophils gathering in small groups within the stratum corneum (Munro's microabscesses).

Intertriginous and groin involvement can be difficult to sort out in the very young. Other causes of diaper dermatitis, including candidiasis, tinea cruris, perianal streptococcus, and irritant dermatitis, should be considered.

Nail involvement without skin changes may warrant a fungal culture or pathologic evaluation of a nail clipping to help differentiate nail changes due to alopecia areata, twenty-nail dystrophy (trachyonychia), and onychomycosis.

Psoriasis must be differentiated from other scaling disorders of the scalp including tinea capitis, seborrheic dermatitis, and atopic dermatitis.

Pustular forms of psoriasis should be differentiated from folliculitis, impetigo, tinea infection, and candidiasis. Palmoplantar psoriasis can mimic dyshidrotic eczema, tinea infection, and infantile acropustulosis in the very young patient.

The differential diagnosis of plaque and guttate psoriasis along with other papulosquamous disorders is listed in Table 2-1.

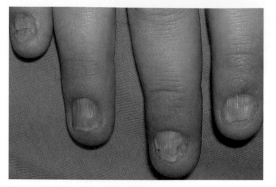

Figure 2-7 Psoriasis of the nails

Etiology

The etiology of psoriasis is not fully understood. Genetic predisposition, immune dysregulation, and environmental factors all contribute. About 30–50% of patients will report a family member with psoriasis. The discovery of the Psor1 gene, linked to chromosome 6, the site of human leukocyte antigen (HLA) class I and II complexes, further supports a genetic cause. Furthermore certain HLA types (B57, Cw6, DR8, DR7, A3) have been variably linked to psoriasis. HLACw6 is associated with onset less than 40 years of age. *Streptococcus* infection is a common trigger for guttate psoriasis and the presence of the HLA Cw0602 allele directly participates in the pathogenesis of streptococcal-associated guttate psoriasis. The role of superantigens in this association is also being considered. Cases have been described following Kawasaki disease as well, like most skin diseases, and stress is a known exacerbating factor for patients with psoriasis. Drugs, such as lithium, beta-blockers, and nonsteroidal anti-inflammatory agents, can also aggravate the condition.

Treatment

Treatment of psoriasis should be tailored towards the age of the child, and the extent and location of the disease. An algorithm for treating psoriasis is given in Table 2-2.

Topical

Topical corticosteroids

Topical corticosteroids are the first-line agents in the treatment of most cases of psoriasis in children. A medium to ultrahigh-potency topical steroid is generally effective for localized lesions. Limiting steroid use to 2 weeks or using a weekday-only regimen can avoid the risk of striae formation and atrophy. This side-effect is of particular concern in the adolescent population, when striae formation is already at its greatest. The face, axilla, and groin areas are at highest risk

for corticosteroid side-effects. Whenever a steroid is placed under occlusion (such as under a diaper), absorption and risk of atrophy increase. Salicylic acid may be added to remove thick, impenetrable scale. A lower-strength steroid should be substituted as lesions flatten and the severity of scaling decreases.

For generalized psoriasis, topical therapies are variably effective. Short-term use of the soak and smear method (tub soaks for 20 min, followed immediately by application of a mid-potency corticosteroid) can be used to help alleviate the severity of symptoms but is limited by the risk of cutaneous absorption and potential for hypothalamic–pituitary–adrenal axis suppression.

For scalp psoriasis specialized formulations suitable for the hair-bearing areas are readily available. Fluocinolone, a mid-to-low-potency steroid, comes in a shampoo (Capex), a solution (Synalar), and oil preparation (Derma-Smoothe F/S). When applied overnight, oils are particularly useful in loosening thick scaling plaques. Oils will make straight hair greasy but may be ideal for patients with coarse or curly hair. They are also a good option for younger children who will not tolerate any burning associated with alcohol-based formulations. Foam preparations containing clobetasol propionate (Olux) or betamethasone valerate (Luxiq) are nongreasy alternatives but may cause brief stinging on any open, excoriated areas.

Intralesional steroid injections may be beneficial for select patients. Triamcinolone injected into the proximal nail bed can improve psoriatic nail involvement. Treatment-resistant thick plaques may also respond to intralesional steroid injection but the risk of local atrophy should be noted.

Calcipotriene Calcipotriene 0.005% (Dovonex) is a vitamin D_3 analog preparation that is available as a cream and solution. Though shown to be effective as monotherapy, it serves as a useful adjunctive therapy in the treatment of psoriasis. Typically an ultrapotent topical steroid ointment is used b.i.d. on weekdays and topical calcipotriene cream is added b.i.d. on the weekends. This combination has a steroid-sparing benefit with the added efficacy of the calcipotriene. Side-effects include local irritation and potential hypercalcemia with systemic absorption. Therefore, calcipotriene should not be applied to greater than 20% body surface area of a child.

Tacrolimus and pimecrolimus Tacrolimus ointment (Protopic) or pimecrolimus cream applied b.i.d. has been used quite successfully for inverse psoriasis where scale is minimal. Areas at greatest risk for steroid atrophy are the ideal sites for use of a topical calcineurin inhibitor. Tacrolimus 0.03% ointment is generally used for children under 12 years of age; and evolving safety

Table 2.1 The differential diagnosis of papulosquamous disorders

	Disorder	Clinical appearance	Distribution	Keys to diagnosis
Common	Psoriasis	Well-demarcated, pink plaques with silvery adherent scale	Localized to scalp, over joints, or generalized	Micaceous scale. Arthritis in 5% of patients
	Pityriasis rosea	Pink-tan papules and oval patches with fine peripheral scale. "Herald patch"	Generalized "Christmas tree" pattern (inverse form uncommon)	Trailing scale. Self resolving in 2–3 months
	Tinea corporis	Annular pink scaling patches and plaques with central clearing	Localized (generalized forms less common)	KOH, fungal culture
	Nummular eczema	Coin-shaped pink scaling patches and plaques. No central clearing	Localized to extremities, more common than generalized	Vesicular evolving to fissured. KOH-negative
	Tinea versicolor	Light tan hypopigmented to darker tan hyperpigmented discrete and confluent patches with very fine scale	Upper back and chest	KOH + short hyphae and yeast forms: "spaghetti and meatballs"
	Seborrheic dermatitis	Light pink, waxy scaling patches and plaques with ill-defined margins	Scalp, eyebrows, nasolabial folds, axilla, and groin; Infantile form often overlaps with atopic dermatitis	Distribution and yellow greasy nature of scale
Uncommon	Pityriasis lichenoides	Varicella-like crusted papules to pink scaling patches, hypopigmented in dark-skinned patients	Generalized trunk and extremities	Consider in cases of suspected pityriasis rosea that do not resolve spontaneously or recur in crops leaving hypopigmentation. Biopsy is key
	Lichen planus	Violaceous papules and plaques with angular borders, annular lesions, and hyperpigmentation in dark-skinned individuals	Localized or generalized	Polygonal papules, distribution
	Discoid lupus erythematosus	Deeper red-purplish plaques with follicular plugging and adherent scale. Annular darker borders with central scarring over time	Sun-exposed areas. Conchal bowl of the ears. Scarring alopecia on the scalp	SLE in 5–10%. Biopsy with immunofluorescence
	Pityriasis rubra pilaris	Well-demarcated yellow-pink plaques with rough sandpaper surface. Follicular papules and islands of sparing within affected areas	Generalized with palm and soles affected	Biopsy often key. Treatment resistant
	Langerhans cell histiocytosis	Pink to tan papules and patches with petechiae and minimal scale	Seborrheic distribution (scalp, axilla, and groin)	Unresponsive to treatments. Biopsy (CD1a +, S100+)
	Secondary syphilis	Reddish-brown papules and plaques with scale, occasionally annular	Generalized, involving palms and soles	Sexual history important. Serologic testing
	Cutaneous T-cell lymphoma	Pink-red to yellowish-copper-colored, minimally scaling patches and plaques. Hypopigmented patches in darker skin	Asymmetric. Localized to generalized. Typically begins in sun-spared areas	Biopsy is key

KOH, potassium hydroxide; SLE, systemic lupus erythematosus.

Table 2.2 Treatment algorithm for psoriasis

	Localized	Generalized
Topical	Medium to high-potency corticosteroids	Medium-potency corticosteroid
	Calcipotriene cream or solution b.i.d. Tazarotene cream Tacrolimus Pimecrolimus Tar Anthralin	Tar baths
Systemic		Phototherapy: UVB/narrow-band UVB Methotrexate Etanercept Cyclosporine Acitretin

UVB, ultraviolet B.

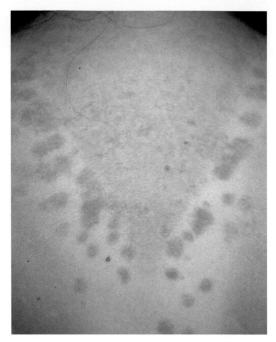

Figure 2-8 Psoriasis. Response to natural sunlight

concerns dictate that use should be intermittent and limited to affected areas only.

Tazarotene This topical retinoid is used for psoriasis and acne vulgaris. It is commercially available in a 0.05% and 0.1% gel and cream (Tazorac). Its use is often limited by irritation but may prove beneficial in select, particularly hyperkeratotic lesions of psoriasis. Concomitant use of a topical steroid may increase tolerability.

Tar Various tar preparations have been used in the treatment of psoriasis for decades. It is available alone in a tar oil (Cutar emulsion), and many over-the-counter shampoo preparations are readily available. Tar can stain plastic bathtubs and parents should be warned accordingly. Preparations incorporating tar, corticosteroid, and/or salicylic acid can be compounded by specialized pharmacies.

Anthralin Skin irritation and staining of the skin are common side-effects with anthralin use and generally limit its use, particularly in children. However, niche uses may be found, particularly in resistant scalp psoriasis (Dritho-Scalp 0.5% cream).

Phototherapy

Most psoriasis responds well to ultraviolet light. The benefits of natural sunlight can be used to the child's advantage during the summer months and many will achieve near clearing just by participating in outdoor activities like swimming (Figure 2-8). Ultraviolet B (UVB) or narrow-band UVB treatment is often employed in older children with extensive psoriasis. Risks include burning, the potential increase in future for photoaging, and the development of skin cancers. Application of moisturizer (such as Eucerin lotion) immediately prior to treatment can enhance penetration of the light by decreasing reflection off the scales. The face and groin should be covered during phototherapy. Sunblock should be applied to areas that do not need treatment. Psoralen plus UVA (PUVA) is not used in children due to prolonged photosensitivity and increased cutaneous malignancy risk.

Systemic therapies

Systemic treatment of psoriasis should be reserved for severe, recalcitrant cases. Methotrexate, cyclosporine, and acitretin have all been used for childhood psoriasis. All systemic treatments come with potential severe risks to the child. Therefore, extensive counseling with the parents and child regarding potential side-effects is mandatory before initiating therapy. Regular laboratory monitoring is necessary. The most commonly used biologic agent in the treatment of psoriasis in children is etanercept (Enbrel), a fusion protein that binds tumor necrosis factor-α and lymphotoxin A inhibiting the inflammatory cascade. Most of its safety data comes from its Food and Drug Administration-approved use in childhood juvenile rheumatoid arthritis.

Pityriasis Rubra Pilaris

- Salmon-colored plaques with follicular papules
- Islands of sparing
- Thick scaling palms and soles

Clinical presentation

Pityriasis rubra pilaris (PRP) is characterized by rough scaling yellow-pink, salmon-colored plaques with follicular prominence and islands of sparing within affected areas (Figure 2-9). The texture is that of a nutmeg grater. Affected areas are sharply delineated from the surrounding unaffected skin. Prominent hyperkeratosis of the palms and soles is common, and dystrophic nails can occur. The Koebner phenomenon occurs in about 10% of patients with PRP. The distribution is symmetric and diffuse, with uncommon progression to erythroderma. Typically, the disorder begins suddenly with a scalp-downward progression.

Subtypes of PRP have been classified according to clinical pattern, prognosis, and age differences. These are listed in Table 2-3. It should be noted that overlap among groups and atypical cases is common.

Itching is variably present, and patients are generally healthy. Although human immunodeficiency virus (HIV) and malignancy have been linked in adults, these associations have not been reported in children.

Diagnosis

A biopsy can be done to confirm the diagnosis of PRP. Typical cases will show follicular plugging, hyperkeratosis with alternating bands of orthokeratosis and parakeratosis, and a superficial perivascular lymphocytic infiltrate.

The differential diagnosis of PRP includes psoriasis, vitamin A deficiency (phrynoderma), inherited palmoplantar keratodermas, subacute cutaneous lupus erythematosus, and dermatomyositis.

Etiology

The etiology of PRP is unknown. Males and females are equally affected and familial cases are well described. There is a bimodal distribution of onset, with most patients presenting in the first and sixth decades.

Treatment

The therapeutic ladder for PRP in childhood typically begins with topical emollients, topical corticosteroids, and topical keratolytic agents (lactic acid or urea preparations). Conservative management may be adequate in localized and self-limited disease. In extensive, chronic cases systemic therapies may be needed. Phototherapy may flare disease in some patients while proving

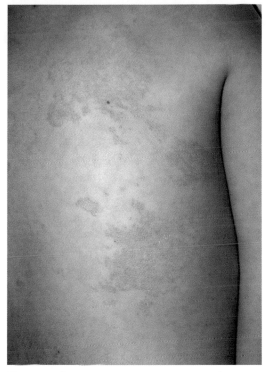

Figure 2-9 Pityriasis rubra pilaris. Follicular prominence with islands of sparing

useful in others. Oral isotretinoin, 0.5–1 mg/kg per day, is most effective, taking 6 months to achieve results. Reported recurrence rates in children are 17%. Methotrexate, cyclosporine, high-dose vitamin A, and azathioprine have also been used with benefit.

Pityriasis Rosea

- Herald patch occurring about 1 week before generalizing
- Salmon-pink patches and thin plaques with central scale
- Christmas-tree distribution
- Spontaneous resolution

Clinical presentation

Patients affected with this common disorder will likely give the history of a single plaque heralding the generalized eruption. This foreshadowing precursor, noted in about 80%, is designated the "mother patch" or "herald patch" (Figure 2-10A). Within about a week, as the initial lesion starts to wane, thin salmon-pink plaques with central scale erupt, following the subtly descending lines of the natural skin folds of the trunk and upper extremities (Langer's lines) (Figure 2-10B). This pattern is commonly known as a "Christmas-tree" distribution given its semblance to the hanging

Table 2.3 Types of pityriasis rubra pilaris

	Type	Course	Clinical appearance
I	Classic adult	80% resolve in 3 years	Abrupt-onset cephalocaudal progression of follicular papules evolving to salmon-colored plaques with islands of sparing. Hyperkeratotic palms and soles
II	Atypical adult	Chronic course	Ichthyosis-like scaling with prominent palmoplantar involvement
III	Classic juvenile	Most resolve in 1 year	Same as type 1 classic adult but with younger age of onset
IV	Circumscribed juvenile	Chronic course	Typical plaques on elbows and knees. Keratoderma of palms and soles. Localized involvement
V	Atypical juvenile	Chronic course	Scleroderma-like palms and soles with hyperkeratosis and minimal erythema. Early childhood onset. Familial cases reported

branches of a fir tree. The face, hands, and feet are typically spared. Oral lesions can occur but are fairly uncommon.

Pityriasis rosea peaks biannually in the spring and fall. Adolescents and younger adults, ages 15–40 years, are most commonly affected. Females are twice as likely to present with the disease as males. A history of a mild systemic prodrome is variable. Mild pruritus is common, with severe pruritus reported in about 25% of cases. Spontaneous resolution of the entire course occurs in 3–8 weeks; and recurrences are very rare. Concurrent lymphadenopathy is more common in African-Americans.

Atypical variants are regularly seen, occurring in about 20%. Papular pityriasis rosea occurs with a greater frequency in children under 5 years of age, in darker-skinned individuals, and in pregnant women. Inverse pityriasis confines itself to the creases of the axillae and groin and, owing to the moist environment, lacks the characteristic scale. A purpuric variant has also been described with petechiae and ecchymoses occurring within the scaling patches. Vesicular pityriasis rosea can mimic varicella.

Diagnosis

The differential diagnosis includes other papulosquamous disorders listed in this chapter. Psoriasis, especially in its guttate form, can be difficult to differentiate from pityriasis rosea. The adherent, silvery scale of psoriasis can usually be distinguished from the finer, centrally located scale of pityriasis rosea. Scalp and nail involvement favor a diagnosis of psoriasis. Pityriasis lichenoides is the closest mimicker of pityriasis rosea. Time is often the best clue in differentiating the two, with pityriasis lichenoides persisting for months to years.

Several medications, most rarely used in children, have been reported to induce a pityriasis rosea-like drug eruption. The list includes arsenicals, barbiturates, bismuth, captopril, clonidine, diphtheria toxin, ergotamine, gold, imatinib, interferon, isotretinoin, ketotifen, levamisole, lisinopril, methoxypromazine, metronidazole, omeprazole, penicillamine, terbinafine, and tripelennamine hydrochloride.

Pathogenesis

Although widely believed to be of a viral origin, seasonality, case clustering, and lack of recurrence due to no clear etiology has ever been elucidated. Human herpesviruses 6 and 7 have often been implicated in the pathogenesis of pityriasis rosea but definitive causation has not been established.

Treatment

Typically pityriasis rosea will resolve spontaneously without treatment over 6–12 weeks. Oral antihistamines and a mid-potency topical corticosteroid can ease symptoms but will not alter the course of disease. In extensive cases, UVB therapy can decrease severity and speed resolution.

Pityriasis Lichenoides

Key Points

- May resemble varicella or pityriasis rosea
- Generally nonpruritic
- Chronic course of months to years

Clinical presentation

Pityriasis lichenoides is often a second-hand diagnosis. The initial diagnoses that are typically entertained include varicella or pityriasis rosea depending on the clinical appearance of the lesions at the time of presentation. However, as both of these conditions are self-limited, the diagnosis of pityriasis lichenoides becomes more obvious over time as new lesions continue to appear and the eruption does not go away in the anticipated timeframe.

The acute form of pityriasis lichenoides, known as pityriasis lichenoides et varioliformis acuta (PLEVA) or Mucha–Habermann disease, is defined by the presence of hemorrhagic crusted papules that can resemble those of chickenpox (Figure 2-11).

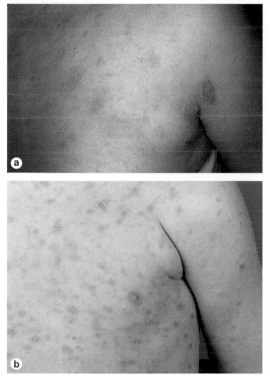

Figure 2-10a Pityriasis rosea. Herald patch amongst thin oval plaques of pityriasis rosea. **b** Pityriasis rosea. Salmon-colored plaques with central scaling

The lesions occur in crops scattered amongst pink, dry scaling patches and thin plaques. Crusted papules often heal with pox-like scarring.

A severe form of the disease is associated with the abrupt onset of hemorrhagic, crusted papules and plaques associated with fever, pneumonitis, myocarditis, or ataxia. This lasts several months then stabilizes to the more classic chronic morphology with resolution of the systemic symptoms.

As the course of the disease lingers on, any thoughts of varicella will fade, and the diagnosis of pityriasis lichenoides will become apparent. With time, the numbers of acute lesions will diminish, being replaced by the pink, dry scaling patches and plaques of the chronic form, pityriasis lichenoides chronica. New crops regularly occur while old lesions heal with hypopigmentation (Figure 2-12). Pityriasis lichenoides does not always progress from acute to chronic lesion types. Patients can have continued crusted papules throughout the course or present with the typical chronic-type pink patches. It is best to consider this disorder as a spectrum of lesion types. Rare progression to cutaneous T-cell lymphoma is controversial but has been reported. Therefore, patients should be followed regularly for any changes in lesion morphology and biopsied when appropriate.

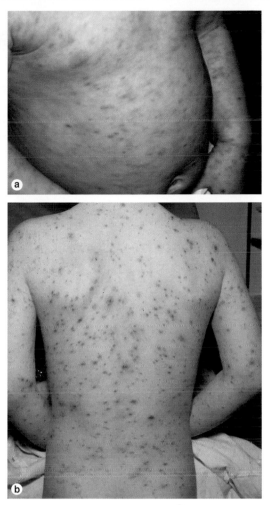

Figure 2-11a Pityriasis lichenoides. Chickenpox-like crusted papules of pityriasis lichenoides et varioliformis acuta. **b** Pityriasis lichenoides

Diagnosis

The background of dyspigmentation, typically hypopigmented macules in various stages of healing, is an excellent distinguishing characteristic useful in differentiating pityriasis lichenoides from guttate psoriasis. The time course will eliminate acute processes, such as varicella or pityriasis rosea. Lymphomatoid papulosis, often presenting with crops of ulceronecrotic papules and nodules, should be considered in atypical cases. The hypopigmented form of cutaneous T-cell lymphoma (mycosis fungoides) poses a particularly difficult differential diagnosis that may require histologic confirmation.

Biopsy will confirm the diagnosis of pityriasis lichenoides, showing epidermal necrosis, hemorrhage, and a wedge-shaped lymphocytic

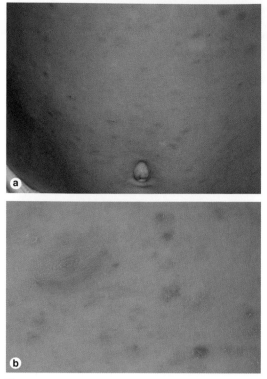

Figure 2-12a Pityriasis lichenoides. Chronic-type lesions with prominent postinflammatory hypopigmentation. **b** Pityriasis lichenoides. Chronic-type lesions

Table 2.4 Treatment of pityriasis lichenoides

Chronic, mild		Acute, severe, scarring
Observation Natural sunlight Mid-potency topical corticosteroid Topical tacrolimus	Erythromycin 40 mg/kg b.i.d. to t.i.d. Azithromycin UVB UVA1	Methotrexate Dapsone PUVA

PUVA, psoralen ultraviolet A; UVA1, ultraviolet A1; UVB, ultraviolet B.

infiltrate. The interface change is vacuolar, with lymphocytes in virtually every vacuole. Vessel lumens are typically packed with neutrophils, and an overlying crust develops depending on the age of the lesion. Erythrocytes are commonly noted within the epidermis. Chronic lesions will show the same histologic morphology with less epidermal change and a less pronounced infiltrate. T-cell gene rearrangement studies have found high rates of clonality in acute-type lesions but not consistently in the chronic form.

Pathogenesis

Pityriasis lichenoides is a T-cell-mediated disorder of unknown etiology. Cytotoxic CD8+ T cells predominate, suggesting a response to an unknown viral pathogen.

Treatment

Treatment of pityriasis lichenoides will depend on the severity of lesions, presence of scarring, presence of symptoms, and the age of the patient. Aggressive therapy is warranted to prevent severe scarring in select cases, while observation, UV light, or natural sunlight may be the best treatment option in young patients with mild, indolent disease. An algorithm for treatment is given in Table 2-4.

Lichen Striatus

Key Points

* Pink to hypopigmented thin dry papules in a linear distribution
* Spontaneous improvement over months to years

Clinical presentation

This is arguably one of the easiest and most fun of the classic pediatric dermatology skin disorders to diagnose. Children under the age of 6 are most commonly affected, though cases in older children and adults are reported. Lichen striatus begins as a suddenly appearing, unilateral linear array of pink to hypopigmented, 1–3-mm papules with mild scaling (Figure 2-13). One or two bands follow the lines of Blaschko. Bilateral involvement is uncommon. As the eruption progresses, the papules can flatten to macules, maintaining the characteristic linear distribution. In darker-skinned patients, hypopigmentation is common. While the limbs are most commonly affected, lichen striatus can appear anywhere. If the eruption involves a limb and extends to the hand, a linear nail dystrophy can occur. The typical course ends spontaneously with resolution occurring in several months to years, with 6 months being the average time course.

Diagnosis

While the diagnosis of lichen striatus is usually made clinically, a biopsy should be performed in atypical cases. A lichenoid infiltrate with a band of necrotic keratinocytes along the dermo-epidermal junction is seen along with a characteristic dense lymphoid infiltrate around the eccrine ducts. The differential diagnosis of a linear eruption in a child includes several atypical variants of common cutaneous diseases, as well as several rare disorders. These are listed in Table 2-5.

Pathogenesis

The etiology of the disorder is unknown, but it probably represents a genetic mosaic of cells predisposed to developing an inflammatory

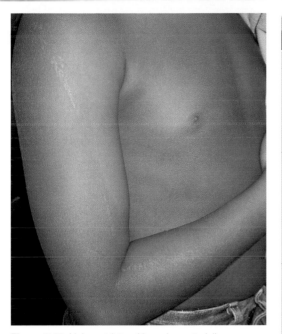

Figure 2-13 Lichen striatus. Hypopigmented, linear papules in lichen striatus on the arm

response to a variety of environmental stimuli. An apoptotic death of these cells could account for the self-limited nature of the eruption. A family history of atopy and reports of affected siblings may be coincidental.

Diagnosis

Treatments are generally ineffective, but trials of a mid-potency topical corticosteroid may be beneficial in flattening the papules or easing pruritus. Topical tacrolimus has been used with good results in facial lesions.

Lichen Planus

Key Points

* Violaceous angular flat-topped papules and plaques on wrists and foot
* Reticulated white network may be visible on surface
* Hyperpigmented in dark-skinned patients
* Variably itchy
* Self-limited over a couple of years

Clinical presentation

Lichen planus is an uncommon pediatric eruption. Lesions typically consist of purple, planar plaques ranging in size from 3 to 10 mm. The wrist and instep of the foot are classic locations (Figure 2-14) but the legs, low back, face, and genitalia are other sites of predilection. Scale may be indistinct, and a reticulated white network, called Wickham's striae, may be seen with magnification. Itch is variable but can be

Table 2.5 Differential diagnoses of linear eruptions

Disorder	Pattern mechanism
Infectious	
Herpes zoster	Dermatomal
Flat warts	Koebner
Thrombophlebitis	Lymphatic
Sporotrichosis	Lymphatic
Cutaneous larva migrans	Random
Inflammatory	
Lichen striatus	Blaschkoid
Linear scleroderma	Segmental
Linear psoriasis	Segmental
Lichen nitidus	Koebner
Lichen planus	Koebner
Incontinentia pigmenti	Blaschkoid
Linear cutaneous lupus	Segmental
Developmental	
Striae distensae	Segmental
Pigmentary demarcation lines	Segmental
Epidermal nevus	Segmental blaschkoid
ILVEN	
Pigmentary mosaicism	Blaschkoid
Miscellaneous	
Phytophotodermatitis	Contact
Contact dermatitis	Contact
Self-induced	Contact

ILVEN, inflammatory linear verrucous epidermal nevus.

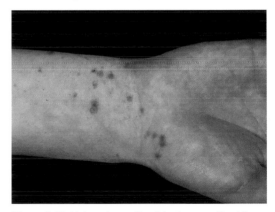

Figure 2-14 Lichen planus. Purplish plaques with white streaks on the wrist

intense. Asymptomatic whitish streaks on the buccal mucosa often accompany the cutaneous lesions. The eruption tends to be self-limited but chronic, lasting 1–2 years or longer.

Diagnosis

A biopsy will confirm the diagnosis and may be needed to rule out other papulosquamous conditions.

Treatment

Topical corticosteroids are the mainstay of treatment but a systemic course of prednisone can be considered for extremely symptomatic cases.

Further reading

Allison DS, el.-Azhari RA, Calobrisi ST, et al. Pityriasis rubra pilaris in children. J Am Acad Dermatol 2002;47:386–389.

Bowers S, Warshaw EM. Pityriasis lichenoides and its subtypes. J Am Acad Dermatol 2006;55:557–572.

Dadlini C, Orlow SJ. Treatment of children and adolescents with methotrexate, cyclosporine, and etanercept: review of dermatologic and rheumatologic literature. J Am Acad Dermatol 2005;52:316–340.

Gelmetti C, Schiuma AA, Cerri D, et al. Pityriasis rubra pilaris in childhood: a long-term study of 29 cases. Pediatr Dermatol 1986;3:446–451.

Gonzalez LM, Allen R, Janninger CK, et al. Pityriasis rosea: an important papulosquamous disorder. Int J Dermatol 2005;44:757–764.

Griffiths WA. Pityriasis rubra pilaris. Clin Exp Dermatol 1980;5:105–112.

Hartley A. Pityriasis rosea. Pediatr Rev 1999;20:266.

Lewkowicz D, Gottlieb AB. Pediatric psoriasis and psoriatic arthritis. Dermatol Ther 2004;17:364–375.

Morris A, Rogers M, Fischer G, et al. Childhood psoriasis: a clinical review of 1262 cases. Pediatr Dermatol 2001;18:188–198.

Patrizi A, Neri I, Fiorentini C, et al. Lichen striatus: clinical and laboratory features of 115 children. Pediatr Dermatol 2004;21:197–204.

Rogers M. Childhood psoriasis. Curr Opin Pediatr 2002;14:404–409.

Romani J, Puig L, Fernandez-Figueras MT, et al. Pityriasis lichenoides in children: clinicopathologic review of 22 cases. Pediatr Dermatol 1998;15:1–6.

Taniguchi Abagge K, Parolin Marinoni L, Giraldi S, et al. Lichen striatus: description of 89 cases in children. Pediatr Dermatol 2004;21:440–443.

3

Acne and related disorders

Albert C. Yan

Acne vulgaris is a chronic skin disorder that involves the pilosebaceous units. It is one of the most common complaints encountered by both primary care clinicians and dermatologists and is estimated to affect some 50 million people in the USA who spend over $2.5 billion each year on a combination of over-the-counter and prescription treatments to treat their condition. Uncommon during early childhood, acne is a nearly universal experience among adolescents, affecting 80–95% of all teenagers. As a chronic disorder that largely remits following the teen years, it may continue to vex a subset of patients into adulthood. Although the primary lesions of acne resolve, postinflammatory dyschromia is not uncommon and some residual permanent scarring may result in a significant subset of patients.

Both the disease and its sequelae may have significant psychosocial impact on patients with acne. Adolescents with the disease may suffer from low self-esteem, social phobias, anger issues, anxiety, and mood disturbances and later, adults may report greater difficulties with unemployment when compared with unaffected individuals.

Acne vulgaris is a common clinical disorder that clearly carries great emotional significance for those who suffer from it. Knowledge of its various clinical presentations, an awareness of potential differential diagnoses, and a thorough understanding of its pathogenesis will help one to combine appropriate skin care measures with both topical and systemic medications in order to design a reasonable and effective treatment regimen for acne patients.

Key Features

- Pilosebaceous distribution (face, ears, neck, chest, shoulders, back, occasionally the scalp)
- Primary lesions
  - Comedones (open or closed)
  - Acneiform papules
  - Acneiform pustules
  - Acneiform nodules
- Secondary lesions
  - Postinflammatory dyschromia

- Hyperpigmentation and dyschromia
  - Scars
- Atrophic ("icepick" or "thumbprint" scars)
- Hypertrophic, papular scars
- Keloidal scars
- Osteoma cutis within acne scars
- Acne-related disorders
  - Follicular occlusion triad: acne conglobata, hidradenitis suppurativa, dissecting cellulitis of the scalp
  - Acne fulminans: severe, acute acne with fever and arthritis
  - SAPHO: synovitis, acne, pustulosis, hyperostosis, osteitis
  - PAPA: pyogenic sterile arthritis, pyoderma gangrenosum, severe acne

Clinical presentation

The primary lesions of acne include: open and closed comedones (Figures 3-1 and 3-2), papules, pustules (Figure 3-3), and nodules ("cysts") (Figure 3-4). Secondary lesions consist of: postinflammatory skin changes of hyper- and hypopigmentation (Figure 3-5), as well as a variety of scar morphologies. Atrophic scars include icepick-type scars which appear as punctate depressions within the skin, while thumbprint or rolling scars are larger, depressed areas. Hypertrophic scars are elevated and approximate the size of the original inflammatory lesion, while keloidal scars – more

Figure 3-1 Open comedones ("blackheads")

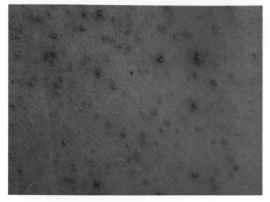

Figure 3-2 Closed comedones ("whiteheads")

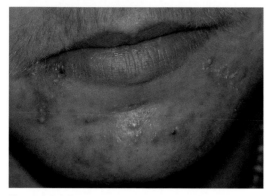

Figure 3-3 Inflammatory acne consisting of papules and pustules

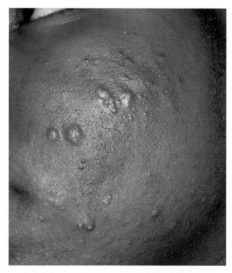

Figure 3-4 Inflammatory acne consisting of nodules and scars

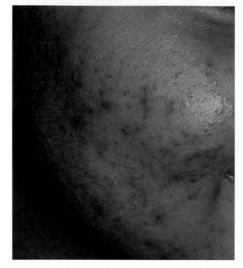

Figure 3-5 Postinflammatory dyschromia consisting of hyperpigmentation

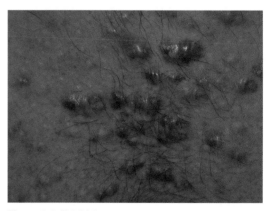

Figure 3-6 Keloidal acne scars

Table 3-1 Primary and secondary lesions of acne	
Primary lesions	Secondary lesions
Comedones (open and closed)	Postinflammatory dyschromia
Papules	Erythema
Pustules	Hyperpigmentation
Nodules ("cysts")	Hypopigmentation
	Scars (atrophic, hypertrophic, keloidal)

commonly encountered on the chest, shoulders, and back – are larger and expand beyond their original areas of inflammation (Figure 3-6). Rarely, small calcified lesions representing miliary osteoma cutis may occur in some individuals with acne scarring.

In patients with mild acne, comedones predominate. Closed comedones ("whiteheads") are small, white papules whereas open comedones ("blackheads") appear black because of exposed melanin from the keratinocytes of the pilosebaceous unit. In moderate acne, a mixture of comedones, papules, and sometimes pustules is noted. Postinflammatory dyschromia and scarring may also be seen in patients with moderate acne. Nodules, postinflammatory changes, and scarring are the hallmark of patients with severe acne (Table 3-1). Although patients with mild (Figure 3-7),

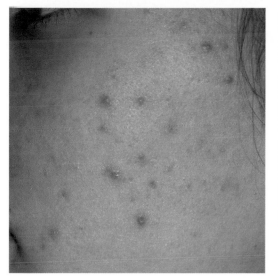

Figure 3-7 Mild acne consisting primarily of comedones

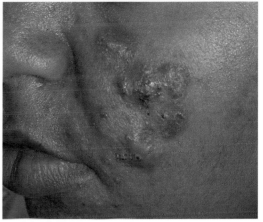

Figure 3-9 Severe acne, comprising inflammatory nodules and extensive scarring

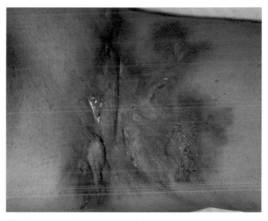

Figure 3-10 Acne inversa (hidradenitis suppurativa)

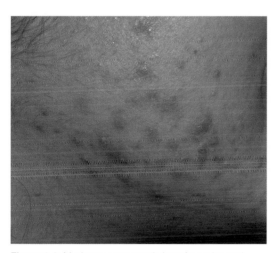

Figure 3-8 Moderate acne consisting of papules and pustules

moderate (Figure 3-8), or severe acne (Figure 3-9) may seek treatment, it is those with the greatest potential for scarring – that is, those with moderate and severe acne – who require the most urgent attention. Longer delays between the onset of acne and obtaining adequate treatment are associated with the greatest degree of scarring.

Because acne derives from the pilosebaceous apparatus, acne lesions are most prominent on the face, chest, shoulders, and back, although other areas such as the neck, scalp, and external auditory canals may be affected as well. Furthermore, some patients may have involvement of other related follicular structures as part of the so-called follicular occlusion complex of acne inversa (Figure 3-10), which consists of: acne conglobata, hidradenitis suppurativa, perifolliculitis capitis abscedens

et suffodiens (PCAS; also known as dissecting cellulitis of the scalp), and pilonidal cysts which may in reality represent developmental anomalies rather than a true acne inversa variant. Acne conglobata is a more severe, idiopathic form of acute, nodulocystic acne which can be disfiguring due to scarring and sinus tract formation. Hidradenitis suppurativa, a follicular disorder associated with apocrine gland abnormalities, presents with nodulocystic lesions in the axillary, inguinal, and perianal areas and in one family has recently been linked to a locus on chromosome 1p21.1-1q25.3. PCAS is an idiopathic follicular disorder that results in a papulopustular and suppurative eruption of the scalp that evolves into scars and sinus tract formation.

Patients with severe acne may also manifest systemic symptoms and signs that have been described as part of a larger systemic syndrome. A variety of acne-associated spondyloarthropathies have been described in association with severe acne:

Acne-related spondyloarthropathy syndromes

Acne inversa with arthritis

Acne fulminans with arthritis

PAPA (pyogenic arthritis, pyoderma gangrenosum, and acne)

SAPHO (synovitis, acne, pustulosis, hyperostosis, osteomyelitis syndrome)

- Severe cases of acne inversa have been associated with spondyloarthropathies.
- Acne fulminans refers to a severe form of inflammatory acne that presents acutely with fever and arthritis and is thought to be related to an exuberant innate immune response to propionibacteria.
- PAPA syndrome describes an autoinflammatory condition in which patients suffer from an erosive pyogenic arthritis, pyoderma gangrenosum, and acne. In some patients, mutations in a gene that serves as a ligand for pyrin, the protein implicated in familial Mediterranean fever, have been associated.
- SAPHO syndrome is an acronym for the idiopathic acne syndrome reported in 1987 by Chamot et al. as "le syndrome acne pustulose hyperostose ostéite" and, alternatively, as synovitis, acne, pustulosis, hyperostosis, osteomyelitis syndrome. Patients with SAPHO present with sterile pustules on the palms and soles. The acne is typically severe, and may include acne fulminans, acne conglobata, or acne inversa, while the synovitis and osteomyelitis are sterile.

Clinicians should be aware that musculoskeletal complaints in acne patients may indicate an underlying systemic disorder that warrants further evaluation (Box 3-1).

Diagnosis

The diagnosis of acne vulgaris is typically an easy one, and generally does not require laboratory studies, imaging studies, or biopsy, except in cases where associated systemic disease is suspected. However, if the review of systems or the physical examination suggests hyperandrogenism as an underlying influence, appropriate laboratory studies for hormonal dysfunction are indicated.

When synovitis or osteomyelitis symptoms occur, appropriate evaluation, including laboratory tests and imaging studies – to rule out an underlying infectious process and to evaluate bones and joints – is essential before attributing these findings to PAPA, SAPHO, or an inflammatory acne variant. In cases of PAPA, a skin biopsy to confirm the presence of pyoderma gangrenosum may be necessary.

Differential diagnosis of acne-like disorders

Acne keloidalis nuchae

Angiofibromas, facial

Folliculitis, secondary to bacteria (Gram-positive and Gram-negative) or yeast

Infantile or toddler acne

Neonatal acne (transient neonatal cephalic pustulosis)

Keratosis pilaris

Perioral (granulomatous) dermatitis

Pseudofolliculitis barbae

Differential Diagnosis (Box 3-2)

- Neonatal acne: this acneiform eruption affects infants and presents during the first 3 months of life. Papules and pustules typically appear on the face, upper chest, and back (Figure 3-11). The eruption is self-limited and heals without scarring. Conventional wisdom has taught that neonatal acne results from the presence in the infant of excess maternal androgens. However, recent evidence indicates that neonatal acne (also referred to as "transient neonatal cephalic pustulosis") is associated with overgrowth of *Malassezia* species and is not in fact a precursor to acne vulgaris. This condition may reflect the relative hyperandrogen state of newborns and may require a seborrheic environment to exist.
- Infantile and toddler acne: this acneiform eruption is characterized by comedones, papules, and nodules which have the potential to leave scars (Figure 3-12). The condition may first present during later infancy or early childhood. Although this form of acne often remits, it may represent a harbinger of later more severe acne during adolescence. Due to the potential for scarring, treatment entails use of traditional acne therapies: topical retinoids, topical benzoyl peroxide (BP), topical or systemic antibiotics (excepting tetracyclines), and, in severe cases, isotretinoin.
- Folliculitis: processes mediated by microorganisms may cause follicular inflammation that may mimic acne vulgaris.
- Gram-positive folliculitis is often characterized by papules and pustules which may involve the face (especially the beard area), chest, back, buttocks, and legs (Figure 3-13) *Staphylococcus aureus* is the organism most commonly implicated. In cases where methicillin-resistant species of *S. aureus* (MRSA) are involved, furuncles, carbuncles, and cellulitis may occur. Drainage is the single

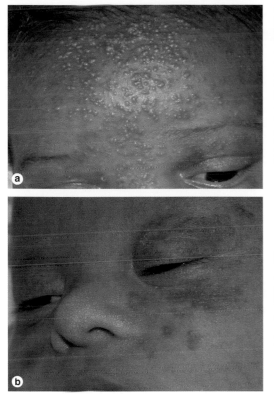

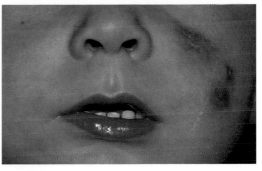

Figure 3-12 Infantile acne – note the inflammatory nodular acne

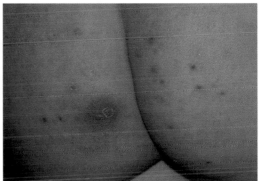

Figure 3-11a, b Neonatal acne – note the papular eruption with no evidence of comedones

Figure 3-13 Gram-positive staphylococcal folliculitis

most important intervention for an MRSA abscess. Staphylococcal carriage is common in the nares. Nasal carriage can be addressed with topical agents, but resistance to mupirocin is common, and newer agents such as retapamulin should be studied in this setting. Staphylococcal carriage is also common in the axillae, groin, and perianal area. These areas may be addressed with topical chlorhexidine, triclosan, or bleach baths (2 tablespoons of bleach per gallon of bath water or about half a cup of bleach per full bathtub of water). When an oral antibiotic is required for an MRSA infection, trimethoprim-sulfamethoxazole, tetracycline derivatives, clindamycin, vancomycin, or linezolid may be appropriate agents depending on the severity of infection, antibiotic sensitivities of the organism, and the age of the patient. Inducible resistance to clindamycin is becoming more common. In areas with a high prevalence of inducible resistance, erythromycin resistance indicates the potential for inducible clindamycin resistance. Strains with inducible resistance may fail in clinical practice despite a lab report indicating that the organism is sensitive to clindamycin. A D-test can be requested to test for inducible resistance.

- Gram-negative folliculitis (GNF): the findings of GNF may resemble those of acne

vulgaris. Inflammatory papules and pustules due to Gram-negative organisms may arise secondary to chronic antibiotic therapy for acne, resulting in overgrowth of *Klebsiella* species, *Escherichia coli*, *Enterobacter* species, and *Proteus* species. Patients with acne-related GNF will often respond to isotretinoin, ampicillin, or trimethoprim-sulfamethoxazole. *Pseudomonas* species may also cause GNF in the context of contaminated closed-cycle water sources, as in the so-called "hot tub folliculitis" or from underlying immunocompromise from human immunodeficiency virus (HIV) disease.

- Pityrosporum folliculitis: like its infantile counterpart, adolescents and adults who develop a papulopustular eruption involving the face, chest, or back areas may suffer from folliculitis secondary to pityrosporum (*Malassezia*) (Figure 3-14A and 3-14B). In contrast to acne vulgaris, comedones are not usually observed. This diagnosis should be considered when patients complain of concomitant pruritus, seborrheic dermatitis, and scalp pustules, worsening with heat and exercise and when they do not respond to typical acne therapies. In fact, some patients may suffer from both acne vulgaris and pityrosporum folliculitis; in these cases, patients may initially show improvement with acne therapy, but may have recalcitrant

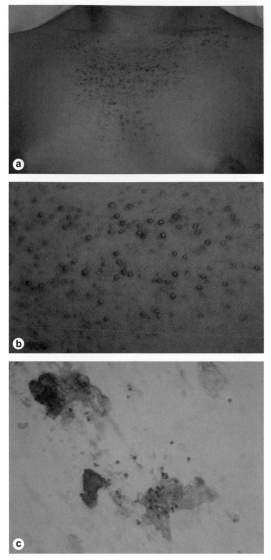

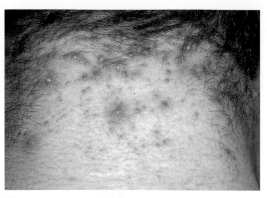

Figure 3-15 Acne keloidalis nuchae

Figure 3-14a, b Pityrosporum folliculitis. **c** Microscopic examination of pityrosporum folliculitis. (Courtesy of Howard Pride, MD)

lesions due to pityrosporum folliculitis. Bacterial Gram stains should be negative, and potassium hydroxide preparations, color stains for yeast (such as chlorazole black), or Tzanck smear will identify the yeast forms (Figure 3-14C) Patients can be successfully treated with topical or oral antifungals, such as selenium sulfide or ketoconazole, but may be aggravated by antibiotics which reduce resident bacterial flora. In adolescents and adults, recommended treatment is 2 weeks of ketoconazole 200 mg daily followed by intermittent use of ketoconazole shampoo or ZNP soap bar.

- Pseudofolliculitis barbae: this condition presents with papules and pustules on closely shaved areas, such as the beard area of the face. Close shaving creates ingrown hairs, which produce a foreign-body reaction and inflamed perifollicular papules and nodules. Remedies include: avoidance of close shaving, use of single-blade razors or electric razors, depilatories, laser hair ablation, discontinuation of shaving, topical retinoids, topical antibiotics, and topical BP.

- Acne keloidalis (folliculitis keloidalis): papules, pustules, and small keloids on the back of the neck and posterior scalp are the telltale signs of this condition (Figure 3-15). Although this may be aggravated by close shaving, the condition is idiopathic and appears to represent an inflammatory scarring alopecia. Treatments include use of topical retinoids, topical BP, as well as topical and systemic antibiotics such as tetracycline derivatives, used more for their anti-inflammatory than their anti-infective properties.

- Perioral dermatitis: perioral (granulomatous) dermatitis is another acneiform eruption in which comedones are absent. Pink to flesh-colored pinpoint papules and pustules manifest in a perioral and periorificial distribution (Figure 3-16). Rarely, extrafacial lesions of this condition may occur. Although idiopathic, many patients report prior use of topical steroids or of other occlusive cosmetic products. Histologically, the lesions show granulomatous changes reminiscent of rosacea. Appropriate treatment consists of discontinuing topical steroid use (if applicable), and use of topical agents such as BP (limited by its irritant potential), erythromycin (particularly the ointment formulation), clindamycin, sodium sulfacetamide, or metronidazole; or systemic antibiotics such as erythromycin or tetracycline derivatives.

- Keratosis pilaris: young children may present with small, perifollicular, keratotic papules on the face, arms, or legs that may be mistaken for early acne vulgaris (Figure 3-17). In this autosomal-dominant condition, follicular openings become

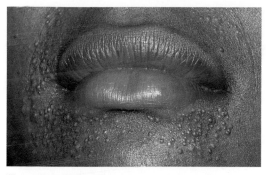

Figure 3-16 Perioral (granulomatous) dermatitis

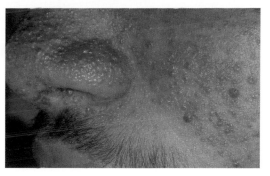

Figure 3-18 Facial angiofibromas of tuberous sclerosis

Figure 3-17 Keratosis pilaris

plugged with keratin. Generally asymptomatic, the facial lesions often resolve spontaneously during late childhood, although lesions on the arms and legs may be more persistent. Active nonintervention is frequently the best course of action, although treatment with keratolytics such as topical ammonium lactate or urea, or topical retinoids such as tretinoin, adapalene, or tazarotene can help moderate the clinical features of this condition.

- Facial angiofibromas: a hallmark of tuberous sclerosis, these flesh-colored to brown-red, rubbery papules typically manifest during the first 5 years (Figure 3-18). Frequently, lesions will cluster around the nasolabial folds. In contrast to acne lesions, facial angiofibromas appear earlier than acne vulgaris, are persistent, and do not respond to conventional acne treatments. Treatment with pulsed-dye laser may help reduce erythema, while carbon dioxide laser resurfacing is more effective at reducing the appearance of these lesions.

Pathogenesis

Acne vulgaris is a disorder of the pilosebaceous unit that is triggered by hormonal factors. Endogenous androgens increase sebum production within the

hair follicle. Abnormal follicular desquamation, possibly aggravated by intracellular retinoid deficiencies, causes the follicle to become clogged, resulting in the development of the microcomedone and comedone.

Bacterial flora resident within the pilosebaceous unit also play a significant role in the transformation of comedonal acne into inflammatory acne. The most important of these is *Propionibacterium acnes*, a commensal anaerobic bacterium that breaks down the accumulated sebum in this lipid-rich environment into free fatty acids and other proinflammatory mediators which stimulate neutrophil chemotaxis and activate neutrophil lysozymes and complement. This eventuates in the formation of inflammatory papules, pustules, and nodules (Box 3-3).

Treatment

Acne patients frequently have implicit or explicit expectations for prompt and rapid improvement of their disease. Devising a treatment plan for patients with acne, therefore, involves communicating: (1) reasonable and realistic expectations for the timeline envisioned for seeing results; (2) the anticipated duration of therapy; (3) a manageable skin care program; (4) an appropriate pharmacologic regimen graded to the severity of the disease; as well as (5) the crucial role of compliance.

Although early signs of acne amelioration may appear as early as 1 week after initiating therapy, most patients will not be able to discern improvement until 4–8 weeks later. Because acne is a chronic condition, patients and their families must understand that treatment is not synonymous with cure. Adolescents and adults with acne may require ongoing treatment for months and sometimes years, with therapy titrated to the degree of disease (Figure 3-19; Table 3-2).

An optimal therapeutic regimen will help reduce aggravating factors that might irritate the skin during treatment. Patients should

BOX 3-3

Key factors in acne pathogenesis

Androgen stimulation or sensitivity

Follicular hyperkeratosis due to abnormal follicular desquamation

Proliferation of *Propionibacterium acnes*

Excess sebum production

Secondary inflammation

avoid scrubbing the face during ablutions because friction can exacerbate acne. Gentle cleansers may be applied using the hands or gentle applicators while avoiding abrasive washcloths. If daily sunscreens or emollients are used, patients should select noncomedogenic products which will often be labeled as such or with terms assuring that they "won't clog pores." Cosmetics should be oil-free and noncomedogenic as well.

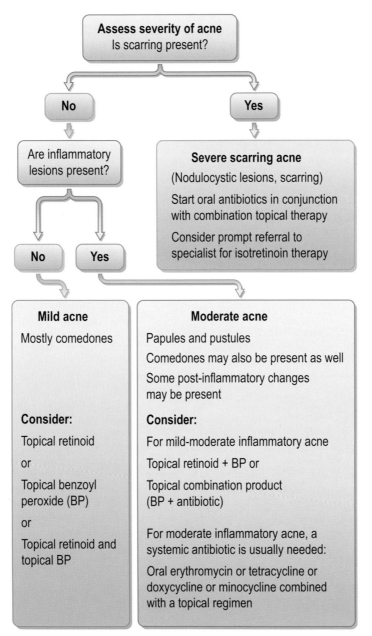

Figure 3-19 Acute therapeutic algorithm for acne

Table 3-2 Conventional therapeutic options and associated mechanisms

Agent	Comedolytic	*Propionibacterium acnes*	Anti-inflammatory	Sebum production
Topical retinoids	+++	–	+	–
Topical benzoyl peroxide	++	+++	–	–
Topical antibiotics	+	++	+	–
Oral antibiotics	++	+++	++	–
Oral contraceptives	+	–	++	+
Oral isotretinoin	++	++	++	+++

Vehicles

Selecting an appropriate vehicle helps to improve patient compliance. A patient who finds a product overly greasy for her already oily skin, or too drying for his combination skin will have difficulty using prescribed choices. Patients with sensitive, dry, or combination skin will generally prefer medicated cleansers, lotions, creams, or even ointments. Those with oily skin often like gels, solutions, or foams that leave less residue behind. For those needing to treat large areas such as the chest and back, cleansers can be applied in the shower, and leave-on products like lotions, gels, solutions, and foams are often easier to spread over more extensive surfaces.

Topical treatments

Topically applied products are ideal as monotherapy for mild acne, and they can also be combined with systemic agents for moderate and severe acne. Topical agents carry less toxicity than their systemic counterparts, and deliver the drug directly to the affected areas.

Topical retinoids

Topical retinoids represent an optimal first-line agent for comedonal acne. Comedones arise as a result of abnormal follicular desquamation, perhaps in response to androgenic hormones or a consequence of low intracellular levels of retinoids. Through their actions on Toll-like receptors and cytokine production, topical retinoids not only help correct follicular hyperkeratosis, they also possess anti-inflammatory properties.

Commercially available topical retinoids include tretinoin (Retin-A, Avita: cream, gel, solution, microsphere gel), adapalene (Differin: gel, cream), and tazarotene (Tazorac: gel, cream). These preparations are often prescribed for nighttime use, because some retinoids are rapidly degraded upon exposure to light and oxygen. Every-day application may result in excessive irritation, and patients should titrate the frequency of application to avoid redness and irritation. For many patients, every-other-day application is a good starting point. Combining older retinoid formulations with simultaneous application of BP is not recommended, since tretinoin is rapidly degraded in the presence of BP. Adapalene and microsphere formulations of retinoid are stable in the presence of BP.

Adapalene, a more selective retinoid receptor agent than its precursor tretinoin, is at its lowest concentration 0.1% less irritating but also somewhat less effective at reducing comedones. A more recent formulation at 0.3% has greater efficacy but also greater irritant potential. Tazarotene, although more irritating than tretinoin, is also more effective at comedolysis. In addition, retinoids can also help accelerate resolution of hyperpigmentation and in those with concomitant postinflammatory dyschromia.

In general, patients are best initiated on low concentrations of tretinoin and at subsequent visits prescribed escalating concentrations as tolerated until the desired response is achieved. Those with sensitive skin or a history of retinoid irritation may prefer adapalene, while those who have failed other retinoids may require tazarotene. For those who have difficulty tolerating this medication, tazarotene can be employed as short-contact therapy. Patients apply it before dinner and wash it off right after dinner; each night, patients may attempt to increase contact times as tolerated. However, it should be noted that tazarotene, despite being a topical agent, carries a pregnancy category X rating and should not be used in females of childbearing age who are likely to become pregnant while on therapy.

Topical antibiotics

The primary rationale for use of topical antibiotics is to address populations of *P. acnes* residing within the pilosebaceous unit. These bacteria produce proinflammatory cytokines that transform simple comedones into more inflammatory papules and pustules and nodules.

A variety of topical antibiotic formulations are available, including: erythromycin (solution, gel, ointment); clindamycin (solution, gel, lotion, pledget); and sodium sulfacetamide (lotion, cream, cleanser, or in combination with sulfur). In addition, erythromycin and clindamycin are available as combination products in which the antibiotic is stabilized with BP. Most of these products are well tolerated and adverse systemic effects are uncommon.

The principal limitations of topical antibiotic monotherapy include their slow onset of action, and the rapid emergence of widespread antibiotic resistance among *P. acnes* populations. These concerns, however, can be reduced when BP is used in concert.

Topical benzoyl peroxide

BP is a lipophilic compound that possesses both mildly comedolytic and potent antibacterial properties. In fact, BP is more active against *P. acnes* than available topical antibiotic preparations. In contrast to topical antibiotics, resistance to BP is not observed among *P. acnes*, likely because BP liberates oxygen which is bactericidal to these mostly obligate anaerobes.

Since the identification of antibiotic-resistant populations of propionibacteria 30 years ago and as the use of antibiotics has become commonplace, recent surveys now document that the majority of *P. acnes* populations have become resistant to at least one or more antibiotics. Fortunately, the use of compounds such as BP can help reduce already extant antibiotic-resistant *P. acnes* populations and appears to reduce the development of new antibiotic-resistant populations, especially when used in conjunction with topical antibiotics.

BP is highly versatile and can be delivered in a variety of vehicles (cleansers, gels, creams, and lotions) in a broad spectrum of concentrations from 2.5 to 10%. Those suffering from chest and back acne may especially benefit from use of BP as a cleanser used in the shower as opposed to a leave-on product which may damage clothing fabrics. The use of these products is limited by the drying qualities of BP, its potential for irritancy and occasionally contact sensitization, as well as its propensity to bleach clothing, towels, and bedding. It may also render ineffective other topical agents used concomitantly, such as topical tretinoin or topical antibiotics unless the products are effectively stabilized. Newer technologies and formulations, however, have addressed some of the irritancy potential by combining urea, hyaluronic acid, panthenol, glycerin, or other humectants and emollients with the active ingredient.

Topical combination products

Topical combination products offer the potential for improved compliance. By combining two products into one, patients may be able to reduce the frequency with which topical medications need to be applied. Because the individual components are stabilized together, the potential for degradation of any one component is reduced. BP has been successfully compounded with erythromycin or with clindamycin into commercially available products (Benzamycin, Benzamycin Pak, Benzaclin, Duac). These combination products may help to reduce the prevalence of propionibacterial antibiotic resistance. Clindamycin has been stabilized with tretinoin and this product has just recently become commercially available. While these combination products may improve compliance, they also tend to be more expensive than their generic counterparts.

Systemic antibiotics

Patients with moderate or severe acne generally require systemic therapy (Table 3-3). As with topical antibiotics, systemic antibiotics help to reduce *P. acnes* populations and some topical antibiotics also possess anti-inflammatory activity.

Erythromycin and its derivatives show activity against *P. acnes*, although the majority of propionibacteria demonstrate resistance to these drugs. However, they remain the mainstay of systemic antibiotic therapy in younger children who are not candidates for tetracycline therapy, due to either documented tetracycline hypersensitivity or the immaturity of dental calcification.

Clindamycin, while frequently employed as a topical agent for acne, is best avoided as a systemic agent because of the risk for pseudomembranous colitis in those receiving the drug. Tetracycline and its derivatives remain the principal systemic antibiotic agents of choice for most adolescents and adults but should be avoided in children under 9 years of age. Permanent staining of teeth is possible with high doses or long-term use of these medications. Tetracycline, doxycycline, and minocycline represent the most popular agents for systemic acne therapy.

Tetracycline is well tolerated, but requires administration on an empty stomach either 1 h before or 2 h after meals. The medication may be prescribed at 250–500 mg per dose and typically given twice daily. Gastrointestinal symptoms and photosensitivity represent the more common side-effects encountered with this agent.

Doxycycline and minocycline can be taken with food and less antibiotic-resistance is noted among *P. acnes* than with tetracycline. Minocycline shows greatest activity against *P. acnes* of any of the tetracyclines. It should not be given concurrently with iron. Doxycycline should not be given concurrently with calcium or dairy products. The rate of photosensitivity is greater with doxycycline than with other tetracycline derivatives and special caution should be taken when prescribing the drug during sunny spring and summer seasons. An enteric-coated form of doxycycline is available for those who experience untoward gastrointestinal symptoms with the generic form. Although doxycycline can be given at 50–100 mg orally once or twice daily, recent data indicate that some patients may also

Table 3-3 Dosage table: systemic agents in acne

Agent	Typical dosage	Important adverse effects
Erythromycin	30–50 mg/kg per day divided q6–8 h	Gastrointestinal upset; pseudomembranous colitis; hepatic dysfunction; drug interactions
Tetracycline	250–500 mg p.o. q6–24 h	Gastrointestinal upset; photosensitivity; hepatic dysfunction; anemia, thrombocytopenia; tooth discoloration
Doxycycline	50–100 mg p.o. q12–24 h Low-dose doxycycline at 20 mg p.o. q12 h may also be useful for less severe inflammatory acne	Photosensitivity; gastrointestinal upset less than with tetracycline; hepatic dysfunction; anemia, thrombocytopenia; tooth discoloration
Minocycline	50–100 mg p.o. q12–24 h An extended-release form is also available at 45–135 mg p.o. q24 h.	Significantly less photosensitivity than with either tetracycline or doxycycline; gastrointestinal upset less than with tetracycline; hepatic dysfunction; anemia, thrombocytopenia; tooth discoloration; urticaria; serum sickness-like reaction; lupus-like reaction; drug hypersensitivity syndrome; drug-induced hyperpigmentation; pseudotumor cerebri
Trimethoprim-sulfamethoxazole	8–10 mg/kg per day trimethoprim divided q12 h	Photosensitivity; marrow suppression; pseudomembranous colitis; urticaria; drug hypersensitivity syndrome; erythema multiforme/Stevens–Johnson syndrome; toxic epidermal necrolysis
Oral contraceptives	Take one pill daily	Menstrual irregularities; bloating; weight changes; thromboembolism; hypertension
Isotretinoin	10–80 mg/day Can be given once daily or divided into q12 h dosing	Xerosis and dry mucous membranes; arthralgias; myalgias; headaches; visual changes; hepatitis; hypertriglyceridemia, leukopenia; pancreatitis; pseudotumor cerebri; mood changes; teratogenicity

respond to low-dose, subantimicrobial dosing regimens. Patients given 20 mg orally twice daily demonstrated approximately 50% improvement in both comedones and inflammatory skin lesions but did not alter the rate of antibiotic resistance among *P. acnes* or other resident bacterial flora. This alternative dosing regimen may be appropriate for some patients with less severe inflammatory acne.

Minocycline also possesses good anti-inflammatory activity and is superior to other tetracyclines in *P. acnes* reduction. The drug is typically given 50–100 mg once or twice daily. Minocycline is less likely than tetracycline or doxycycline to be associated with photosensitivity or gastrointestinal upset. However, patients using minocycline are more likely to complain of vertigo, tinnitus, or minocycline-induced mucocutaneous dyspigmentation (Figure 3-20). Serum sickness-like reactions; drug-induced systemic lupus erythematosus-like reactions; vasculitis; pneumonitis with eosinophilia; autoimmune hepatitis as well as severe drug hypersensitivity syndromes have been reported. A sustained-release minocycline formulation (Solodyn) can reduce the incidence of vertigo and tinnitus. Safety data to date show no increased incidence of antinuclear antibody prevalence with this formulation.

Patients who fail or cannot tolerate tetracycline derivatives may benefit from treatment with trimethoprim-sulfamethoxazole. Little antibiotic resistance to this drug is noted among propionibacteria, and trimethoprim-sulfamethoxazole can be highly effective for recalcitrant cases of inflammatory acne. Its use, however, is limited by the relatively greater frequency of associated adverse effects, which include photosensitivity, marrow suppression, drug hypersensitivity syndromes, erythema multiforme major/Stevens–Johnson syndrome, and toxic epidermal necrolysis.

Hormonal control

Acne is a pathogenic process that is fundamentally driven by androgenic hormones. Female patients may benefit from treatment designed to antagonize circulating androgens. Specifically, oral contraceptives may help reduce acne through a variety of

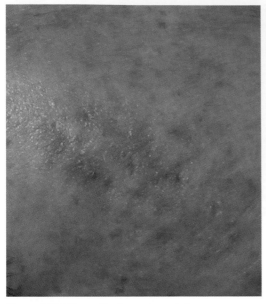

Figure 3-20 Minocycline hyperpigmentation

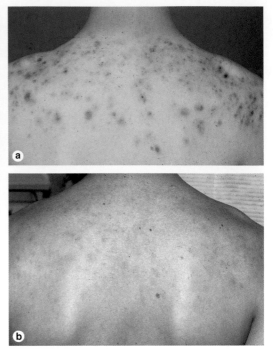

Figure 3-21 a Before and **b** after isotretinoin therapy

mechanisms: pharmacologic doses of estrogens and progestins may produce a feedback inhibition on secretion of pituitary gonadotropins while also increasing the production of sex hormone-binding globulin which binds circulating androgens.

Currently, three oral contraceptives carry approval by the Food and Drug Administration (FDA) for acne: Ortho Tri-cyclen (norgestimate/ethinyl estradiol), Estrostep (norethindrone acetate/ethinyl estradiol/ferrous fumarate), and dorspirenone/ethyl estradiol (Yaz/Yasmin). Preliminary studies have indicated that other agents containing low doses of ethinyl estradiol, such as desogestrel/ethinyl estradiol (Desogen), should also act similarly to reduce acne. Oral contraceptives are not recommended in patients who are pregnant, those who smoke, as well as those with high blood pressure, hypercoagulable states, complicated migraines, or certain malignancies.

Spironolactone, a diuretic, may also represent a useful adjunct to acne therapy due to its antiandrogenic properties. It is particularly useful in treating postadolescent acne and polycystic ovary disease.

Isotretinoin

Isotretinoin is a systemic retinoid that is indicated for the treatment of severe, nodulocystic acne. The drug's various mechanisms of action on acne make it an almost ideal therapeutic choice for severe acne. Isotretinoin reduces follicular hyperkeratosis, possesses anti-inflammatory effects, secondarily reduces *P. acnes* populations, and, most importantly, decreases sebum production. Patients with severe nodulocystic acne who have failed a combination of topical and systemic therapies often show significant improvement with isotretinoin. In fact, the majority of patients can expect a long-term remission, if not cure, of their disorder following a typical 5–6-month course or 120–150 mg/kg cumulative dose (Figure 3-21).

However, its use is limited by its potential side-effect profile. A potent teratogen, isotretinoin has been associated with a retinoid embryopathy that is characterized by craniofacial, cardiac, central nervous system, growth delays, and other anomalies. In addition, mood changes – including depressive symptoms and anger – have been attributed to isotretinoin, although larger studies have not indicated a definitive association. From our collective clinical experience, it appears that this phenomenon may occur among a subset of patients – perhaps among those already predisposed to mood disorders – although it remains unclear which patients in particular may be susceptible a priori.

Because of the concerns regarding the drug's teratogenicity, the manufacturers of isotretinoin in cooperation with the FDA implemented a new monitoring program in 2006 in an effort to reduce pregnancies among female patients of childbearing age who are receiving isotretinoin. This intensive program involves registration of all patients receiving isotretinoin, prescribing clinicians, and dispensing pharmacists; monthly laboratory monitoring, and verification of contra-ception counseling.

Surgery, lasers, and lights

When patients complain of "scars," it is important to clarify on examination whether these represent true scars ("icepick," "thumbprint," or rolling, papular, hypertrophic, or keloidal) or whether they actually represent postinflammatory dyschromia characterized by erythema, hypopigmentation, or hyperpigmentation.

Patients may be reassured that dyspigmentation typically improves with time. Bleaching agents – such as topical retinoids, hydroquinones, or combination products that may also include topical steroids – may help accelerate the resolution of excess pigment, but may also create irritation or secondary unintended dyspigmentation. However, true scars indicate permanent skin changes. Simple surgical methods such as subcission may help reduce the appearance of thumbprint scars by lysing underlying adhesions. Scars may also be ameliorated using the pulsed-dye, ND:Yag, and carbon dioxide lasers, while other studies suggest a potential role for radiofrequency techniques.

Other therapies

A variety of novel therapeutic options have appeared on the horizon. Oral dapsone has been used for patients with severe, recalcitrant acne vulgaris. A topical dapsone formulation has shown some modest efficacy and is being evaluated by the FDA for approval. Likewise, recent trials involving 5α-reductase inhibitors have been disappointing. Investigations are currently under way into the utility of targeting prostaglandins, interleukins, peroxisome proliferator-activated receptors, and Toll-like receptors. In addition, ultraviolet-free intense blue light devices have been developed which target propionibacterial porphyrins and have also shown safety and efficacy, although these devices are not yet widely used. Whether these therapies will prove safe and effective, and whether clinicians will choose to add them to the therapeutic arsenal, remains to be seen.

Summary

Acne vulgaris is one of the most common pediatric dermatologic disorders. A disease of the pilosebaceous apparatus, acne is characterized by comedones, papules, pustules, and nodules, and acne which can result in postinflammatory skin changes, including findings of dyschromia, scarring, and sinus tract formation. Severe cases can also occur as part of a larger systemic syndrome, and in these cases, may frequently be associated with spondyloarthropathies. Familiarity with the typical clinical features of acne vulgaris can help differentiate this disorder from other acneiform or follicular diseases. In combination with an understanding of the disease pathogenesis, safe and effective treatment in the form of topical and systemic medications can be appropriately prescribed.

Further reading

Ayers K, Sweeney SM, Wiss K. *Pityrosporum* folliculitis: diagnosis and management in 6 female adolescents with acne vulgaris. Arch Pediatr Adolesc Med 2005;159:64–67.

Bernier V, Weill F, Hirigoyen V, et al. Skin colonization by *Malassezia* species in neonates: a prospective study and relationship with neonatal cephalic pustulosis. Arch Dermatol 2002;138: 215–218.

Bickers DR, Saurat JH. Isotretinoin: a state-of-the-art conference. J Am Acad Dermatol 2001;45: S125–S128.

Cunliffe WJ, Baron SE, Coulson IH. A clinical and therapeutic study of infantile acne. Br J Dermatol 2001;145:463–466.

Eady EA. Bacterial resistance in acne. Dermatology 1998;196:59–66.

Goldsmith LA, Bolognia JL, Callen JP, et al. American Academy of Dermatology Consensus Conference on the safe and optimal use of isotretoin: summary and recommendations. J Am Acad Dermatol 2004;50:900–906.

Gollnick H, Cunliffe W, Berson D, et al. Management of acne: a report from a Global Alliance to Improve Outcomes in Acne. J Am Acad Dermatol 2003;49:S1–S38.

Koo JY, Smith LL. Psychologic aspects of acne. Pediatr Dermatol 1991;8:185–188.

Leyden JJ. The evolving role of *Proprionibacterium acnes* in acne. Semin Cutan Med Surg 2001; 20:139–143.

Neubert U, Jansen T, Plewig G. Bacteriologic and immunologic aspects of gram-negative folliculitis: a study of 46 patients. Int J Dermatol 1999;38: 270–274.

Plewig G, Kligman AM. Acne and Rosacea. New York: Springer-Verlag, 1993.

Sapadin AN, Fleischmajer. Tetracyclines: nonantibiotic properties and their clinical implications. J Am Acad Dermatol 2006;54:258–265.

Skidmore R, Kovack R, Walker C, et al. Effects of subantimicrobial-dose doxycycline in the treatment of moderate acne. Arch Dermatol 2003; 139:459–464.

Tan J. Hormonal treatment of acne: review of current best evidence. J Cutan Med Surg 2004;8(Suppl 4):11–15.

Webster G. Acne rulgaris: state of the science. Arch. Dermatol. 1999;135:1101–1102.

Wilkinson DS, Kirton V, Wilkinson JD. Perioral dermatitis: a 12-year review. Br J Dermatol 1979; 101:245–257.

4

Infections and infestations

Howard B. Pride

Introduction

Infectious diseases cause the majority of acute pediatric office visits and account for a large proportion of pediatric dermatology. The enormity of this topic could constitute a textbook in itself so this chapter will deal with the entities most commonly encountered in a pediatric dermatology practice. Treatments will be discussed in a general fashion and readers should know their own local epidemiology, particularly regarding bacterial sensitivities to antibiotics. The *Sanford Guide* (www.sanfordguide.com) is an excellent pocket-sized reference for dosing of antibacterials. The American Academy of Pediatrics' *Red Book* (www.aap.org) is an invaluable resource, particularly when making decisions regarding isolation procedures and permission to attend day care and school.

Bacterial infections

Impetigo

Key Points

* Honey crust or flaccid bullae with collarette of scale
* Caused by *Staphylococcus aureus*, with some being *Streptococcus pyogenes*
* Confirm with bacterial culture
* Topical mupirocin or systemic antibiotics effective against *Staphylococcus aureus*

Clinical presentation

Impetigo is a very common superficial skin infection caused most commonly by *S. aureus* and, less often, *Streptococcus pyogenes* (group A *Streptococcus*). It is more common in the summer and may spread like wildfire in crowded or unsanitary environments. Traditionally the condition has been categorized in two forms, bullous and nonbullous impetigo, but this distinction has become less important over time since *Staphylococcus aureus* is the dominant pathogen in both.

Nonbullous impetigo starts as a small vesicopustule with a seropurulent exudate that forms a golden (honey-colored) crust (Figure 4-1). The face, particularly around the nose, is a favorite location, but other exposed areas of the upper and lower extremities are also commonly involved. Bullous impetigo begins as a large, flaccid vesicle or bulla that ruptures quickly, leaving a collarette of scale (Figure 4-2). The intertriginous areas of the groin and axillae are most frequently involved but any body area can demonstrate lesions. Blisters are so superficial that they tend to break with minimal friction so none may be seen on physical exam. Skin disorders, especially eczema, may become secondarily impetiginized, and findings of impetigo may be subtler in this setting. Increased oozing and crusting (Figure 4-3) along with an unexplained worsening of the underlying condition may be the only clues. Chickenpox, scabies, and bug bites all have the tendency to become secondarily infected.

Children with impetigo are otherwise well with only mild complaints of discomfort unless large surfaces are involved. There are generally no systemic complaints and no fever. Painless adenopathy is common. *Streptococcus pyogenes* infection may be associated with glomerulonephritis but the strains that cause impetigo are not associated with rheumatic fever.

Ecthyma is a deeper infection that looks like bullous impetigo at the outset but develops a central, well-marginated ulceration with elevated margins and a crust (Figure 4-4). There is a surrounding rim of erythema. The extremities, particularly the lower extremities, are involved. It may be caused by both *Staphylococcus aureus* and *Streptococcus pyogenes*. This is distinguished from ecthyma gangrenosum, which is caused by *Pseudomonas aeruginosa* sepsis and presents with punched-out necrotic ulcers.

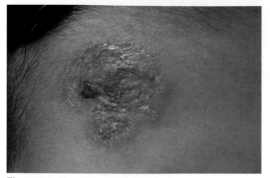

Figure 4-1 Nonbullous impetigo. Golden, honey-colored crust typical of impetigo

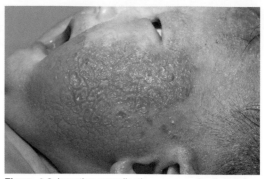

Figure 4-3 Impetigo complicating eczema. Oozing and crusting overlying pre-existing atopic dermatitis

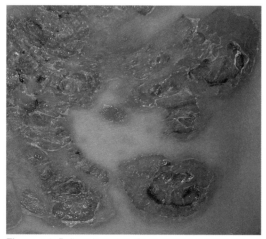

Figure 4-2 Bullous impetigo. Denuded superficial blisters that leave a collarette of scale

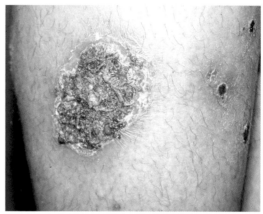

Figure 4-4 Ecthyma. (Courtesy of Richard Vinson, MD)

Diagnosis

Impetigo can usually be diagnosed clinically but a bacterial culture will confirm the diagnosis, and antibiotic sensitivities may be helpful in directing antibacterial treatment. Methicillin-resistant *Staphylococcus aureus* (MRSA) is discussed below and is rapidly becoming an important pathogen. The blisters of herpes simplex are deeper and tend to maintain their integrity with friction. A Tzanck smear, culture, direct fluorescent antibody (DFA) testing or polymerase chain reaction (PCR) testing will help rule out this diagnosis. Tinea can be confirmed with a fungal culture and potassium hydroxide (KOH) examination. An acute contact or nummular dermatitis may mimic impetigo but itch will dominate the clinical picture. Pemphigus foliaceus and subcorneal pustular dermatosis may be indistinguishable from impetigo. They can be secondarily colonized, but will have a minimal response to antibiotics. Biopsy may be necessary to make the correct diagnosis.

Secondarily infected dermatitis may pose a diagnostic dilemma, and culture is valuable in this circumstance. Many of these patients will improve with topical steroid preparations, even without antibiotics.

Pathogenesis

All cases of bullous impetigo and most cases of nonbullous impetigo are caused by *S. aureus*. *Streptococcus pyogenes* may be a co-invader but is the sole pathogen in fewer than 5% of cases. The infection is spread rapidly from person to person or from fomites (objects).

Treatment

Localized disease can be treated with topical mupirocin three times daily or with topical retapamulin. Fusidic acid is an appropriate alternative topical treatment but is not available in the USA. Nonlocalized disease should be treated systemically with a first-generation cephalosporin such as cephalexin (40 mg/kg per day) or dicloxacillin (30–40 mg/kg per day). Dicloxacillin suspension has an undesirable taste and is not a good choice for children who will not swallow pills. Resistance to erythromycin limits its use unless bacterial sensitivities confirm efficacy.

Azithromycin, clindamycin, and fluoroquinolones are alternatives. Ecthyma should be treated systemically.

It is important that patients, families, and health care providers practice good hygienic measures, washing with soap and water, an antibacterial cleanser, or an alcohol-based hand sanitizer. Fomites should be thoroughly cleaned.

Frequent recurrences of impetigo may indicate bacterial carriage in the nares, axillae, or groin, and this should be confirmed with culture. Mupirocin inside the nose three times daily for a week is commonly adequate, but resistance is emerging and off-label use of retapamulin or teatree oil cream may have a role in this setting. Oral rifampin together with a beta-lactam or clindamycin alone will clear most mucous membrane carriage but is seldom necessary.

Other *Streptococcus* infections

Key Points

* *Streptococcus pyogenes* has varied cutaneous presentations, including ulcers, crusts, perianal erythema, and blistering fingers
* Diagnosis confirmed by culture
* Treat with dicloxacillin or cephalexin

Clinical presentation

Blistering distal dactylitis is characterized by a painful, superficial blister on the volar distal tip of one or more fingers and, less frequently, toes (Figure 4-5).

Perianal streptococcal dermatitis consists of superficial, well-marginated, flat, nonindurated, confluent erythema extending from the anus outward to the perianal skin (Figure 4-6). Boys outnumber girls and the typical age is 7 months to 10 years with a mean age of about 4–5 years. Only 13% have a symptomatic pharyngitis but 60% have a positive throat culture. The rash may be moist, dry and scaling, or psoriasiform. Girls may have an associated vulvovaginitis with a bright red, edematous, tender introitus and vaginal mucosa. Penile involvement may occur as balanitis (Figure 4-7).

Skin folds may develop streptococcal intertrigo. Bright red, moist erythema is noted in the neck folds, axillae, or groin (Figure 4-8). There may be a foul odor.

Scarlatina is a fine, sandpapery erythematous rash associated with streptococcal pharyngitis or soft-tissue infection in children 2–10 years of age. Fever, sore throat, strawberry tongue, and adenopathy will precede the rash by about 2 days. The exanthem starts at the base of the neck, face, and upper back and spreads downward over the next couple of days. It is characteristically harder to see than a viral rash and can sometimes be best appreciated by feeling the fine sandpaper texture. Erythema is most notable in skin folds where petechiae (Pastia's lines) may form. The rash fades over a week and is followed by sheets of desquamation that may last days to weeks.

Cellulitis presents as ill-defined erythema, warmth, edema, and pain in a child who may have systemic symptoms of fever, chills, and malaise. While a leading edge of the erythema can be determined, this edge is not raised or sharply demarcated from the adjacent normal skin. Bullae and petechiae may be noted in dependent limbs. Portals of entry for the infection include an abrasion, ulcer, body piercing, toe web fissure, insect bite, or surgical wound. Venous and lymphatic damage from past surgeries, trauma, thromboses, or congenital vascular malformations may result in chronic limb edema and serve as predisposing factors for cellulitis.

Erysipelas is a superficial form of cellulitis characterized by the abrupt onset of fever, chills, and malaise followed by the development of a warm, shiny, bright red, confluent, indurated, tender plaque with elevated, sharply defined margins. The lower extremity is the most common location, but the face and, less commonly, other areas can be affected.

Diagnosis

The clinical picture in each of these entities may be sufficient to make the correct diagnosis. Direct swabs of blistering dactylitis, perianal *Streptococcus*

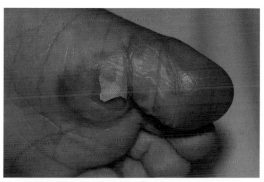

Figure 4-5 Blistering dactylitis. Painful, superficial blister on the great toe

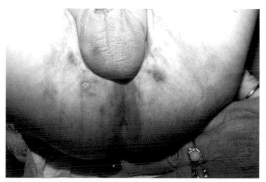

Figure 4-6 Perianal streptococcal dermatitis. Bright red erythema and mucoid drainage in perianal area

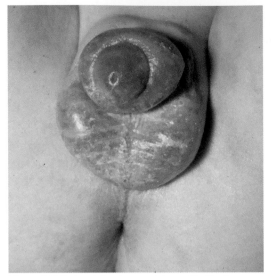

Figure 4-7 Perianal streptococcal dermatitis. Penile involvement with balanitis

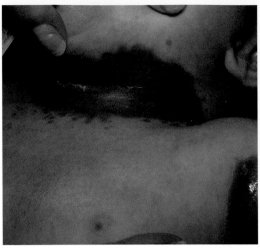

Figure 4-8 Streptococcal intertrigo. Bright red, moist erythema is noted in the fold of the neck

and streptococcal intertrigo will usually be positive. The diagnosis of scarlatina will be supported by a positive throat culture but a culture of the exanthem will not be positive since the rash is toxin-mediated. Deep tissue cultures with a biopsy may be positive in cellulitis and erysipelas but this degree of invasiveness is not generally needed and the condition is appropriately treated based on a clinical diagnosis. Surface cultures will not usually grow.

Herpes simplex may look very similar to distal dactylitis. Tzanck smear, DFA, or PCR will help confirm this diagnosis. Frictional intertrigo, *Candida* infection, and psoriasis may look like perianal *Streptococcus* and streptococcal intertrigo. A KOH scraping will fail to demonstrate *Candida*. Patients with a negative bacterial culture and negative KOH may benefit from a trial of a low-potency topical steroid and barrier cream before jumping to a biopsy. An allergic contact dermatitis may mimic cellulitis and erysipelas, but itch will be the dominant symptom and patients will not typically be ill.

Pathogenesis

S. pyogenes is the organism responsible for all of these entities, although other strepto-coccal species or *Staphylococcus aureus* may occasionally produce a similar clinical picture. *Klebsiella pneumoniae* and *Yersinia enterocolitica* may cause cellulitis. *Haemophilus influenzae* B is rarely seen in the postimmunization era but this organism can cause a cellulitis or erysipelas-like picture.

Scarlet fever is caused by streptococcal pyrogenic exotoxins and does not represent direct skin infection.

Treatment

Perianal *Streptococcus*, streptococcal intertrigo, and distal dactylitis may be treated with penicillin. Mupirocin may be used topically as an adjunct. Since *Staphylococcus aureus* may be a secondary or primary pathogen, the use of dicloxacillin or cephalexin is prudent.

Dicloxacillin and cephalexin are good choices for most patients with cellulitis or erysipelas. Oral clindamycin, quinolones, or macrolide antibiotics may offer substitutions for uncomplicated infections in patients allergic to dicloxacillin and cephalexin. Patients who are very ill, show rapid progression, have worsening symptoms despite good outpatient therapy, are vomiting too much to take oral medications, have very unstable social networks, or are immunocompromised should be admitted to hospital for supportive therapy and intravenous cefazolin or nafcillin.

Folliculitis, Furuncles, Carbuncles

Key Points

* Papulopustules with central hair
* Deeper nodules indicate furuncles and carbuncles
* Treat with drainage ± antibiotics directed toward *S. aureus*

Clinical presentation

Small, 2–4-mm papules and pustules with a central protruding hair shaft characterize folliculitis (Figure 4-9). Magnification facilitates the observation of a follicularly centered process. Lesions are usually grouped and are most common on the face, chest, back, buttocks, thighs, and axillae. Itch and/or pain are sometimes present.

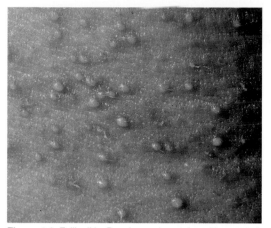

Figure 4-9 Folliculitis. Papules and pustules with a central protruding hair shaft

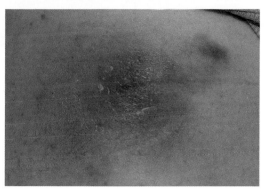

Figure 4-10 Carbuncle. Multiloculated nodule representing fusion of several furuncles (boils)

Friction, maceration, shaving, heat, and occlusion may all play a role in the origin or spread of the lesions and immunosuppression increases the likelihood of infection. Deep, tender folliculitis of the beard is called sycosis barbae.

A furuncle, or boil, is a deeper infection of the follicular unit that has spread into the surrounding tissue. Furuncles may occur anywhere but favored sites are the buttocks, groin, thighs, and neck and ears. A carbuncle (Figure 4-10) is simply the fusion of several furuncles. Pain is the primary symptom and lesions may spontaneously rupture with purulent drainage.

Diagnosis

A culture of an intact pustule or draining nodule growing *Staphylococcus aureus* confirms the diagnosis, although clinical suspicion should lead to empiric therapy while awaiting cultures. Gram-negative organisms may be seen in facial lesions of teenagers treated with oral antibiotics for acne and *Pseudomonas aeruginosa* is responsible for folliculitis after hot tub exposure. Acne vulgaris or *Pityrosporum* folliculitis will have negative bacterial cultures and will usually be suspected clinically. Molluscum contagiosum may look like a primary folliculitis but is usually an easy clinical diagnosis. Keratosis pilaris may appear pustular but close inspection will reveal a rough keratotic core rather than a true pustule. This can be a challenging differential requiring culture.

A ruptured epidermoid cyst will look exactly like a furuncle. Drainage of keratinaceous material and the history of a preceding cyst are helpful differentiating features. Hidradenitis suppurativa and acne conglobata (see Chapter 3) are recognized by their clinical presentation and negative cultures.

Pathogenesis

S. aureus is the cause of most cases of folliculitis and furunculosis. Trauma to the skin such as shaving and waxing and an environment that is warm, occluded, or subject to friction favor its growth. Immunosuppression increases the likelihood of infection but most patients are completely healthy. Isotretinoin therapy for acne predisposes to *S. aureus* infections.

Treatment

Drainage of individual lesions and washing the skin with antibacterial cleansers containing chlorhexidine or benzoyl peroxide and topical mupirocin may be all that is needed for a very limited infection, and washes may help prevent recurrences. Antibiotics effective against *S. aureus* such as dicloxacillin and cephalexin are indicated for widespread folliculitis or deeper infections such as sycosis barbae and furunculosis. Abscesses need to be drained surgically. When a furuncle has solid induration rather than fluctuance, warm compresses are helpful.

Recurrent bouts of infections indicate carriage of *S. aureus*, usually in the nares but also in the axillae, perianal region, and groin. Culture should be performed in these areas and topical mupirocin applied to the nares and chlorhexidine soap wash to the body. Because of its broad antimicrobial properties dilute bleach may also be a helpful adjunct to reducing recurrent staphylococcal infections. Bathing in a formulation of two teaspoons of standard bleach per gallon (4.5 litres) of water (approximately 1/8–1/4 cup of bleach per tub of water) once or twice weekly for 5–10 minutes may reduce staphylococcal carriage and provides a less expensive alternative to chlorhexidine.

Painful or rapidly evolving abscesses are suspicious for community-acquired (CA) MRSA. Most strains remain sensitive to sulfa and drainage remains the primary intervention for the primary lesion (see below). The carrier state is addressed as with methicillin-sensitive *S. aureus*.

Staphylococcal Scalded-Skin Syndrome

Key Points

* Tender red desquamation in young children
* *S. aureus* toxin
* Admit for support and antibiotics

Clinical presentation

Staphylococcal scalded-skin syndrome (SSSS) is mainly a disease of infants and preschool children. It is sometimes referred to as Ritter disease in infants. Early symptoms include irritability, malaise, fever, and a marked tenderness to the skin, and there may be a preceding pharyngitis, conjunctivitis, or rhinitis. A site of primary infection such as a purulent draining umbilical stump may be noted, but usually the source of infection is not obvious. Erythema begins at the head and neck and rapidly spreads over a matter of hours. The face and flexures tend to be the most involved. Erythema transitions to a wrinkled desquamation and prominent scaling with radial fissuring around the mouth (Figure 4-11). In more severely affected patients, flaccid blisters and erosions will leave a denuded, glistening cutaneous surface (Figure 4-12) and light friction to intact skin will result in a sheared epidermal surface (Nikolsky sign). Conjunctivitis and dry lips may be present but severe mucous membrane involvement as seen in toxic epidermal necrolysis is conspicuously absent. Uneventful healing takes place over 1–2 weeks, but the mortality rate associated with SSSS may be as high as 5%.

Diagnosis

The diagnosis of SSSS must be suspected on the basis of clinical findings and treatment instituted prior to confirmatory tests. Frozen-section pathology of a desquamating sheet of skin will differentiate SSSS from the very dangerous toxic epidermal necrolysis. The same technique can be performed on biopsy tissue but with a greater degree of invasiveness for the patient. Cultures of blisters or denuded skin will be negative since these lesions are caused by staphylococcal toxin rather than by direct *S. aureus* infection. Cultures should be obtained from the eyes, nose, throat, axillae, groin, blood and from any suspected focus of infection such as a wound or surgical site.

The early phase of SSSS may resemble a drug eruption, viral exanthem, or scarlatina but the differential diagnosis also includes burns, Kawasaki disease, epidermolysis bullosa, and pemphigus foliaceus.

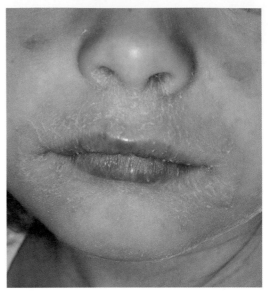

Figure 4-11 Staphyloccal scalded-skin syndrome. Radial fissuring around the mouth

Pathogenesis

SSSS is caused by toxin-producing *S. aureus*, most commonly phage group II, strains 55 and 71. The exfoliative toxin is a serine protease that targets desmoglein 1, an epidermal adhesion molecule, and results in a split at the granular layer of the epidermis. Pemphigus foliaceus is characterized by autoantibodies to this same adhesion molecule, accounting for the somewhat similar appearance of the two entities.

Older children and adults have acquired neutralizing antibodies to the staphylococcal toxin, accounting for the rarity of SSSS in this age group. Adults with kidney failure are at risk of developing SSSS since they are not capable of clearing the toxin, and mortality is very high in this population.

Treatment

All children, unless very minimally involved, should be admitted to hospital for supportive care of temperature control, electrolyte and fluid balance, and aggressive analgesia. Bland emollients such as petrolatum should be frequently and copiously applied and gentle tubbing done to remove debris.

Intravenous or oral antibiotics directed against *S. aureus* should be started as soon as the diagnosis is suspected. There have been reports of MRSA causing SSSS but this has usually been in the adult population with other complicating medical problems. Coverage with dicloxacillin or cephalexin should be sufficient but should be governed by the incidence of MRSA in the local area.

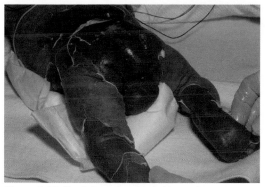

Figure 4-12 Staphyloccal scalded-skin syndrome. Denuded, glistening cutaneous surface

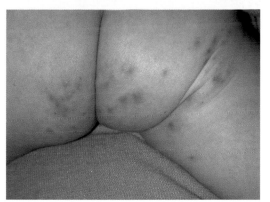

Figure 4-13 Methicillin-resistant *Staphyloccus aureus* (MRSA). Deep seated nodules and abscesses typical of MRSA in the diaper area

Methicillin-Resistant *Staphyloccocus aureus*

Key Points

* Generally presents with spontaneous abscesses
* The primary treatment for an abscess remains drainage
* Most strains remain sensitive to trimethoprim-sulfamethoxazole, tetracyclines, and clindamycin

Clinical presentation

MRSA infection used to be a condition of institutionalized or chronically hospitalized individuals. It is now widespread in the community, accounting for the majority of *S. aureus* isolates in emergency departments and increasing steadily in frequency everywhere.

MRSA infections may be indistinguishable from their methicillin-sensitive counterparts, although there is a distinct tendency toward abscess formation caused by the presence of the Panton–Valentine leukocidin (PVL) gene. The diaper area, in particular, is prone to deep-seated nodules and abscesses (Figure 4-13) and MRSA should be suspected in this setting. Wrestlers, football players, especially those playing on artificial turf, and other athletes who have abraded skin are at particular risk, and an abscess in this setting is highly suggestive of MRSA infection. Children with atopic dermatitis and other chronic skin conditions have been increasingly noted to be colonized and/or infected with MRSA.

Many children will self-resolve, even without antibiotics effective against MRSA, especially when abscesses are drained or drain spontaneously. Long-lasting hyperpigmentation is the rule and permanent scarring is likely. Deep, systemic infections causing sepsis, pneumonia, and osteomyelitis can be fatal.

Diagnosis

The presence of a painful rapidly evolving abscess, although not diagnostic, is very suggestive of MRSA. Culture of an infected site is diagnostic and it is wise to culture sites of colonization as well. It is very important to understand the epidemiology of staphylococcal infections in one's own geographic area. The differential diagnosis is the same as for a furuncle.

Pathogenesis

Most cases of MRSA infection are now CA-MRSA in children who are in good health with none of the traditional risk factors of chronic disease, multiple hospitalizations, and previous courses of antibiotics. The community-acquired strains are genetically distinct from the hospital-acquired strains with quite different antibiotic sensitivities. Methicillin resistance is the result of mutations in the *mecA* gene that, for CA-MRSA, is generally packaged in a novel type IV staphylococcal cassette cartridge. One clone, currently called USA 300, dominates in the USA. The PVL toxin is lethal to neutrophils and is specifically associated with soft-tissue infections, particularly abscesses.

Treatment

Any abscess requires surgical drainage. Antibiotic sensitivities will evolve so it is imperative that practitioners know the trends in their own area. Currently, the tetracycline family of antibiotics and trimethoprim-sulfamethoxazole are good choices for uncomplicated infections. Clindamycin is an alternative but inducible resistance from erythromycin has weakened its reliability and fluoroquinolone resistance is common. Serious limb- or life-threatening infections should be treated in the hospital setting with intravenous vancomycin, oral linezolid, or other newer antibiotics. There is evidence that treatment with linezolid is superior to vancomycin in this setting and has relatively few complications, but linezolid should not be used for simple, uncomplicated infections.

The common phenomenon of MRSA colonization in chronic skin diseases has led to increasing use of topical therapies. Mupirocin and retapamulin are reasonable treatments for limited areas, but *S. aureus* resistance to mupirocin is becoming more common. Sodium hypochlorite (Clorox bleach) added to the tub at a concentration of 2–4 tablespoons per tub is an excellent, well-tolerated method of reducing colonization and recurrent infections. Chlorhexidine wash is a good alternative but may be irritating to eczema-prone skin.

Pitted Keratolysis

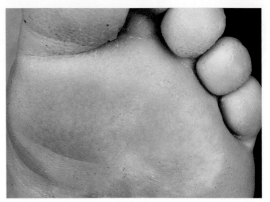

Figure 4-14 Pitted keratolysis. Depressed patches on the plantar foot

Key Points

* Superficial pits on the plantar foot with foul odor ("toxic sock syndrome")
* *Corynebacterium* species, *Micrococcus sedentarius*, or *Dermatophilus congolensis*
* Clindamycin or erythromycin topically

Clinical presentation

Pitted keratolysis is a superficial infection, seen almost exclusively on the weight-bearing areas of the plantar foot and around the toes. It is more common in males, particularly those whose feet are excessively sweaty, in a wet environment, or in boots for long periods. It is associated with a noxious, socially isolating odor and slimy texture but is otherwise asymptomatic. Small, 1–2-mm, noninflamed craters that coalesce into larger depressed patches are noted on exam (Figure 4-14).

Diagnosis

The diagnosis is often obvious upon entering the exam room when a rancid, suffocating odor can be immediately detected. The examination is usually diagnostic, although a KOH scraping may help differentiate tinea pedis. Culture and superficial shave biopsies are seldom needed. Plantar warts can be excluded by paring with a scalpel blade.

Pathogenesis

Pitted keratolysis is a superficial infection of the stratum corneum with *Corynebacterium* species, *Micrococcus sedentarius*, or *Dermatophilus congolensis*. The stratum corneum is digested by proteolytic enzymes produced by the organisms.

Treatment

Various topical regimens work very well. Clindamycin or erythromycin in a 2% solution and mupirocin are effective. Aluminum chloride (Drysol or Certain Dry) will help control sweating and patients should try to keep their feet dry as much as possible. Oral

erythromycin, clindamycin, and tetracycline are effective but not usually necessary.

Erythrasma

Key Points

* Pink-brown patch in skin fold
* Coral pink fluorescence
* Topical clindamycin or erythromycin

Clinical presentation

Erythrasma is a superficial bacterial infection seen mostly in the skin folds of the groin and axillae but it may also be seen in the gluteal cleft (Figure 4-15), inframammary region, abdominal fat folds, and the interdigital spaces of the toes. It is seen equally in both sexes and incidence increases with age. It is usually asymptomatic but itch may occur, especially in the groin. The rash consists of a sharply defined pink to brown patch with scant scaling. Woods light examination reveals the very characteristic coral-pink fluorescence (Figure 4-16).

Diagnosis

Diagnosis may be delayed since most cases are assumed to be tinea, *Candida*, or frictional intertrigo. A negative KOH examination is helpful but previous treatment with antifungal agents may decrease reliability. A Woods light exam will demonstrate coral-pink fluorescence which is striking when positive. Tinea versicolor looks somewhat like erythrasma, although it is not common in skin folds. KOH should rule this out. Concomitant tinea versicolor and erythrasma have been reported. Psoriasis, seborrheic dermatitis, and a nonspecific dermatitis may occur in skin folds.

Pathogenesis

Erythrasma is a superficial skin infection with *Corynebacterium minutissimum*, a Gram-positive rod that produces porphyrins, accounting for its fluorescence. Warmth and moisture will aid its growth.

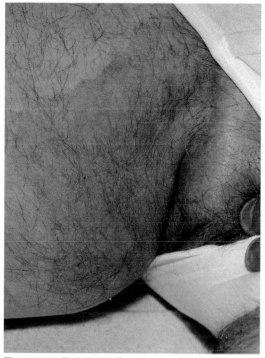

Figure 4-15 Erythrasma. Brownish scaling patch typical of groin erythrasma

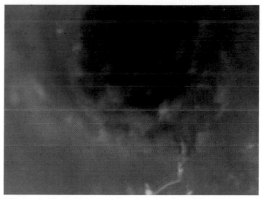

Figure 4-16 Erythrasma. Coral-pink color of fluorescence under a Woods light

Treatment

Topical clindamycin or erythromycin works very well. Oral clindamycin, erythromycin, or tetracycline may be easier if extensive areas are involved. Topical aluminum chloride has been used, but may not be well tolerated in skin folds.

Pseudomonal Infections

Key Points

- Cause of folliculitis in hot tubs
- Ears are particularly prone to infection
- Green nails
- Life-threatening ecthyma gangrenosum in immunocompromised children

Clinical presentation

Hot tub folliculitis consists of edematous, red papules and pustules, usually on the trunk and proximal extremities, occurring after exposure to an improperly chlorinated hot tub or spa (Figure 4-17). Tub toys and sponges, particularly if left in a mesh container in the tub, may be responsible for this condition in infants and young children. The follicular origin of the papulopustules is not usually obvious on exam. Patients may complain of malaise and have a low-grade fever but are typically well. Itch is the usual symptom but the lesions may hurt. An associated otitis externa may coexist with the folliculitis

and there are reports of painful plantar nodules representing neutrophilic eccrine hidradenitis in association with hot tub folliculitis.

The external ear is particularly prone to infections with *Pseudomonas aeruginosa*. An excruciatingly painful otitis externa may result from swimmers leaving moisture in the external auditory canal.

Surgeries performed on the ear may become secondarily infected with *P. aeruginosa* and there have been reports of ear piercing, particularly if done through the cartilage of the ear, becoming infected.

P. aeruginosa may impart a greenish-black discoloration to nails (Figure 4-18) that have undergone separation from the nail bed (onycholysis). It is more common when hands spend long periods in a moist environment. *Candida* or other fungi may be co-colonizers.

Severe *P. aeruginosa* toe web space infections may occur in chronically moist or hyperhidrotic feet (Figure 4-19). Tinea pedis may be the original infection with eventual overgrowth of Gram-negative organisms. A characteristic pseudomonal odor can usually be detected.

Chronic wounds are prone to secondary infection with *P. aeruginosa* and these are particularly seen in epidermolysis bullosa, burn wounds, neuropathic ulcers in patients with spina bifida, and ulcerated hemangiomas of infancy.

Ecthyma gangrenosum is a very severe infection seen in immunocompromised patients. An edematous vesicopustule rapidly becomes hemorrhagic and evolves into a punched-out ulcer with a black eschar surrounded by violaceous edema (Figure 4-20). Children are bacteremic and usually clinically septic.

Diagnosis

Culture will confirm the presence of *P. aeruginosa* but clinical suspicion will lead to the correct diagnosis in most cases. The history of hot tub

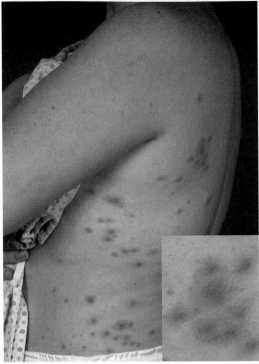

Figure 4-17 Hot tub folliculitis. Large, edematous follicular papules and pustules developing after hot tub use

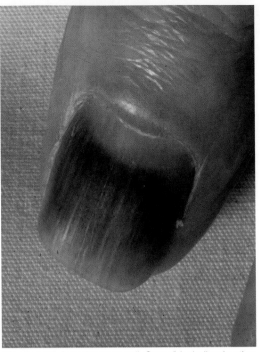

Figure 4-18 *Pseudomonas* nail. Green/black discoloration from pseudomonal colonization under an oncholytic nail plate

exposure suggests *P. aeruginosa* folliculitis and the lesions are more substantive than those of *S. aureus* folliculitis. Bug bites and nodular scabies might be considered. Any infection of the external ear should lead to the suspicion of *P. aeruginosa*. Contact dermatitis from antibiotic eardrops will itch but may pose a diagnostic challenge.

The descriptive terms of "fruity," "sweet," or "grape-like" have been applied to the odor of *P. aeruginosa*. Interpretation of these descriptors is in the nose of the beholder, but there is no mistaking the distinctive character of this aroma once it has been experienced. This in conjunction with the moist maceration and the extreme inflammation associated with toe web infections should suggest *P. aeruginosa* rather than tinea, which may be a coexistent infection, or dermatitis.

Ecthyma gangrenosum must be diagnosed quickly and treatment instituted prior to the availability of blood and cutaneous cultures. A Gram stain from beneath the black eschar may demonstrate Gram-negative rods, giving an immediate clue to the diagnosis. A punch biopsy for histologic evaluation and culture may be needed to rule out a myriad of other bacterial and fungal (*Aspergillus* or *Mucor*) pathogens, pyoderma gangrenosum, or Sweet syndrome.

Pathogenesis

P. aeruginosa is a Gram-negative, aerobic rod found throughout the environment. It is particularly fond of warm water. It may be part of the normal flora of the skin, especially the ear canal, groin, and axillae. It produces pyocyanin, which accounts for its green color.

Treatment

Most pseudomonal infections can be easily treated with local measures. Soaks with acetic acid (made by adding one half-cup of white vinegar to 1 quart (approx. 1 litre) of water) are helpful, inexpensive, and easy to apply, especially for the toe webs or under fingernails.

Hot tub folliculitis is a self-limited infection that does not require treatment. Benzoyl peroxide soap washes and topical antibiotics may be of some modest help. The hot tub needs to be emptied, cleaned, and appropriately chlorinated. Tub toys and sponges can be cleansed with bleach but are best thrown away.

Eardrops that contain gentamicin, tobramycin, or ciprofloxacin may be used for otitis externa, under green nails, or for toe web infections. Severe infections, especially wounds or piercing infections of the ear, should be treated systemically with ciprofloxacin since significant cartilage deformity may result. Onycholytic nails are best trimmed aggressively to remove pockets where moisture will collect.

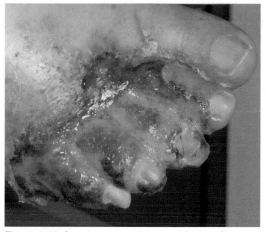

Figure 4-19 *Pseudomonas* web space infection. Seeping and moist web spaces

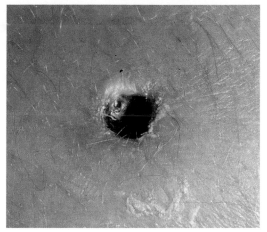

Figure 4-20 Ecthyma gangrenosum. Punched-out ulcer with black eschar

Patients with ecthyma gangrenosum need to be admitted to hospital for intravenous antibiotics and supportive care. Antipseudomonal therapy must not be delayed while awaiting cultures. Necrotic tissue may require debridement.

Lyme disease

Key Points

- Erythema chronicum migrans after a tick bite
- Diagnose clinically: titers my be negative with early rash
- Doxycycline or amoxicillin

Clinical presentation

Lyme disease is so common in southern New England that the average layperson can easily make an accurate diagnosis, but it is virtually nonexistent in some other areas of the country. Additional endemic areas include southeastern New York, New Jersey, eastern Pennsylvania, eastern Maryland, Delaware, Wisconsin, and Minnesota and, less commonly, northern California.

Most cases occur in April through October with a peak in June and July. All ages may be affected but it is most common among children aged 5–9 years.

The characteristic rash of Lyme disease, erythema chronicum migrans, starts as a red papule that expands to an ever-widening circle 5–30 cm in size. It may be confluently red or have a pale interior and is usually asymptomatic with, at most, mild itch. The spirochetal infection is spread from a tick bite, that likely went unnoticed, 1–2 weeks prior. The bite may leave a vesicular or necrotic center to the rash. Systemic symptoms such as fever, malaise, headache, neck stiffness, myalgia, and arthralgia may accompany the eruption.

Early dissemination, characterized by multiple smaller annular erythematous patches (Figure 4-21),follows several weeks later and represents spirochetemia. Systemic symptoms may accompany this stage, which may be associated with nerve palsy, meningitis, conjunctivitis, and arthralgia. Late disease is very uncommon in treated children and consists of recurrent pauciarticular arthritis.

Diagnosis

Early localized disease with erythema chronicum migrans must be diagnosed clinically since serologic studies are negative during this stage. It is recognized readily in highly endemic areas but may pose a challenge when the disease is unsuspected. Other annular erythemas such as tinea, urticaria, erythema multiforme, erythema marginatum of rheumatic fever, and subacute cutaneous lupus erythematosus, may be entertained in the differential diagnosis. Biopsy may be helpful in confusing cases.

Most patients with early disseminated disease and virtually all with late disease will have positive serologic tests. A two-step approach to testing is recommended, with the initial screen being a sensitive enzyme immunoassay or immunofluorescent antibody assay. Positive tests are then confirmed with Western blot analysis. In an endemic area, a positive blood test does not necessarily mean current infection.

Pathogenesis

The spirochete, *Borrelia burgdorferi*, is transferred by an infected deer tick, either *Ixodes scapularis* in the east and midwest or *I. pacificus* in the west. *Amblyomma americanum* is a secondary vector, especially for southern erythema migrans. The larval ticks are very small and bites may go unnoticed for days. Roughly 72 h of attachment is needed to transfer infection.

Treatment

Early localized and early disseminated disease is best treated with doxycycline 100 mg twice daily for 10–21 days in children aged 8 years and older.

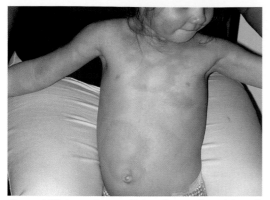

Figure 4-21 Lyme disease. Polycyclic, annular patches of erythema chronicum migrans

Younger children may be treated with amoxicillin 50 mg/kg per day (maximum 500 mg 3 times daily) or cefuroxime 30 mg/kg per day. Erythromycin and azithromycin are less effective substitutes.

Protective clothing, repellents, and daily skin inspection are wise preventive measures in highly endemic areas.

Viral Infections

Much of general pediatrics revolves around the treatment of viral infections and the overwhelming majority of viral rashes are minimally symptomatic, nonspecific in presentation, self-limited, and harmless. They therefore constitute a huge part of a pediatric practice but make up only a small proportion of a pediatric dermatology practice. Some viral infections such as chickenpox have a more characteristic presentation and many have a known etiologic cause, leading to a much more enlightened diagnosis and prognosis. Warts and mollusca contagiosa are an unavoidable viral nuisance that no pediatric practice can evade. Cutaneous viral infections more than compensate in vastness for what they may lack in consequence.

Morbilliform Exanthems

Key Points

* Nonspecific presentation, just like a drug rash
* Symptomatic treatment

Clinical presentation

The adjective morbilliform (measles-like) has lost much of its descriptive meaning. The rarity of measles infection makes it possible that a practitioner will never see a case of measles in a career. Nonspecific drug eruption-like rash is probably a better analogy for the typical viral exanthem and conjures a more concrete mental image than the descriptor morbilliform.

Children with a morbilliform rash may have had a preceding viral prodrome but it is surprisingly common to have had no preceding symptoms that can be recalled. The rash consists of blanchable, erythematous macules and papules with a diffuse and symmetric distribution. Pruritus is variable. The duration of the rash may be as short as several days or may last several weeks. Resolution in 1–3 weeks is the norm.

True measles begins with fever, cough, nasal congestion, and conjunctivitis. Koplik spots, punctate white-gray papules on an erythematous base located on the buccal mucosa, appear 2 days before the rash. The exanthem starts at the hairline and behind the ears and spreads downward.

Diagnosis

There is no diagnostic test to confirm a viral exanthem. A drug eruption will be indistinguishable clinically, and the confusion will be compounded if the child has been treated with an antibiotic for the viral prodrome. The initial rash of Kawasaki disease may look morbilliform but other mucocutaneous signs and very high fevers will help with this diagnosis.

Pathogenesis

A myriad of viral agents can cause a morbilliform rash and there is seldom any benefit to hunting down a specific etiology. The rash may result from an immunologic response to the virus or by direct infection of the skin by the virus.

Treatment

Reassurance and time are the only treatments that are necessary. Some modest relief of itch may be obtained with the use of an oral antihistamine such as diphenhydramine or hydroxyzine. Topical steroids are not very effective and the large surface area makes their use impractical. Oatmeal (Aveeno), menthol-containing creams (Sarna), or bland emollients may be soothing.

Parvovirus Infections

Key Points

* Slapped cheeks and lacy rash in fifth disease
* Anemia, arthritis, and arthralgia
* Purpuric socks and glove syndrome
* Fetal hydrops in some pregnancies

Clinical presentation

Fifth disease or erythema infectiosum occurs mainly in the winter and spring and is characterized by bright red macular erythema of the cheeks ("slapped cheeks") (Figure 4-22). A generalized eruption of lacy, reticulated, macular erythema

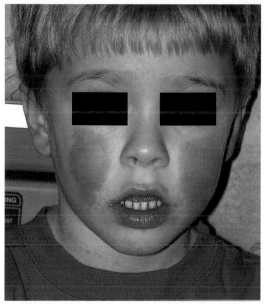

Figure 4-22 Fifth disease. Bright red "slapped cheeks"

then follows (Figure 4-23). Sun exposure may worsen the rash, which may last several weeks. Arthritis and arthralgia may be present with or without the rash, particularly in older individuals. The knees, ankles, wrists, and elbows are the most regularly affected joints. Anemia is common and may be profound in those with inherited hemoglobinopathies or those on chemotherapy.

Pregnant women who become infected may pass the infection to their unborn child, leading to a profound anemia, fetal hydrops, and death. Pregnancies in the first two trimesters are at greatest risk. Greater than 50% of adult women are seropositive for parvovirus and the risk of a seronegative adult becoming infected after exposure is about 50%. The percentage of pregnancies lost as the result of an infection is not known, but is less than 10%. Children with the rash of fifth disease are no longer infectious and pregnant women need not avoid children with the exanthem.

The papular-purpuric gloves and socks syndrome is characterized by the rapid onset of erythema and edema of the palms and soles that subsequently become petechial and purpuric with a sharp line of margination. Petechiae may be found elsewhere, including the oral mucosa. Children may complain of pain, burning, or itch.

Diagnosis

Parvovirus infections may be confirmed by an elevation of immunoglobulin (Ig) M antibody titers 1–2 weeks following the illness, but this is seldom necessary or helpful. The classic clinical picture of fifth disease is readily diagnostic. Scarlatina, viral exanthema, and drug eruption are part of the differential diagnosis. The combination

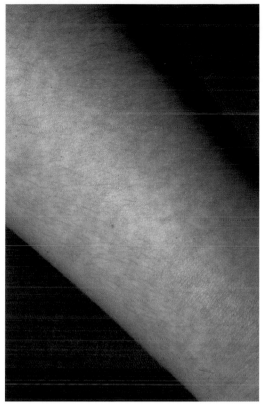

Figure 4-23 Fifth disease. Lacy exanthem of erythema infectiosum

of a rash and arthritis may suggest systemic lupus erythematosus, Henoch–Schönlein purpura, or juvenile rheumatoid arthritis.

The papular-purpuric gloves and socks syndrome may look like Rocky Mountain spotted fever or early meningococcemia. These very serious, life-threatening infections must be considered in the ill-appearing, febrile child with this presentation.

Pathogenesis

Parvovirus B19 is a single-stranded DNA virus spread via the respiratory route.

Treatment

No specific treatment is available. Sun and heat avoidance are important in not worsening the rash. Nonsteroidal anti-inflammatory agents are helpful for the arthritis. Serial ultrasounds are used to follow an infection during pregnancy, and intrauterine transfusion may be performed for fetal hydrops.

Roseola (Exanthem subitum)

Key Points

- High fever in a well-appearing child followed by rash
- Human herpesvirus-6B and 7

Clinical presentation

Roseola starts with a high fever in a child 6 months to 3 years of age. Despite the impressive fever, children are remarkably well with, at most, mild upper respiratory symptoms or abdominal pain. The fever resolves after 3–5 days, and the exanthem appears immediately thereafter, lasting about a week. It is composed of erythematous, nonpruritic macules and papules concentrated on the neck and trunk. Edema of the eyelids and an enanthem of erythematous papules on the soft palate are sometimes seen. Febrile seizures may accompany the rise in fever.

Diagnosis

The clinical picture of a rash following a high fever in a well-appearing child is enough to seal the diagnosis. Confirmatory viral titers are seldom necessary or helpful. Other viral rashes, scarlatina, or drug eruptions are in the differential diagnosis.

Pathogenesis

Roseola is caused by infection with human herpesvirus-6B or 7. They are double-stranded DNA viruses spread via the respiratory route. Almost everyone is infected at some point in early childhood, although not everyone develops the rash of roseola.

Treatment

No specific treatment is available. Acetaminophen may be used for the high fever.

Hand, Foot, and Mouth Disease and Herpangina

Key Points

- Painful mouth erosions
- Oval blisters paralleling skin surface lines on the palms, soles, and buttocks
- Coxsackievirus A and B, echovirus, and enterovirus

Clinical presentation

Hand, foot, and mouth disease (HFMD) is an enteroviral infection occurring mostly in the late summer and early fall. Fever and malaise precede the characteristic mucocutaneous outbreak. The enanthem consists of vesicles that rupture, leaving painful erosions and ulcers on an erythematous base, usually on the buccal mucosa and tongue but also on the palate, uvula, and tonsils (Figure 4-24). The oral lesions of herpangina are even more painful and located on the soft palate, tonsils, pharynx, and uvula.

The exanthem of HFMD consists of grayish, oval vesiculopustules located on the palms, soles, buttocks, and perineum (Figure 4-25). The vesicles tend to run parallel to skin surface lines. The rash fades over a week.

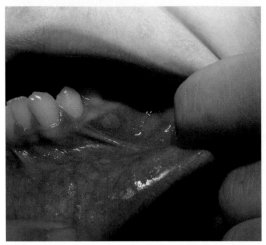

Figure 4-24 Hand, foot, and mouth disease. Painful erosions and ulcers on the gingival mucosa

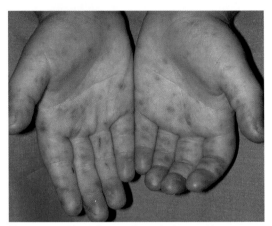

Figure 4-25 Hand, foot, and mouth disease. Linear grayish blisters on the palms

Diagnosis

The clinical picture, particularly during an epidemic, is diagnostic. Viral culture can be performed but is not of great practical benefit. Herpes simplex virus (HSV) infection can be ruled out with negative DFA. Erythema multiforme has blisters on the hands but they are characteristically targetoid rather than oval. Biopsy may be helpful in confusing cases but is seldom needed.

Pathogenesis

HFMD and herpangina are the result of infections with coxsackievirus A and B, echovirus, and enterovirus, all single-stranded RNA viruses. Spread is via the fecal–oral route or via respiratory droplets.

Treatment

Analgesics are helpful for the mouth pain, which can be very severe. Intravenous rehydration may be needed for children who are unable to drink fluids.

Gianotti–Crosti syndrome

Clinical presentation

Gianotti–Crosti syndrome (GCS) is a distinctive viral exanthem, initially described in association with hepatitis B infection. Children range in age from 3 months to 16 years of age but the vast majority are less than 4 years. Some have a viral prodrome of an upper respiratory or gastrointestinal infection but this is quite variable.

The rash is characterized by the sudden onset of multiple monomorphous, planar, red-brown 2–5-mm papules and papulovesicles on the face, buttocks, and extensor surfaces of the extremities (Figure 4-26). Individual papules may coalesce into larger plaques. The trunk is strikingly spared or minimally involved. Papules may develop where the skin has been traumatized (Koebner phenomenon). Lesions last from several weeks to several months and resolve without scarring. Adenopathy and hepatosplenomegaly may be present.

Diagnosis

The clinical picture, particularly the absence or scarcity of truncal lesions, is highly diagnostic. Biopsy will help rule out lichen planus, lichenoid drug eruption, papular eczema, bug bite reaction, keratosis pilaris, Langerhans cell histiocytosis, urticaria pigmentosa, and erythema multiforme, but this procedure is only necessary in atypical cases. Epstein–Barr serologies may indicate an acute infection and liver enzymes may be elevated but laboratory tests are not routinely needed.

Pathogenesis

The earliest reports out of Europe indicated a direct causal link between GCS and hepatitis B virus. This is seldom the case in the USA and now, with the advent of more universal hepatitis B vaccination, Epstein–Barr virus is the most common causal agent worldwide. Other infections associated with GCS include hepatitis A and C, cytomegalovirus, human herpesvirus-6, coxsackievirus, rotavirus, parvovirus, molluscum contagiosum virus, respiratory syncytial virus, echovirus, mumps, parainfluenza virus, human immunodeficiency virus (HIV), *Bartonella henselae*, streptococci, *Borrelia burgdorferi*, and *Mycoplasma pneumoniae*. Immunizations have been implicated but may be guilty by association since young children are frequently receiving vaccinations.

Treatment

No treatment is necessary. Oral antihistamines and mid-potency topical steroids may offer modest relief of pruritus.

Asymmetric Periflexural Exanthem

Clinical presentation

Asymmetric periflexural exanthem is sometimes referred to by its tongue-twisting name of unilateral laterothoracic exanthem. The similarities to a nonspecific morbilliform exanthem in history, examination, and disease progression, are striking and it is possible that this represents a unique presentation of the same entity.

Most cases occur in the first 3 years of life, with a mean of about 2 years of age. There is a predominance of girls. There may be evidence of a preceding viral infection but most children are well at the time of presentation with the rash. Duration of the exanthem is usually 3–6 weeks but may be as long as 4 months.

The eruption begins unilaterally close to the axilla, thorax or, less commonly, the groin folds. It spreads centrifugally, with new patches appearing on the opposite side of the body and at distal sites, often separated by normal skin. At the time of

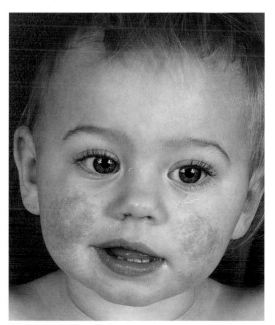

Figure 4-26 Gianotti–Crosti syndrome. Monomorphous, planar papules also on the face

presentation, the rash may already be bilateral and the unilateral origin will need historical confirmation from the parent.

The rash consists of discrete, erythematous papules, often surrounded by a pale halo. Coalescence of lesions may occur and sometimes a circinate, annular, or reticulate pattern may develop. Excoriations and lichenification are notably absent. After 1–2 weeks, the rash becomes more scarlet fever-like or eczematous and eventually ends with a fine, branny desquamation.

Diagnosis

The diagnosis is made on clinical grounds. Routine laboratory studies are normal. The absence of a diffuse symmetric distribution, so characteristic of exanthems, may lead the differential diagnosis away from a viral process, and atopic dermatitis, acute contact dermatitis, scabies, scarlet fever, miliaria, and atypical pityriasis rosea may be considered. Biopsy is seldom needed or helpful.

Pathogenesis

The cause of the rash is unknown, although it is strongly suspected to be a reactive process in response to a viral infection. The fact that this is a condition of younger children and the lack of recurrence imply the development of immunity. There are a few reports of similarly affected family members, suggesting an infectious agent. It is likely that this rash is not specific to a single viral agent.

Treatment

No treatment for periflexural exanthem is needed, although mild pruritus may be improved with oral antihistamines and bland emollient creams. Topical steroids help some children but are mostly ineffective.

Varicella/Zoster

Key Points

- Vesicles on an erythematous base, dew drop on a rose petal
- Chickenpox with polymorphous papules, vesicles, and crusts
- Shingles (zoster) with dermatomal distribution
- Tzanck smear, culture (DFA) or PCR for diagnosis
- Symptomatic treatment, antiviral agents in some circumstances

Clinical presentation

Chickenpox represents a primary infection with varicella virus. The institution of routine immunization in 1995 has dramatically decreased the incidence of this infection, which was a nearly universal childhood rash in the preimmunization era. As a result, the epidemiology of chickenpox has shifted from a disease dominated by children less than 10 years of age to a condition with a high proportion of adolescents and adults. The overall incidence in all ages has, however, decreased as a result of immunization.

Low-grade fever and malaise may precede the rash, which begins on the scalp and trunk as crops of red papules that form vesicles on an erythematous base, the so-called dewdrop on a rose petal. The lesions form crusts and then eventually heal while new lesions are simultaneously forming in a more generalized distribution (Figure 4-27). The polymorphous nature of chickenpox lesions with the coexisting presence of papules, vesicles, and crusts is one of this condition's most characteristic features (Figure 4-28). Mucous membranes may be involved.

Uneventful healing is usually complete by the end of 2 weeks but some of the lesions may leave depressed or hypertrophic scars. The eruption may be particularly severe with underlying skin diseases such as eczema, skin trauma, or sunburn, in the setting of immunocompromise and with the use of oral or inhaled corticosteroids. Teenagers and adults tend to have a more difficult and complicated course.

Chickenpox may be complicated by secondary skin infections with *Staphylococcus aureus* or *Streptococcus pyogenes*, pneumonia, thrombocytopenia, and various central nervous system abnormalities, including encephalitis, cerebellar ataxia, aseptic meningitis, transverse myelitis, and Guillain–Barré syndrome. Reye syndrome is seldom seen since the elimination of aspirin use in children.

Infection during the first two trimesters of pregnancy may lead to congenital varicella syndrome with resultant birth defects or fetal death. Maternal infection 5 days prior to delivery or 2 days after delivery may lead to devastating infections in the newborn infant who carries no protective maternal antibodies.

Immunization offers a high level of immunity against primary varicella infection. Natural experiments in immunity occurring in elementary schools around the country indicate about 70–85% efficacy in preventing infection and nearly 100% efficacy in preventing a severe infection. Breakthrough cases are usually blunted in terms of the number of lesions and the length of time to healing and seem to be more common in children whose immunizations were given greater than 5 years prior to the outbreak. The American Academy of Pediatrics now recommends a second dose of the vaccine.

Varicella virus establishes latency within the dorsal root ganglia and reactivation results in shingles (zoster). Unilateral, grouped, monomorphous vesicles form within the

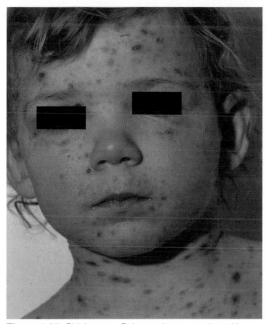

Figure 4-27 Chickenpox. Polymorphous eruption with papules, vesicles, pustules, and crusts

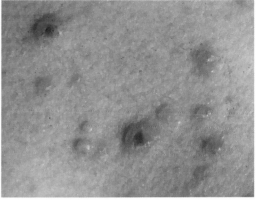

Figure 4-28 Chickenpox. Vesicles, pustules, and crusts of chickenpox

and scabies. A biopsy is seldom needed but may be helpful in the setting of unexplained pain associated with the nonspecific urticarial lesions of subtle shingles.

Pathogenesis

Varicella/zoster virus is in the herpes family of double-stranded DNA viruses. It is spread via direct skin contact and via the respiratory route. It is highly contagious, with nearly all susceptible members of a household becoming infected. The incubation period is about 14 days.

Shingles requires direct contact with skin lesions. It occurs much more commonly among children with underlying immunodeficiency or malignancy, especially lymphoma, but the majority of children with shingles are completely healthy. A hunt for underlying diseases is not warranted on the basis of uncomplicated shingles.

Treatment

Symptomatic treatment is all that is generally necessary. Itch may be helped with oral antihistamines, oatmeal baths, calamine lotion, bland emollients, Domeboro soaks, and menthol-containing lotions (Sarna). Secondary infection must be recognized and treated with antibiotics for *Staphylococcus aureus*. Acetaminophen (never aspirin) may be used for fever and discomfort.

The American Academy of Pediatrics' *Red Book* suggests treating those older than 12 years of age, those with chronic cutaneous or pulmonary disease, those receiving long-term salicylate therapy, and those receiving short, intermittent, or aerosolized steroid therapy. Acyclovir at a dose of 80 mg/kg per day in 4–5 divided doses for 7–10 days is the accepted therapy but valacyclovir and famciclovir may be reasonable alternatives. Very sick individuals require intravenous acyclovir and supportive care in a hospital setting. The nuances

boundaries of 1–3 dermatomes (Figure 4-29). The eruption is generally accompanied by pain, which often consists of a dull constant burning interspersed with jabs of lancinating, knife-like pain. Lesions on the nasal tip indicate involvement of the nasociliary branch of the trigeminal nerve and may be associated with ocular complications such as keratitis. Ophthalmologic consultation should be obtained in this circumstance.

Pain may precede the rash or may be accompanied by nonspecific urticarial papules, making diagnosis quite challenging. Postherpetic neuralgia may last for months after the vesicles have disappeared but this is far more common among the elderly.

Shingles may occur in those who have received varicella vaccine, but the frequency is less than in those who develop natural varicella. Many immunized individuals with shingles will be found to have wild-type varicella virus, indicating a subclinical infection at some time in the past.

Diagnosis

The correct diagnosis is usually obvious but may be confirmed by culture (DFA) or PCR. The base of lesions should be scraped vigorously. A positive Tzanck preparation (Figure 4-30) will confirm the diagnosis immediately but requires some skill and experience in interpretation. The differential diagnosis includes impetigo, folliculitis, herpes simplex infection, HFMD, pityriasis lichenoides,

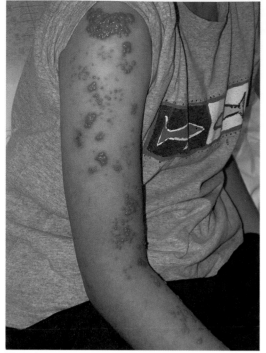

Figure 4-29 Zoster. Grouped blisters in a C5 dermatomal distribution

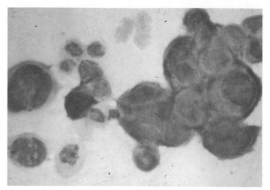

Figure 4-30 Tzanck preparation. Multiple giant cells with multinucleation of the far left cell nucleus

of treating every possible scenario are beyond the scope of this book and the *Red Book* is the best source of comprehensive guidelines.

Herpes Simplex Virus Infections

Key Points

- Grouped vesicles on an erythematous base
- HSV-1 usually mucocutaneous lesions
- HSV-2 usually genital lesions
- Tzanck smear, culture (DFA), or PCR for diagnosis
- Acyclovir, famciclovir, and valacyclovir

Clinical presentation

The classic herpetic lesions consist of grouped vesicles on an erythematous base (Figure 4-31) that coalesce into larger vesicles, bullae, pustules, and erosions that crust. The resultant geographic lesions have scalloped borders and generally heal without scarring. Several different clinical pictures are recognized by location and setting.

Primary gingivostomatitis occurs mainly in infants and young children and may be asymptomatic or involve fever, malaise, irritability, adenopathy, and pain on swallowing. The mucous membranes of the mouth and lips show erythema, ulcerations, exudates, and crusting but not usually intact vesicles. Breath may be fetid. Dehydration may result from refusal to drink.

Primary cutaneous herpes can occur anywhere but is most common on the face (Figure 4-32) and upper extremities. Classic herpetic lesions may be preceded by systemic symptoms and pain or may be asymptomatic. Herpetic whitlow consists of deep, tender vesicles and pustules on the finger (Figure 4-33) and is probably acquired when young children put their hands in an infected individual's mouth.

Primary genital herpes is predominantly a sexually transmitted condition. Females may have widespread areas of the labia, vagina, and cervix with grouped blisters leading to very painful ulcerations associated with itching, dysuria, and vaginal discharge. Males may have urethritis and dysuria. Scarring and adhesions can occur in both sexes. Sexual abuse must be entertained in any prepubertal child with genital herpes.

Eczema herpeticum refers to herpes simplex infection complicating a primary skin condition, usually atopic dermatitis. Fever, malaise, and extreme discomfort are the norm. Extensive punched-out erosions and crusting may dominate the clinical presentation (Figure 4-34) and the scarcity of vesicles may delay diagnosis.

Recurrent disease may occur in all locations but recurrences are noted for decreased severity and duration. A prodrome of tingling, burning, or pain may herald the onset of a new outbreak. Sun exposure, illnesses, and stress might serve as trigger factors.

Diagnosis

Culture (DFA) will confirm the diagnosis of herpes simplex and will distinguish type 1 from type 2 infections as well as identify varicella virus or other viruses such as cytomegalovirus or coxsackievirus that are in the differential diagnosis. A Tzanck smear will often be positive but requires expertise in interpretation and it will also be positive in varicella infections. Facial lesions of herpes simplex are frequently misdiagnosed as impetigo. Blistering

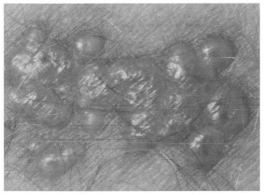

Figure 4-31 Herpes simplex. Grouped vesicles on an erythematous base

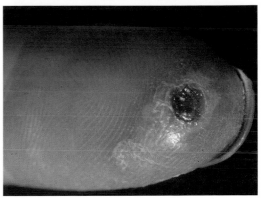

Figure 4-33 Herpetic whitlow. Deep blisters on the fingertip

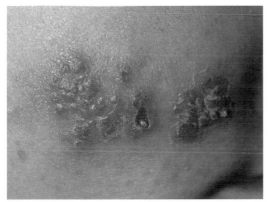

Figure 4-32 Herpes simplex. Primary cutaneous herpes simplex on the cheek

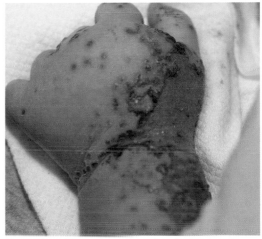

Figure 4-34 Eczema herpeticum. Punched-out erosions and crusting

distal dactylitis from *Streptococcus pyogenes* mimics herpetic whitlow and culture is diagnostic. Orf (sheep pox) and milker's nodules (pseudocowpox) are parapoxvirus infections acquired through contact with infected animals and may look just like herpetic whitlow. Allergic contact dermatitis may resemble herpes but itch will be the dominant symptom. Erythema multiforme may coexist with herpes simplex and may be impossible to distinguish clinically on the oral mucosa.

Eczema herpeticum must be suspected by its sudden onset, systemic symptoms, significant pain, characteristic punched-out lesions, and positive culture but the assumption of secondary impetiginization or simply a severe flare of the underlying atopic dermatitis may delay correct diagnosis.

Pathogenesis

Herpes simplex is a double-stranded DNA virus. Type 1 classically causes mucocutaneous disease and type 2 genital disease but this distinction has blurred over time. Infection occurs by direct contact and may occur during a time of asymptomatic shedding. The incubation period is about 1 week. Once infection has occurred, the virus establishes latency in the dorsal root ganglion.

Treatment

Asymptomatic or minimally symptomatic outbreaks of herpes simplex can be treated with bland emollients such as petrolatum and oral analgesics, but primary outbreaks are often severe enough to warrant therapy. Acyclovir, famciclovir, and valacyclovir are available for oral use and offer equal efficacy although the decreased bioavailability of acyclovir makes dosing very inconvenient. Famciclovir and valacyclovir should be safe in children but have not been well studied, are not Food and Drug Administration (FDA)-approved and are not available in liquid preparations. Recurrent outbreaks can be treated episodically, especially if a prodrome warns of an eruption. Topical therapy with penciclovir or acyclovir is minimally effective.

All but the mildest cases of eczema herpeticum should be treated in the hospital setting with supportive wound care and intravenous acyclovir.

Severe frequent mucocutaneous or genital outbreaks, recurrent eczema herpeticum, recurrent HSV-associated erythema multiforme, and outbreaks in immunosuppressed individuals may be treated with daily suppressive dosing.

The *Red Book* offers detailed indications and dosing for multiple HSV infection scenarios.

Warts and Condylomata Acuminata

Key Points

- Human papillomavirus (HPV) infection
- Verrucous papules and plaques on hands and feet, other areas
- Most infections self-limited, "do no harm"
- Salicylic acid, tape, immunotherapy, cryotherapy, laser, excision

Clinical presentation

Common warts (verruca vulgaris) are a nearly universal cutaneous infection of childhood and adolescence and are the bane of every pediatric practice. Lesions consist of rough, hyperkeratotic, callus-like papules that coalesce into larger plaques and are easily recognized as warts by patients and parents. Black dots representing thrombosed vessels are characteristic and may be referred to as "seeds" by the patient (Figure 4-35). Warts are usually located on the hands and feet but may be in any location. They may have finger-like (filiform) projections on the face, mucous membranes, and hair-bearing skin. Pain on pressure-bearing areas and embarrassment are common symptoms, but warts are mostly an asymptomatic nuisance.

Flat warts (verruca plana) are small, 2–4-mm flesh-colored-to-red-brown, flat-topped papules with a less warty surface and may be very subtle (Figure 4-36). Magnification is helpful for examination. The face and legs are common locations but they may be found anywhere. Autoinoculation by scratching or shaving may be demonstrated by a marked linear distribution.

Condylomata acuminata (singular form is condyloma acuminatum) are red to brown warty papules in the genital or perianal regions (Figure 4-37). Fusion of lesions into large plaques may lead to vegetating, moist, fissuring, and bleeding lesions, particularly in the perianal region. These are typically sexually transmitted in adolescents and adults. While preadolescent children with condylomata require some suspicion for child abuse, most children likely acquire their condylomata via maternal inoculation at birth.

Diagnosis

Diagnosis of common warts is almost always obvious. Calluses may look like warts and paring with a scalpel blade to a point of punctate bleeding is very characteristic of a wart. Knuckle pads and granuloma annulare may mimic warts but lack the warty surface and the black dots.

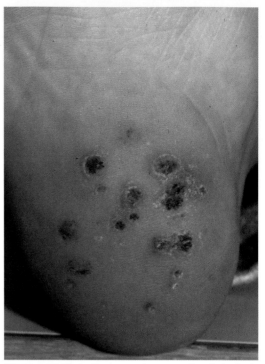

Figure 4-35 Warts. Verrucous plaques on the plantar foot with characteristic black dots

Flat warts may be more difficult to diagnose clinically. Mollusca contagiosa, keratosis pilaris, folliculitis, acne, benign cephalic histiocytosis, granuloma annulare and syringomas may mimic flat warts. Biopsy may, on rare occasions, be needed.

Condylomata acuminata may pose a diagnostic challenge. Mollusca contagiosa tend to look more warty and less umbilicated in the skin folds of the groin or buttocks and are easy to confuse with condylomata. Finding a few typical mollusca in other body areas is very helpful. Midline skin tags are fairly common in infants. Wart-like papules (pseudoverrucous papules) may be seen in the perianal region of children with chronic diarrhea or fecal incontinence. Confusion over the correct diagnosis can be settled with a skin biopsy but a clinical diagnosis can usually be made.

Pathogenesis

All warts are caused by HPV obtained by direct contact, perhaps through damaged or abraded skin. Common warts are caused by HPV types 1, 2, 4, and 7, flat warts by HPV types 3, 10, and 28 and condylomata mainly by HPV types 6 and 11, but also types 16, 18, 30, and others. HPV associated with condylomata have a concerning risk of inducing cervical dysplasia but the exact risk in children is not known. Females should certainly have screening performed as they enter adolescence.

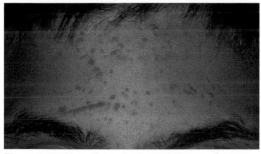

Figure 4-36 Warts. Brown flat-topped plaques of verruca plana demonstrating linear inoculation

The association of condylomata acuminata and sexual abuse is a can of worms for most practitioners. Condylomata are seldom the result of sexual abuse, and there is little chance of finding a definitive sign or symptom diagnostic of abuse, even in children suffering from sexual abuse. Very young children who have, in all likelihood, acquired the warts perinatally, could possibly still be abused and older children with genital warts in whom the suspicion of abuse is appropriately high may not be suffering abuse. It is immensely important to enlist the help of an experienced abuse team in obtaining the history and completing an appropriately thorough physical exam with the aid of colposcopic observations.

Treatment

It is important to educate parents and patients about the viral, self-limited nature of warts. It is often a revelation that warts will self-resolve, usually in 1–2 years, and the option of ignoring the warts may look much more appealing with this information. The pain and morbidity of the treatments should not outweigh the discomfort of the warts, and it is usually inappropriate to treat an unwilling child with painful techniques at the parent's insistence. Judgment is required in marching up the ladder of therapeutic interventions and practitioners need to remember to do no harm, especially when there is some failure rate to all treatments, even very aggressive techniques.

Salicylic acid-containing preparations and/or tape occlusion should form the first line of therapy. Duct tape has been found to be effective for many children, even without a medication applied beforehand. If these measures fail, then watchful waiting is usually the best option.

Topical immunotherapy (see treatment of alopecia areata, Chapter 11) consists of sensitization with 2% solution of squaric acid or diphenylcyclopropenone and then treatment with a dilute solution, usually about .001%, to perpetuate a low-grade contact dermatitis. Spread of the allergen from fingers to other areas of the body and face is problematic. *Candida* antigen works by the same T-cell-mediated immunologic mechanism but must be injected.

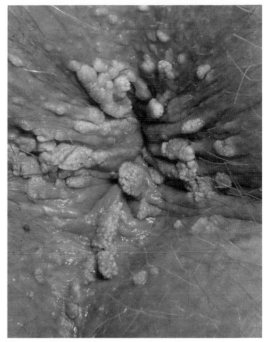

Figure 4-37 Condylomata acuminata. Brown warty papules in the perianal region

Topical imiquimod (Aldara) is a way of stimulating local immunity and painlessly treating warts, although it may not penetrate thick callus. It is not terribly effective, is very expensive, and is not FDA-approved in children or for common warts. Topical 5% fluorouracil cream (Efudex), especially under tape occlusion, may be helpful.

Oral cimetidine at a dose of 30–40 mg/kg per day has anecdotal evidence of efficacy when used for about 8 weeks in young children. It is not FDA-approved for this indication, but it may be considered in desperate situations. The mechanism is probably immunologic but is unknown.

The blistering agent cantharidin is more useful in treating mollusca contagiosa but may help some warts. A solution mixed in collodion is applied to each wart and left in place for 8–10 hours and then ever-increasing periods of time thereafter. It is painless in the office but induces a tender blister later in the day. Cure rate is low and a crateriform ring wart may result.

Cryotherapy with spray or cotton swab application of liquid nitrogen or other cryogen is effective if done repetitively but should be reserved for motivated, older children who will tolerate painful procedures. A 10-s freeze, preferably repeated with about a 5-s freeze, should be done to each wart. Tenderness and some blistering are expected if this is done with the appropriate degree of aggressiveness. Treatment sessions are repeated every 2–3 weeks for a total of 3–5 treatments. Patients or parents may use an over-the-counter cryogen spray consisting of dimethyl ether and propane (Wartner wart removal system). This technique seems to be better tolerated but less effective than liquid nitrogen.

Pulsed dye laser is about as effective as liquid nitrogen and the pain level is roughly equivalent. The relative lack of morbidity after treatments makes this modality particularly well suited for the treatment of plantar warts.

Surgical removal should be reserved for recalcitrant, symptomatic warts that have failed other modalities. Pointed scissor extraction followed by vigorous curettage may be facilitated by first performing electrodesiccation. Scarring is inevitable and about 1 in 4 warts will recur. Surgical removal should not be done on the plantar surface except for rare, extreme circumstances since scarring may lead to permanent debility. Flat warts are generally too numerous and elusive to consider a surgical approach.

The treatment of condylomata acuminata is similar to that for common warts. There is some evidence that children who are untreated fare just as well as those who receive treatment so "do no harm" is again the mantra. Topical imiquimod or podophyllotoxin gel 5% (Condylox) both cause local irritation but are fairly well tolerated. Aggressive therapies should be done with great reserve, possibly under general anesthesia.

The immunosuppressed population with warts poses a tremendous challenge. Control and comfort are much more appropriate goals than cure.

Mollusca Contagiosa

Key Points

- Umbilicated papules clustered in flexural areas
- Self-limited poxvirus infection that can be left untreated
- Cantharidin treatment or curettage

Clinical presentation

Mollusca contagiosa (singular is molluscum contagiosum) are extremely common in preschool and elementary school-age children. The scarcity in adults, even parents with very close contact with their infected children, suggests nearly universal exposure and long-lasting immunity to the virus.

Discrete, dome-shaped, flesh-colored to erythematous papules, frequently with a central umbilication, are characteristic. They may look like pustules on casual examination but are solid to palpation. They may be located anywhere but are common in the axillae, sides of the trunk, abdomen, face, thighs, and buttocks (Figure 4-38). They may appear like skin tags in intertriginous areas. Secondary infection or a host

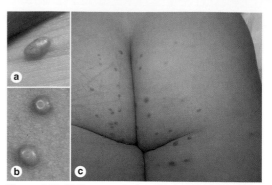

Figure 4-38 Mollusca contagiosa. Typical location on the buttock. **a** Bottom left shows obvious umbilicated papule but the upper left **b** is a more subtle tag-like papule

inflammatory response to the virus may result in large, erythematous, painful papules or pustules. Surrounding dermatitis is very common and may be difficult to treat until the lesions are gone. Lesions around the eye may cause conjunctivitis.

Diagnosis

Clinical diagnosis is usually very easy, although finding mollusca within a sea of keratosis pilaris may be challenging. Folliculitis, skin tags, warts, and milia can usually be excluded on clinical grounds. Dermatitis may dominate the clinical picture and the individual mollusca may be hidden within the scaling erythema of atopic dermatitis. Very large mollusca may look like epidermoid cysts. A KOH smear of a molluscum examined microscopically is diagnostic but requires some experience and is seldom necessary (Figure 4-39). Biopsy is rarely needed and the pathologic diagnosis of mollusca is usually a surprise finding when some other entity was suspected.

Pathogenesis

Mollusca contagiosa are caused by a DNA poxvirus. Infection is usually spread via person-to-person contact but may spread via fomites. Spontaneous resolution is the rule in 6–12 months.

Treatment

No treatment is necessary. Low-potency steroid creams will improve the associated dermatitis. Salicylic acid, tretinoin, and benzoyl peroxide have all been used but the resultant irritation is a poor tradeoff for the low efficacy. Imiquimod has had anecdotal modest success, although its irritancy and high cost are limiting. Cantharidin left on for 4 h is well tolerated and distinctly more effective for treating mollusca than common warts. Cryotherapy or removal with a curette after topical anesthesia may be appropriate for older children with few warts. Pockmark scars may result with or without treatment.

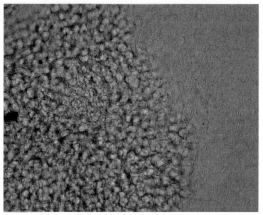

Figure 4-39 Mollusca contagiosa. Potassium hydroxide examination showing infected cells to the left with shiny, refractile appearance compared to normal cells on the right

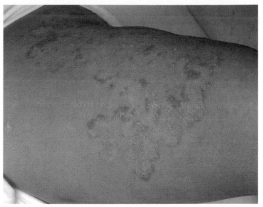

Figure 4-40 Tinea corporis. Annular scaling patch with central clearing and a darker leading edge

Fungal Infections

Tinea

Dermatophytes are fungal organisms belonging to the three genera of *Microsporum*, *Trichophyton*, and *Epidermophyton*. They invade and cause infections in the keratinized tissues of skin, hair, and nails. The zoophilic organisms *M. canis* (cats and dogs) and *T. verrucosum* (cows and horses) are acquired from animals whereas the anthropophilic organisms *T. mentagrophytes*, *T. tonsurans*, *T. rubrum*, and *E. floccosum* primarily infect humans and are spread through person-to-person contact. The infection is labeled by the prefix tinea, followed by the Latin name for the anatomical location such as tinea pedis for dermatophyte infection of the foot. Ringworm is the familiar but misleading slang for dermatophyte infections. Tinea capitis is a common and troublesome infection of the scalp hair that will be discussed separately.

Key Points

- Annular scaling erythema with central clearing and a darker leading edge
- KOH preparation and culture
- Various topical antifungal creams and selective use of oral griseofulvin

Clinical presentation

Tinea corporis is a dermatophyte infection of the body. The classic lesion is a pruritic, red, annular scaling patch or plaque with central clearing and a darker leading edge (Figure 4-40). There may be multiple lesions and coalescence will give polycyclic, scalloped borders. The lesions may be very inflammatory, especially with zoophilic organisms, and pustules may dominate. Treatment with topical steroids results in a nonclassic presentation termed tinea incognito that may challenge correct diagnosis and lead to a deeper hair follicle invasion known as Majocchi granuloma (Figure 4-41).

Tinea faciei is an infection of the face, and tinea barbae that of the beard. Pustules and papules may dominate in the beard.

Tinea cruris or jock itch involves the upper medial thighs and is seen almost exclusively in teenage or older men. Warmth, moisture, and friction aid in its development. The scrotum is characteristically spared but may be red and lichenified due to rubbing.

Tinea pedis, or athlete's foot, has three different presentations that may coexist. Interdigital tinea (Figure 4-42) consists of fissuring and scaling between the toes. Inflammatory or bullous tinea pedis (Figure 4-43) consists of multiloculated, erythematous vesicles and bullae, usually on the arch but also the heel. Moccasin tinea pedis (Figure 4-44) has fine powdery scaling on the weight-bearing areas with a sharp line of demarcation at the lateral edge of the foot. A tinea infection of the hand will almost always be accompanied by tinea pedis and is referred to as tinea manuum.

An id reaction (dermatophytid) refers to an immunologic reaction to the causative dermatophyte that may manifest as vesicles on the hands and feet or as a dermatitic rash elsewhere.

Diagnosis

A KOH preparation (Figure 4-45) of scale scrapings is invaluable in making a diagnosis of tinea. The blister roof should be examined in bullous tinea. The necessity of heating the slide can be avoided by the addition of dimethylsulfoxide to the KOH and stains such as chlorazol black E may enhance visualization of the fungal hyphae. Both can be purchased from medical supply stores. The condenser of the microscope should be closed as much as possible to allow

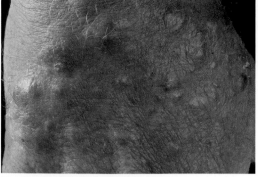

Figure 4-41 Majocchi granuloma. Nodules and papules indicating deeper hair follicle tinea invasion

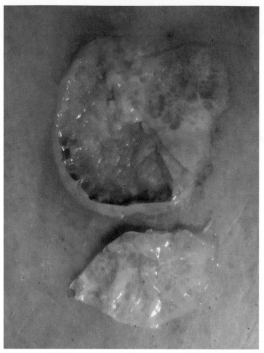

Figure 4-43 Tinea pedis. Bullous variety of tinea pedis with multiloculate bulla. Potassium hydroxide specimen should be from the blister roof

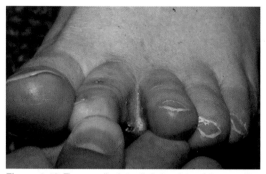

Figure 4-42 Tinea pedis. Interdigital variety of tinea pedis

for good depth of field. Interpretation of a KOH preparation requires some practice but eventually becomes quite easy and its value is immense.

Fungal culture will confirm the diagnosis but results may not be available for many days so treatment decisions will need to be made prior to the availability of a positive culture. Dermatophyte test media provides an easily interpreted culture method that can be performed and read in the outpatient clinic setting, but sending the culture to a hospital laboratory may be less cumbersome in a busy clinic. Scraped specimens can be placed directly on to Sabouraud's agar or a routine moistened culture swab can be vigorously rubbed over the lesion and sent much the same as a bacterial culture. A culture of *M. canis* is particularly valuable because it indicates the presence of an infected animal, usually a kitten, which needs to be removed or treated. A culture growing *T. tonsurans* suggests that someone in the household has tinea capitis.

All forms of tinea can be mistaken for any of the entities in the papulosquamous group of disorders (see Chapter 2), particularly psoriasis, seborrheic dermatitis, pityriasis rosea, nummular dermatitis, and pityriasis lichenoides chronica. Granuloma annulare is frequently mistaken for tinea, although the reverse is seldom true. Tinea in sun-exposed areas, particularly tinea faciei,

may look like lupus erythematosus. Tinea barbae may be mistaken for a bacterial or herpes simplex infection. Erythrasma, lichen simplex chronicus, and *Candida* intertrigo may look like tinea cruris. Involvement of the scrotum speaks against tinea. Juvenile plantar dermatosis or sweaty-sock feet is often mistaken for tinea pedis. The absence of toe web involvement, the generally younger age of the patient, and negative KOH will suggest dermatitis.

Majocchi granuloma (fungal folliculitis) poses a particular challenge since the KOH evaluation will sometimes be negative and even a surface culture may not grow. A biopsy may be needed in puzzling cases.

Pathogenesis

The six dermatophytes mentioned above account for the vast majority of tinea infections. Keratinases produced by the organisms aid in their invasion.

Treatment

A plethora of topical antifungal agents are available as brand-name and generic preparations. The azole antifungals are fungistatic and clotrimazole and miconazole creams are relative bargains in this category. Others include econazole, ketoconazole, oxiconazole, and sulconazole. The allylamines are fungicidal and should theoretically be more effective, but they are also more expensive. Terbinafine, butenafine, and naftifine belong to this group. Ciclopirox is a hydroxy pyridone that is also

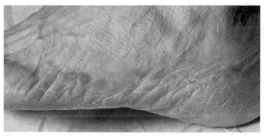

Figure 4-44 Tinea pedis. Moccasin variety of tinea pedis

fungicidal. Topical treatments should be continued for 1 week past clinical clearing.

A combination cream containing betamethasone dipropionate (a high-potency corticosteroid) and clotrimazole has no place in treating any dermatophyte infection and, arguably, has no therapeutic indication for any skin disease except chronic paranychia. Nystatin preparations will only kill yeast and are not useful for tinea.

Tinea barbae, Majocchi granuloma, inflammatory tinea pedis, and any documented infection resistant to topical therapy are best treated systemically with griseofulvin or any of the newer oral antifungal agents. The length of treatment will need to be assessed clinically but 2–4 weeks should be anticipated.

Id reactions will improve as the tinea infection is treated. A topical steroid can be used as long as the diagnosis is correct, but steroids should not be used directly on the fungal infection.

Tinea Capitis

Key Points

- Hair loss with scaling and adenopathy
- *Trichophyton tonsurans* and *Microsporum canis*
- KOH with spores in or on hair shaft, no hyphae
- Must be treated with oral antifungal agent, griseofulvin

Clinical presentation

Hair loss due to broken hairs, itch, and scaling erythema are the hallmarks of tinea capitis (Figure 4-46). Adenopathy is almost always present but is a nonspecific finding. Broken hairs may form black dots but papules, pustules, and crusts develop as the areas of alopecia become more inflammatory. A kerion is an edematous, boggy, tender nodule that represents a heightened inflammatory response (Figure 4-47). Permanent scarring may result. Diffuse, powdery scaling without hair loss may be the only manifestation of tinea capitis and poses a difficult diagnostic challenge. An id reaction consisting of a nonspecific erythematous or dermatitic eruption on the trunk and extremities may occur and is often mistaken for an allergic drug rash from antifungal therapy.

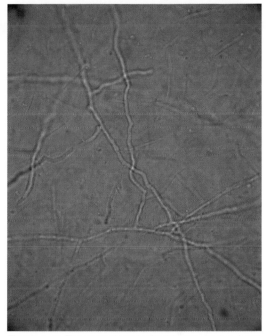

Figure 4-45 Tinea potassium hydroxide preparation. Long hyphae visible overlying keratinocytes

Diagnosis

Obtaining and interpreting scalp scrapings require more experience and expertise. A KOH preparation will demonstrate fungal spores within or outside an infected hair shaft (Figure 4-48), but hyphae on scale will be scant or absent. Scraping with a scalpel blade or curette obtains more hairs than using a toothbrush or cotton-tip swab but may be frightening to young children. Using the least painful and nonthreatening technique first and then trying a scalpel blade second is helpful in reassuring anxious patients.

Examination with a Woods light will reveal green fluorescence within the hairs of patients infected with *M. canis* but not *T. tonsurans*. Care must be taken not to interpret the whitish fluorescence seen with lint and scale as a positive finding.

Obtaining a culture is important not only for establishing the diagnosis but also for identifying the specific organism. The growth of *M. canis* indicates that there is an animal in the environment that needs to be located and treated. *M. canis* is also a much more stubborn organism to treat, requiring longer and, perhaps, higher dosing. The organism is resistant to terbinafine. A good culture can be quickly and easily obtained by using a sterile toothbrush or a moistened routine culture swab that is aggressively rubbed on many areas of affected scalp. The specimen can be plated directly on to culture media or sent to the lab in much the same fashion as a bacterial culture.

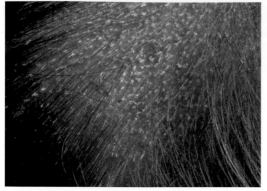

Figure 4-46 Tinea capitis. Alopecia, broken hairs, and scaling

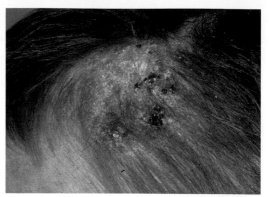

Figure 4-47 Tinea capitis. Edematous, boggy, tender nodule

Alopecia areata and trichotillomania form the main differential diagnosis. Seborrheic dermatitis, psoriasis, discoid lupus, and lichen planopilaris may be mistaken for tinea capitis. Biopsy may be needed if these entities are entertained and the fungal culture is negative. A kerion looks like a folliculitis or abscess and *Staphylococcus aureus* may in fact be grown from a kerion as a secondary invader. A biopsy may be needed but usually KOH exam and culture of scrapings and plucked hairs will establish a fungal origin.

Pathogenesis

T. tonsurans accounts for the majority of tinea capitis, particularly in urban areas of the USA. Transmission is from person to person or through fomites such as shared combs and hats. *M. canis* is common in suburban and rural areas and must spark the search for an infected cat or dog, frequently a stray kitten.

Treatment

Tinea capitis cannot be satisfactorily treated with topical agents alone. Oral therapy with griseofulvin at a dose of 20–25 mg/kg per day is the treatment of choice. A liquid suspension of 125 mg/teaspoon is available for young children. Use of an ultramicrosized pill will enhance absorption and the dose can be decreased to about 16–20 mg/kg per day. The medicine should be taken with a fatty food such as whole milk or ice cream. Headache and stomach upset are fairly common side-effects but generally this treatment is very well tolerated and safe. An allergic reaction is possible but a rash during treatment is likely to be an id reaction that does not necessarily warrant stopping the medication. Duration of therapy should be no shorter than 6–8 weeks and total duration of therapy should be determined by a negative physical exam and, perhaps, negative reculture. *M. canis* will require extended treatment, generally 3–5 months and sometimes longer.

Laboratory monitoring is not needed for healthy children whose treatment is within the usual 6–8-week time frame. Liver function studies and blood counts should be considered for extended courses or for children with other complicating illnesses.

Alternative oral therapies, including terbinafine (62.5 mg < 20 kg, 125 mg 20–40 kg, 250 mg > 40 kg or a target of about 5–6 mg/kg per day), itraconazole (5 mg/kg per day) and fluconazole (6 mg/kg per day), are treatments that match the efficacy of griseofulvin with the advantage of short courses of 2–3 weeks. They are not FDA-approved for this indication. *M. canis* is sluggishly responsive to these antifungal agents as well, with particular resistance to terbinafine.

Topical antifungal agents and sporicidal shampoos such as ketoconazole, zinc pyrithione, or selenium sulfide may serve as adjunctive treatment, especially to decrease shedding.

Onychomycosis

Onychomycosis is the broad term given to any fungal infection of the nail whereas tinea unguium specifically refers to a dermatophyte invasion of the nail.

Key Points

- Thick, brown nails with subungual debris
- *Trichophyton rubrum*, sometimes *T. mentagrophytes*, *Epidermophyton floccosum*, *Candida albicans*
- Culture must be done correctly, false negatives
- Treatment tailored to symptoms

Clinical presentation

Onychomycosis is far more common in the older population but does occur in children and adolescents. It is probably underrecognized. Pain may be the presenting symptom but the nails are mostly a cosmetic concern. Yellow-brown

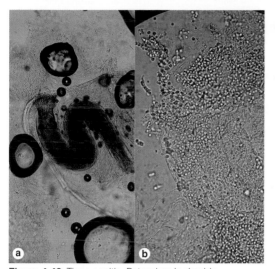

Figure 4-48 Tinea capitis. Potassium hydroxide preparation showing a dystrophic hair **a** and close-up showing fungal spores **b**

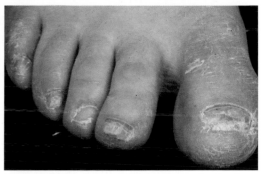

Figure 4-49 Onychomycosis. Yellow-brown discoloration, thickening, and crumbly subungual debris of tinea infection of the nail

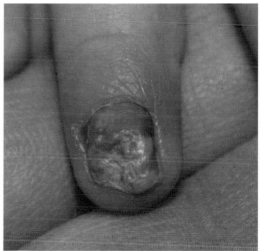

Figure 4-50 Onychomycosis. Infant infected with *Candida albicans*

discoloration, thickening, and crumbly subungual debris are characteristic (Figure 4-49) but the infection can be on the proximal rather than the distal tip and the superficial variety of onychomycosis gives an opaque white discoloration that can be scraped with a scalpel blade. Tinea pedis will often coexist with onychomycosis and is probably the source of infection in most. Trauma to the nail offers a portal of entry.

Infants with onychomycosis are usually infected with C. *albicans* acquired via intrauterine or vaginal transmission (Figure 4-50).

Diagnosis

What may appear to be a straightforward diagnosis of onychomycosis may in fact be psoriasis, lichen planus, traumatic dystrophy, twenty-nail dystrophy, or a congenital abnormality such as pachyonychia congenita. The diagnosis should be proven before systemic therapy is considered.

It is imperative to include subungual debris in the sample. Crumbling subungual debris should be scraped free with a small curette and sent for fungal culture. KOH examination can be performed but interpretation is difficult, even to very experienced eyes, and may be falsely negative. A nail clipping including a generous amount of subungual debris can be sent to pathology for histologic examination and staining with periodic acid–Schiff to demonstrate fungal elements.

Pathogenesis

T. *rubrum* is the most common dermatophyte but T. *mentagrophytes* or E. *floccosum* may be causative. C. *albicans* may be seen in infants with or without other features of cutaneous

candidiasis. Molds such as *Aspergillus, Alternaria, Scopulariopsis,* and many others may grow from the distorted nail but pathogenicity is unsure. As a general rule, only dermatophytes and C. *albicans* should be considered pathogenic unless cultures from differing locations taken at different times consistently grow the same organism.

Treatment

Onychomycosis does not need to be treated if asymptomatic. Filing, sometimes with the aid of a Dremel tool, and sculpting may give acceptable cosmetic results and relieve pressure points causing pain. Practitioners and parents need to weigh the risks and expense of systemic treatment against the modest cure (65–75%) and high recurrence rate (50%). Griseofulvin requires very long courses and should not be considered in this setting due to its low efficacy. Terbinafine (62.5 mg < 20 kg, 125 mg 20–40 kg, 250 mg > 40 kg or a target of about 5–6 mg/kg per day), itraconazole (3–5 mg/kg per day up to 200 mg/day) and fluconazole (3–6 mg/kg per day up to 300 mg/day) can be given daily for 3 months for toenails and 2 months for fingernails. Longer courses probably offer greater cure rate. Creative pulse dosing regimens have been designed whereby the medicine need only be taken 1 week of each month or 1 day out of each week but studies are scant in the pediatric age group. None of these antifungal agents is FDA-approved for children with onychomycosis.

Topical therapy has an outside chance of working since children's nails grow fairly rapidly. Very vigorous paring and filing in association with a topical antifungal agent are safe and worth considering prior to initiating systemic therapy. Ciclopirox lacquer (Penlac) or bifonazole in 40% urea (Mycospor Onycho-Set) is of modest benefit.

Infants with *Candida* in the nails will frequently self-resolve as the abnormal nail plate grows out.

Tinea Versicolor

Key Points

- Hypopigmented or hyperpigmented patches on the trunk and neck of teenagers
- Spaghetti and meatballs on KOH exam
- *Malassezia* yeasts
- Topical or oral antifungal agents with topical prophylaxis afterwards

Clinical presentation

This common eruption generally affects teenagers and young adults but may occasionally be seen in younger children. It is usually asymptomatic but may be mildly pruritic. Slightly scaling macules and patches develop on the trunk and neck and appear pink-to-brown on white skin (Figure 4-51) and hypopigmented on dark skin (Figure 4-52). As they coalesce, the patches become geographic and polycyclic. The fine, powdery scale may not be readily appreciated until the skin is gently scraped.

Diagnosis

The clinical picture is usually obvious but a KOH scraping will reveal typical stubby hyphae and spores (macaroni and meatballs: Figure 4-53). Woods light of unwashed skin purportedly gives an orange fluorescence but this is seldom a useful test. Postinflammatory hypopigmentation and vitiligo make up the main differential diagnosis in the hypopigmented form. Seborrheic dermatitis or reticulated and confluent papillomatosis may look like the hyperpigmented form.

Pathogenesis

Lipophilic yeasts of the *Malassezia* genus are part of the normal postpubertal flora and are responsible for the eruption. Growth is aided by sebum and warmth and affected individuals may possess some genetic factor that accounts for their susceptibility.

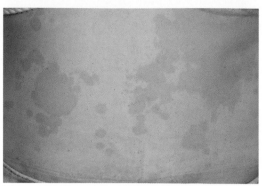

Figure 4-51 Tinea versicolor. Pink-to-brown macules and patches on white skin

Treatment

Multiple topical regimens exist, although the large surface may make topical therapy unwieldy and impractical. Any of the azole antifungal agents such as clotrimazole can be used. Selenium sulfide lotion or shampoo, ketoconazole shampoo, and zinc pyrithione may be applied in the shower for 10–15 min, but compliance with this regimen is no doubt low. A single overnight application of selenium sulfide lotion is generally effective. Oral treatment with a singe dose of fluconazole or ketoconazole may be curative. A popular regimen uses 400 mg oral ketoconazole with a repeated dose in 1 week. Patients must be reminded that the pigmentary abnormalities will not normalize for several weeks.

Recurrence is the norm so some prophylactic measure should be instituted after treatment is complete. Washing with a zinc pyrithione soap bar (ZNP) 1–2 times per week is an easy method of prophylaxis, but any of the topical treatments mentioned above can be performed on an inter-mittent basis.

Candidal Infections

Key Points

- Beefy red with satellitosis in skin folds
- KOH with spores
- Reduce friction and moisture
- Topical antifungal agents, sometimes oral agents

Clinical presentation

Skin folds favor the growth of *Candida* so the rash of cutaneous candidiasis tends to occur in the axillae, groin folds, and under large breasts or bellies. A diaper provides the perfect environment for growth. The pruritic and tender rash is beefy-red with edema, oozing, crusting, and pustule formation. Small macules form outside the confluent erythema (satellitosis) and frequently have a collar of scaling (Figure 4-54). A "yeasty" odor may be present.

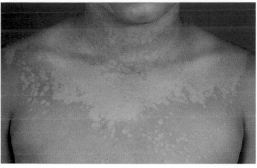

Figure 4-52 Tinea versicolor. Hypopigmented macules and patches on white skin

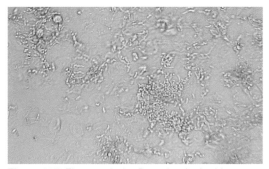

Figure 4-53 Tinea versicolor. Potassium hydroxide preparation showing clusters of spores and stubby hyphae (macaroni and meatballs)

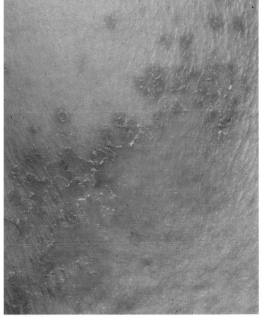

Figure 4-54 *Candida*. Small macules outside the confluent erythema (satellitosis) with a collar of scaling

Thrush refers to the development of a curd-like exudate on the oral mucosa, usually in infants. It is easily removed with a cotton swab or tongue depressor, leaving a glistening red base.

Angular cheilitis consists of fissures and crusts that develop at the corners of the mouth. It is common in children with braces and especially in acne patients receiving isotretinoin therapy. *Candida* from the oral mucosa is a secondary invader after fissures develop.

Diagnosis

A KOH preparation will demonstrate hyphae and clusters of spores. *Streptococcus pyogenes* infection (perianal *Streptococcus* or streptococcal intertrigo), impetigo, inverse psoriasis, seborrheic dermatitis, contact dermatitis, and frictional intertrigo may look like cutaneous *Candida* and, to confuse the differential diagnosis further, may be a cohabitant with any of these disorders.

Formula or food may look like thrush. Herpes simplex infection, erythema multiforme, geographic tongue, and the rare conditions of lichen planus and leukoplakia should be considered in the differential diagnosis.

Angular cheilitis may rarely indicate riboflavin, pyridoxine, or zinc deficiency.

Pathogenesis

C. albicans is part of the normal flora of the mouth, gastrointestinal tract, and cutaneous surfaces. An environment of warmth, moisture, and maceration and host factors of immunosuppression, diabetes, and antibiotic use favor its overgrowth and infectivity.

Treatment

Cutaneous candidiasis can be treated with any of the host of creams used for the treatment of tinea. Reducing friction and moisture is more easily said than done, particularly in obese individuals, but may be accomplished with the use of powders or thick, zinc oxide-containing barrier creams. Diapers should be changed frequently or removed altogether. Decreasing oral and gastrointestinal colonization with oral nystatin may be helpful.

Nystatin suspension applied with a cotton swab or facecloth, followed by a 1–2 ml oral dose 4 times daily is effective. Children may suck on clotrimazole troches as long as there is not a risk of aspiration. Rarely, oral fluconazole may be needed for mucocutaneous infection but severe, unrelenting, documented infection that does not respond to simple measures should prompt a search for an underlying reason such as HIV, chronic mucocutaneous candidiasis, or other immunosuppressive disorder.

Angular cheilitis can be treated with a nystatin/triamcinolone ointment combination and lubrication.

Infestations

Scabies

Key Points

* Severe itch with lesions on fingers, web spaces, wrist, axilla, and groin
* KOH with mites and eggs
* *Sarcoptes scabiei*
* 5% permethrin cream or lindane lotion

Clinical presentation

Incessant, severe itch, especially at nighttime, is the hallmark of scabies. The hands, particularly the interdigital spaces, wrists, axillae, abdomen, genitals, and female breasts are typically involved. Infants will have prominent involvement of the palms, soles, and scalp (Figure 4-55). Papulovesicles may be obscured by secondary excoriations, lichenification, and impetiginization. The classic lesion of scabies is the burrow, a serpiginous microvesicle with a tiny black dot at the tip seen with magnification. A good burrow can be hard to find, although they tend to be numerous in infants and those previously treated with topical steroids.

Nodular scabies represents a bug bite-like hypersensitivity to the scabies mite and consists of red-brown edematous 5–20-mm papules and nodules on the penis, scrotum, axillae, waist, and buttocks (Figure 4-56).

Norwegian or crusted scabies occurs in institutionalized, elderly, or immunosuppressed individuals and represents infestation with thousands of mites. Thick, ichthyotic crusting, especially of the hands, dominates the picture and pruritus is surprisingly scant (Figure 4-57).

Diagnosis

A scraping from a burrow will be diagnostic, demonstrating mites (Figure 4-58), intact eggs, or egg fragments on microscopic exam with mineral oil or KOH. Feces (scybala) will only be seen with oil. Taking advantage of the thick stratum corneum of the palms and soles facilitates vigorous scraping without pain and a better diagnostic yield. If no burrow can be found, a blind scraping of nonspecific lesions from the interdigital spaces and wrists may be positive but the yield decreases without a burrow.

Atopic dermatitis is the main differential diagnosis but impetigo, bug bites, viral exanthem, and dermatitis herpetiformis may look like scabies. In fact, any pruritic disorder may be part of the differential. Infants with prominent hand and foot vesicles without burrows and a negative scraping probably have infantile acropustulosis.

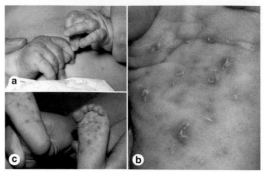

Figure 4-55 Scabies. Prominent vesicles and papules on the hands and feet of an infected infant

Pathogenesis

Scabies is caused by the mite, *S. scabiei*. The female mite is transferred to her new host via skin-to-skin contact and burrows into the stratum corneum to begin laying eggs that hatch and emerge as larvae in 15 days. The incubation period from the time of contact to the time of first symptoms is 3–6 weeks, faster in cases of reinfestation. The mite will survive for about 2 days away from its human host.

Treatment

Overnight application of permethrin 5% cream is the treatment of choice. All family members and close contacts should be treated, even if not symptomatic. A single application from the neck downward has a high cure rate when performed thoroughly and completely. It must be stressed that every square centimeter of the body needs to be covered, even if there are no lesions present. Night linens and bed clothing should be washed in hot water. A repeat application in 1 week is reasonable for those with significant infestations. Some epidemiologic data suggest a link between pyrethroids or other insecticides and leukemia. Well-designed studies are urgently needed to confirm or refute the association.

Lindane lotion offers a cure rate similar to permethrin. Neurotoxicity has been reported in very young children, particularly with massive overuse, and it should not be used in children less than 4–5 years of age or pregnant women. Solutions of precipitated sulfur, crotamiton, and benzyl benzoate have some purported efficacy but are not part of mainstream treatment.

Very stubborn cases, epidemics in institutions, and crusted scabies can be treated with oral ivermectin at a dose of 200 µg/kg. Scale in crusted scabies can be removed with tubbing and use of keratolytic agents such as salicylic acid. Ivermectin should be avoided in children less than 15 kg and in pregnant women.

Patients should be re-examined about 2 weeks after completing therapy when postscabies irritation and dermatitis should have settled. Residual lesions

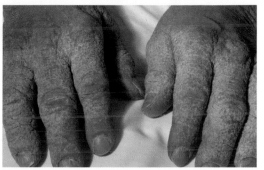

Figure 4-57 Scabies. Crusted, hyperkeratotic lesions of Norwegian scabies

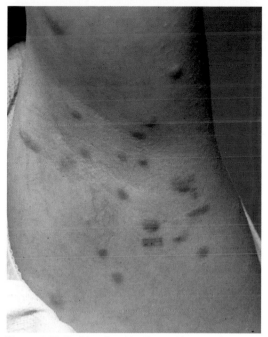

Figure 4-56 Scabies. Bug bite-like, red-brown edematous papules and nodules of nodular scabies

should be rescraped and a low-potency topical steroid can be used if this is negative. Nodular scabies can be treated with topical or intralesional steroids once scabies treatment is complete.

Pediculosis

- Itch, excoriation, and adenopathy
- Nits and lice are diagnostic
- *Pediculus humanus capitis* (head) and *Pthirus pubis* (pubic region)
- Permethrin, pyrethrins, malathion, suffocation treatment

Clinical presentation

Pediculosis capitis represents a louse infestation of the scalp that is most common in elementary school-aged girls and is very uncommon in those of African descent. Itch is the main symptom and opalescent nits can be seen attached to the hair. Specks of fecal material may be noted on the scalp. The postauricular and occipital regions are the most affected areas and may have excoriations, crusts, and signs of secondary impetiginization. Adenopathy is common. It is difficult to find a louse since they are only 1–2 mm in size and move quickly. Wetting the hair may momentarily immobilize lice. Vigorously and repetitively combing wet hair with an underlying white sheet of paper or pillowcase may cause some live lice to fall and be seen.

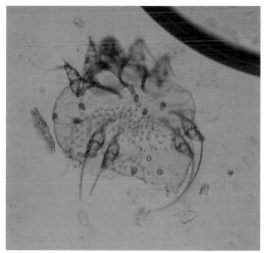

Figure 4-58 Scabies. Potassium hydroxide preparation showing an adult mite, slightly tilted

The nits are laid close to the scalp and grow upward as the scalp hair grows at a rate of 1 cm per month. Microscopic inspection of nits will indicate if they are full or empty. The age and activity of an infestation can be judged in this fashion.

Pediculosis pubis ("crabs") refers to an infestation of the pubic region and is frequently sexually transmitted. A high percentage of infestations are associated with other sexually transmitted diseases. The louse may be seen grabbing the base of pubic hairs or hairs on the chest, abdomen, thighs, buttocks, axillae, and eyelashes. Nits will be seen as in pediculosis capitis and dominate the clinical picture with infestation of the eyelashes.

Diagnosis

Visual inspection of a louse is diagnostic but the finding of viable nits close to the skin suggests active infection. The use of a magnifying glass and good lighting are helpful in making the diagnosis.

Hair casts, fragments of hairspray, and the *Trichosporon* infection white piedra may look like nits. Psoriasis, seborrheic dermatitis, and tinea capitis might be mistaken for pediculosis infestation.

Pathogenesis

Scalp infestations are caused by *Pediculus humanus capitis*, an elongated organism with antennae and three pairs of clawed legs (Figure 4-59). *Pthirus pubis* is the pubic louse. It is broader and square-shaped with two pairs of legs sporting large crab-like claws and a front pair of legs that are much smaller. Spread is via person-to-person contact but may take place on fomites such as shared hats.

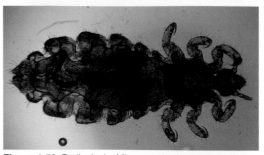

Figure 4-59 Pediculosis. Microscopic view of *Pediculus humanus capitis*, showing elongated torso and three pairs of clawed legs

Treatment

Several agents are available for treating pediculosis capitis. Cure through manual removal is possible if done vigorously and repetitively but is work-intensive and unrealistic for most families.

Topical agents should be applied to dry hair and the use of cream rinse or conditioners should be stopped. Permethrin in a 1% cream rinse applied for 5–10 min is generally effective although resistance has been documented. Permethrin 5% cream is more difficult to apply to the scalp, but can be used on wet hair. The higher concentration may overcome some knock-down resistance with prolonged application. Several products contain pyrethrins, natural extracts from chrysanthemums (caution in those with allergy), and piperonyl butoxide. Use and efficacy levels are similar to permethrin. Cross-resistance is common. Prescription malathion (Ovide) is relatively new to the US market after being unavailable for many years. Resistance is currently very low but will no doubt rise with more extensive use. It is expensive, is indicated for overnight application, has a bad odor, hurts if it gets in the eyes, and is flammable. Lindane should rarely be used, as better options are available.

Suffocation therapy with oils, petrolatum, pomades, and mayonnaise has some efficacy but is very messy. Shrink-wrap suffocation by application of Cetaphil cleanser followed by drying with a hairdryer is an intriguing technique that has yet to stand the test of time. Better louse asphyxiators are under investigation.

Ivermectin has been creatively mixed into shampoos or vegetable oil with some anecdotal efficacy but is not commercially available as a topical agent. A single oral dose offers about 75% cure when combined with vigorous nit removal.

Oral trimethoprim-sulfamethoxazole for 2 weeks with or without topical agents has been effective. The louse ingests the antibiotic as part of a blood meal with subsequent death of necessary louse gut flora and resultant malnutrition.

Purported treatment failures should raise suspicion of noncompliance, concomitant use of cream rinse with treatments, reinfection, persistent nonviable nits without active infection, or incorrect diagnosis.

Pubic lice can be treated with any of the treatments mentioned above. Generic permethrin 5% cream is well tolerated and effective. A thick coat of petrolatum 2–3 times daily can be used for eyelash infestation.

Further reading

Bacterial infections

Deresinski S. Methicillin-resistant *Staphylococcus aureus:* an evolutionary, epidemiologic, and therapeutic odyssey. Clin Inf Dis 2005;40: 562–573.

Elston D. Community-acquired methicillin-resistant *Staphylococcus aureus.* J Am Acad Dermatol 2007; 56:1–16.

Iwatsuki K, Yamasaki O, Morizane S, et al. Staphylococcal cutaneous infections; invasion, evasion and aggression. J Dermatol Sci 2006; 42:203–214.

Kowalski TJ, Berbari EF, Osmon DR. Epidemiology, treatment, and prevention of community-acquired methicillin-resistant *Staphylococcus aureus* infections. Mayo Clinic Proc 2005;80:12–18.

Patel GK, Finlay AY. Staphylococcal scalded skin syndrome: diagnosis and management. Am J Clin Dermatol 2003;4:165–175.

Shapiro ED, Gerber MA. Lyme disease: fact versus fiction. Pediatr Ann 2002;31:170–177.

Silvestre JF, Betlloch MI. Cutaneous manifestations due to *Pseudomonas* infection. Int J Dermatol 1999;38:419–431.

Takama H, Cuce LC, Souza RL, et al. Pitted keratolysis: clinical manifestations in 53 cases. Br J Dermatol 1997;137:282–285.

Viral infections

Brandt O, Abeck D, Gianotti R, et al. Gianotti–Crosti syndrome. J Am Acad Dermatol 2006;54: 136–145.

Coustou D, Masquelier B, Lafon ME, et al. Asymmetric periflexural exanthem of childhood: microbiologic case-control study. Pediatr Dermatol 2000;17:169–173.

Hambleton S. Chickenpox. Curr Opin Infect Dis 2005;18:235–240.

Smolinski KN, Yan CY. How and when to treat molluscum contagiosum and warts in children. Pediatr Ann 2005; 34:211–221.

Torrelo A. What's new in the treatment of viral warts in children. Pediatr Dermatol 2002; 19:191–199.

Vásquez M. Varicella infections and varicella vaccine in the 21st century. Pediatr Infect Dis J 2004; 23:871–872.

Waggoner-Fountain LA, Grossman LB. Herpes simplex virus. Pediatr Rev 2004;25:86–93.

Ward KN. Human herpesviruses-6 and 7 infections. Curr Opin Infect Dis 2005;18:247–252.

Yourn NL, Brown KE. Parvovirus B19. N Engl J Med 2004;350:586–597.

Fungal infections

Gupta AK, Skinner AR. Onychomycosis in children: a brief overview with treatment strategies. Pediatr Dermatol 2004;21:74–79.

Gupta AK, Batra R, Bluhm R, et al. Skin diseases associated with Malassezia species. J Am Acad Dermatol 2004;51:785–798.

Hay RJ. The management of superficial candidiasis. J Am Acad Dermatol 1999;40:S35–S42.

Huang DB, Ostrosky-Zeichern L, Wu JJ, et al. Therapy of common superficial fungal infections. Dermatol Ther 2004;17:517–522.

Roberts BJ, Fallon Friedlander S. Tinea capitis: a treatment update. Pediatr Ann 2005; 34:191–200.

Romano C, Papini M, Ghilardi A, et al. Onychomycosis in children: a survey of 46 cases. Mycoses 2005;48:430–437.

Infestations

Chosidow O. Scabies. N Engl J Med 2006; 354:1718–1727.

Huynh TH, Norman RA. Scabies and pediculosis. Dermatol Clin 2004;22:7–11.

Ko CJ, Elston DM. Pediculosis. J Am Acad Dermatol 2004;50:1–12.

Vascular birthmarks in children

5

Albert C. Yan

Vascular anomalies are among the most common birthmarks encountered by the pediatric clinician. The prompt and accurate diagnosis of a vascular birthmark can at times provide the clinician with essential clues to potential underlying extracutaneous complications. For instance, patients manifesting port-wine stains of the face may expect highly different prognoses from those exhibiting facial segmental hemangiomas or those having arteriovenous malformations.

Because the literature has been obfuscated by the use of imprecise terms for vascular birthmarks, particular attention should be paid to using terms that best reflect our current pathogenetic and histologic understanding of these disorders. In 1982, Mulliken and Glowacki proposed a classification scheme to describe vascular anomalies based on their biologic characteristics, and in 1992 and 1996, the International Society for the Study of Vascular Anomalies updated its framework to encompass additional clinical, imaging, and histologic characteristics in order to differentiate better between tumors (including infantile hemangiomas (IH), kaposiform hemangioendothelioma, pyogenic granuloma) and malformations (including capillary, venous, and arteriovenous malformations) (Table 5-1). Vascular tumors are defined as typically dynamic lesions that grow, change, and exhibit cellular proliferation whereas malformations – though capable of evolution – tend to grow with the patient and show significantly less mitotic activity.

Salmon Patch(Nevus Simplex, "Angel's Kiss," "Stork Bite")

Key Points

- Common birthmark with facial lesions that often fade by a year of age
- Often have midline or symmetric distribution on the face, scalp, posterior neck
- Most require no intervention

The salmon patch is a common vascular birthmark that is noted in approximately 30–40% of newborns. Affected infants present at birth with faint, blanchable erythematous macules that are located most often on the glabella, posterior scalp, and nape of the neck, but can also be seen on the eyelids, philtrum, and occasionally the lateral forehead areas (Figure 5-1A). The majority of these lesions fade by 1–2 years of age, although the nuchal lesions may persist into the early school age period. These birthmarks are benign, isolated findings and are not associated with extracutaneous manifestations. Occasionally, lesions on the scalp or posterior neck can eczematize (Figure 5-1B), but usually respond to low-potency topical corticosteroid agents. Rarely, salmon patches on the face persist into school age and can be referred for treatment with an appropriate vascular laser.

Hemangiomas and Tumors

Infantile Hemangioma (Hemangiomas of Infancy, Capillary Hemangioma, Strawberry Hemangioma, Cavernous Hemangioma)

Key Points

- IHs are rarely visible at birth
- Hemangiomas show a characteristic growth pattern of proliferation, plateau, and involution
- IHs stain positively for a number of markers – Glut-1, Lewis Y, merosin, FcγRII – that can help differentiate it from other vascular tumors
- Lesions that occur at certain anatomic sites may pose a risk for specific complications: periocular, perioral/beard/parotid, nasal tip, midline lumbosacral, perineal
- Segmental hemangiomas of the face or perineum may be associated with extracutaneous manifestations as part of PHACES, PELVIS/SACRAL syndromes (see below for definitions)
- Multiple cutaneous lesions can be associated with visceral hemangiomatosis

Table 5-1 International Society for the Study of Vascular Anomalies classification scheme for vascular anomalies

Tumors	Malformations (high-flow and low-flow)
Infantile hemangioma	Capillary malformation
Pyogenic granuloma (lobular capillary hemangioma)	Venous malformation
Kaposiform hemangioendothelioma	Lymphatic malformation
Tufted angioma	Arteriovenous malformation
RICH	Complex combined malformations
NICH	CMTC

CMTC, cutis marmorata telangiectatica congenita; NICH, noninvoluting congenital hemangioma; RICH, rapidly involuting congenital hemangioma.

- IHs are *not* associated with Kasabach–Merritt phenomenon
- Early pharmacologic intervention for problematic hemangiomas may prevent long-term sequelae

IHs are common vascular tumors composed of vascular endothelial cells that occur in approximately 4–10% of infants. Although approximately 2–3% may present at birth, the majority manifest initially with only faint, premonitory, blanchable, erythematous macules which, within a few weeks after birth, begin to develop into more prominent lesions. For still unknown reasons, hemangiomas arise 2.5–4 times more often among female than among male infants. Other risk factors for the development of IH recently identified by the Hemangioma Interest Group include: low birthweight, multiple gestation, advanced maternal age (> 30 years of age), pre-eclampsia, and placental abnormalities, such as placenta previa or abruption.

Hemangiomas are clonal tumors of vascular endothelial cells. Recent studies have noted the remarkable resemblance in the expression of surface markers of IH and placental tissue. Both tissues stain for the glucose transporter, Glut-1, as well as Lewis Y, merosin, and FcγRII, potentially indicating a common progenitor. Glut-1 has emerged as a useful and reliable marker for IH since it is expressed at all stages of hemangioma evolution, thereby helping to differentiate IH from other vascular tumors, including the pyogenic granuloma (lobular capillary hemangioma), kaposiform hemangioendothelioma (Figure 5-2), and other similar-appearing tumors such as the infantile fibrosarcoma (Figure 5-3), all of which are Glut-1 negative.

The terms superficial ("strawberry"), deep ("cavernous"), and mixed have been applied to hemangiomas to reflect their clinical morphology (Figure 5-4), while their configuration can best be described as localized, segmental, and indeterminate (Figure 5-5).

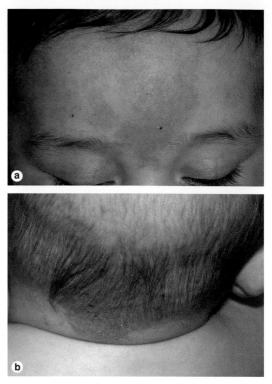

Figure 5-1a Salmon patch on the glabellar area. **b** Nuchal salmon patch with secondary eczematization

IHs undergo a characteristic evolution. Proliferation of a typical hemangioma occurs during the first 6–9 months after birth; growth then slows during a "plateau" phase during which the hemangioma grows along with the child; and after 1 year of age, involution then begins to occur. While the majority of hemangiomas involute satisfactorily without intervention, 20–50% of hemangiomas leave residua in the form of telangiectasia, fibrofatty tissue, or atrophy (Figure 5-6), so that, when counseling parents, it is important to explain the difference between expected *involution* and possible *resolution*.

When confronted with an IH, most clinicians can appropriately provide reassurance that the hemangioma will involute over time as, in most cases, active nonintervention represents the best approach for managing this type of birthmark. However, certain clinical situations may warrant either closer follow-up or therapeutic intervention (Table 5-2).

Incomplete involution

IHs arising at certain anatomic locations tend to involute incompletely. Nasal tip hemangiomas pose a risk for underlying developing cartilage and often require eventual surgical excision (Figure 5-7). Lip and parotid hemangiomas commonly leave residua in the form of fibrofatty tissue and selected lesions may benefit from steroid or later surgical revision (Figure 5-8). Pedunculated hemangiomas often fail to regress completely and likewise benefit from surgical excision.

Amblyopia

Periocular hemangiomas (Figure 5-9) may produce irreversible visual acuity loss in the ipsilateral eye by one of several mechanisms: directly obstructing vision (deprivation), pushing the affected eye out of alignment (strabismus), or simply by inducing an astigmatism by putting

pressure on the globe (anisometropia). Because rapidly proliferating hemangiomas have their greatest growth during the first 6–9 months coinciding with early visual development, prompt pharmacologic or surgical intervention may be necessary to preserve vision.

Airway involvement

IHs that occur on the lower face – particularly the preauricular, cheek, perioral, chin, anterior neck, or oral mucosa in the so-called "beard distribution" – have been associated with concomitant airway hemangiomas in a supraglottic or subglottic location (Figure 5-10).

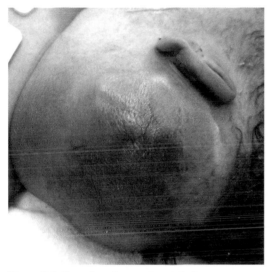

Figure 5-2 Kaposiform hemangioendothelioma

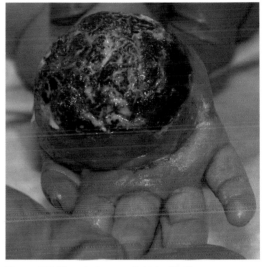

Figure 5-3 Ulcerated congenital infantile fibrosarcoma with silver sulfadiazene

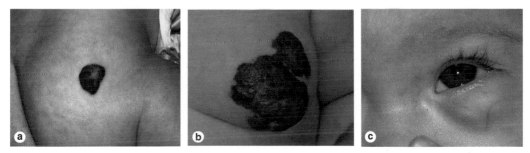

Figure 5-4a Superficial hemangioma, **b** Mixed hemangioma, **c** Deep (subcutaneous) hemangioma

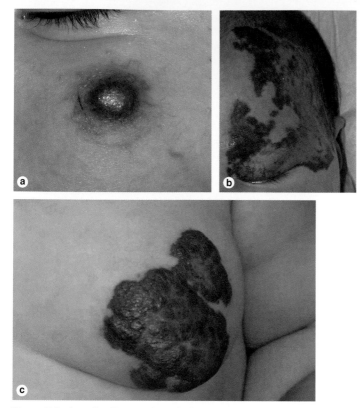

Figure 5-5a Localized hemangioma, **b** Segmental hemangioma, **c** Indeterminate hemangioma

Table 5-2 Hemangiomas – when to worry	
Issue	**Concern**
Periocular location	Amblyopia
Perioral/beard location	Airway hemangioma
Nasal tip/parotid/lip location	Incomplete involution
Presacral midline location	Spinal dysraphism
Facial segmental	PHACES; hypothyroidism
Perineal segmental	PELVIS/SACRAL
Multiple cutaneous	Visceral hemangiomatosis
Hepatic	Hypothryoidism

PELVIS, perineal hemangiomas occurring in association with external genital anomalies, lipomyelomeningocele, vesicorenal abnormalities, imperforate anus, and skin tag; PHACES, posterior fossa brain malformations, facial hemangiomas, arterial anomalies, coarctation of the aorta and cardiac abnormalities, structural eye malformations, and sternal clefting or supraumbilical raphe; SACRAL, spinal dysraphism, anogenital, cutaneous, renal and urologic anomalies, associated with an angioma of lumbosacral localization.

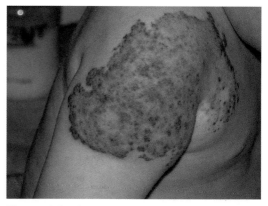

Figure 5-6 Involuting hemangioma with residual telangiectasia and some fibrofatty tissue

Ulceration

Hemangiomas located at sites prone to friction, such as the scalp, the parotid and lip areas, and especially on the perineum, may ulcerate (Figure 5-11). Ulcerated hemangiomas are painful and may predispose the child to poor feeding and infection. Treatment with local

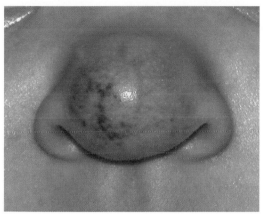

Figure 5-7 Nasal tip hemangioma

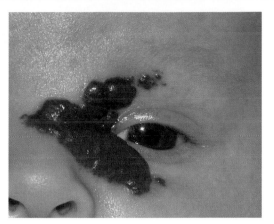

Figure 5-9 Periocular hemangioma

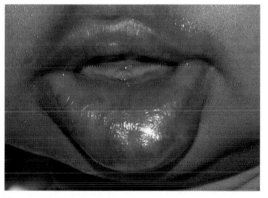

Figure 5-8 Lip hemangioma that will require surgical revision

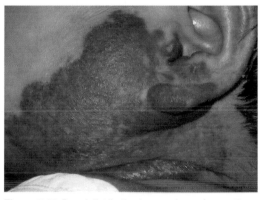

Figure 5-10 Beard distribution hemangioma, frequently associated with airway hemangioma

wound care, topical and oral antibiotics, topical becaplermin gel, systemic steroid, and pulsed-dye laser may be helpful in managing this complication. Local and systemic analgesia may also be necessary for children with very painful, ulcerated hemangiomas.

Visceral hemangiomatosis

The presence of multiple cutaneous hemangiomas may be a marker for associated visceral hemangiomas, typically involving the liver, spleen, or intestinal tract. Hepatic hemangiomas, particularly large or multiple lesions, have been linked to acquired infantile hypothyroidism. Vascular shunts have also been observed with visceral hemangiomas that can cause high-flow states, hepatosplenomegaly, and associated congestive heart failure in affected infants. Symptomatic children may require systemic steroid therapy, interventional radiological embolization, or surgical resection.

Spinal dysraphism

As with other midline congenital abnormalities, midline hemangiomas of the lumbosacral area may indicate underlying occult spinal dysraphism or tethered-cord syndrome (Figure 5-12). This is in contradistinction to Cobb syndrome in which a cutaneous arteriovenous malformation or other vascular anomaly is associated with spinal angiomatosis and resulting neurologic sequelae.

Syndromic hemangiomas

Posterior fossa brain malformations have been described in conjunction with segmental facial hemangiomas, arterial anomalies (including absent unilateral carotid arterial circulation or intracranial anomalies), coarctation of the aorta and cardiac abnormalities, structural eye malformations, and sternal clefting or supraumbilical raphe as part of the PHACES syndrome (Figure 5-13).

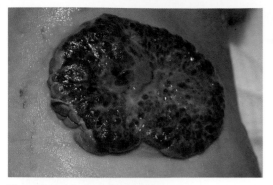

Figure 5-11 Ulcerated hemangioma

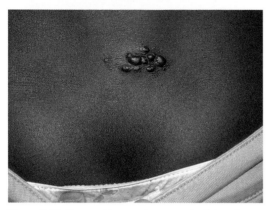

Figure 5-12 Presacral hemangioma, a potential marker for underlying spinal dysraphism

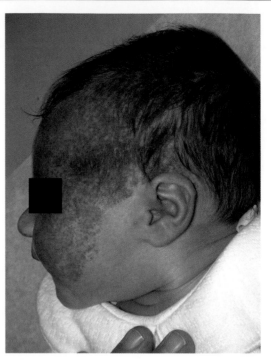

Figure 5-13 A facial segmental hemangioma as part of posterior fossa brain malformations, facial hemangiomas, arterial anomalies, coarctation of the aorta and cardiac abnormalities, structural eye malformations, and sternal clefting or supraumbilical raphe (PHACES) syndrome

While IHs occur with high frequency among infant girls, PHACES syndrome is strongly correlated with female gender, with a female-to-male ratio of 9:1. Although some children may manifest multiple features represented by the PHACES acronym, most affected children manifest facial segmental hemangioma in association with just one other extracutaneous feature of the syndrome. Children with PHACES are potentially also at risk for thyroid dysfunction and cerebrovascular disease. PELVIS syndrome has been applied to the conjunction of perineal hemangiomas (that are also typically segmental) occurring in association with external genital anomalies, lipomyelomeningoccle, vesicorenal abnormalities, imperforate anus, and skin tag (Figure 5-14). Another recent report attaches the name SACRAL syndrome to this phenomenon, representing the issues of spinal dysraphism, anogenital, cutaneous, renal and urologic anomalies, associated with an angioma of lumbosacral localization.

Kasabach–Merritt phenomenon

While Kasabach and Merritt reported in 1940 that capillary hemangiomas could predispose to a syndrome of microangiopathic hemolytic anemia, thrombocytopenia, congestive heart

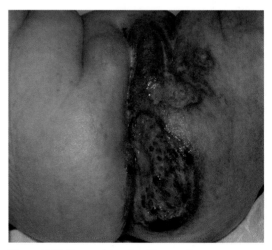

Figure 5-14 Segmental perineal hemangioma as part of PELVIS syndrome (perineal hemangiomas occurring in association with external genital anomalies, lipomyelomeningocele, vesicorenal abnormalities, imperforate anus, and skin tag)

failure, and visceral hemorrhage, subsequent studies have clearly documented that the syndrome described by Kasabach and Merritt does not occur with typical IHs. Kasabach–Merritt phenomenon is a complication associated with other vascular tumors such as kaposiform hemangioendothelioma and tufted angioma.

The appropriate treatment of a particular IH depends in large part on its potential for causing complications. Most hemangiomas are amenable to expectant management. Those at risk for causing functional impairment or that threaten life warrant timely pharmacologic, interventional radiology, or surgical intervention.

Evaluation

In general, the diagnosis of an IH is made on clinical grounds. Although in the perinatal period, the premonitory manifestations of an IH may resemble a salmon patch or port-wine stain, the hemangioma will show typical signs of proliferation within the first month. If in doubt about the diagnosis, having the child return for a follow-up visit in 2–4 weeks is a reasonable approach.

Hemangiomas that arise in the periocular area may be associated with underlying extraconal and intraconal involvement. If visual acuity deficits, frank strabismus, or restricted extraocular movements are noted, ultrasound or magnetic resonance imaging (MRI) should be considered to determine the extent of periocular involvement. Children with more extensive involvement may require pharmacologic therapy at higher doses or for longer durations.

Because beard-area hemangiomas may be linked with airway involvement, infants with proliferating hemangiomas in this distribution should be evaluated by an otolaryngologist, and imaging of the neck considered.

In infants with midline hemangiomas overlying the presacral area, imaging should be performed to rule out underlying spinal dysraphism. For centers with experienced pediatric radiologists, ultrasound can be performed for those under 6 months of age. For older children, MRI is recommended.

Because of their association with PHACES syndrome, large facial segmental hemangiomas should be evaluated for other extracutaneous manifestations. Given the features of PHACES, MRI and angiography of the brain, cardiology consultation, echocardiography, and/or cardiac MRI, ophthalmologic consultation, and CT of the chest for clinically apparent sternal malformations can be considered. Likewise, for PELVIS or SACRAL syndrome, appropriate imaging studies include ultrasound, computed tomography (CT), or MRI of the abdomen and pelvis.

If a vascular lesion appears atypical and is showing signs of rapid growth, fixation to underlying tissue planes, and ulceration, a malignancy should be considered on the differential diagnosis along with other vascular anomalies. In these instances, imaging studies such as Doppler ultrasound, CT scanning, MRI and angiography, and biopsy should be considered to assist in diagnosis.

Treatment

Corticosteroids possess potent antiangiogenic activity and are particularly useful for treating rapidly proliferating hemangiomas occurring in critical anatomic areas. Oral corticosteroids, typically given as oral prednisolone or intravenous methylprednisolone at 2–3 mg/kg per day, are often used to manage periocular, airway, or nasal tip hemangiomas to decrease the rate of proliferation. Appropriate weekly monitoring for hypertension, growth parameters, signs of immunosuppression or hypothalamic–pituitary–adrenal axis suppression and other potential adverse effects is essential. Prophylactic administration of an H2-blocker may help prophylaxis against gastrointestinal complications. Some have advocated weekly antibiotic prophylaxis with trimethoprim-sulfamethoxazole for children on chronic corticosteroid therapy in order to prevent *Pneumocystis carinii* infection, although this practice remains controversial. Topical steroids are of limited benefit but can be used in selected instances where systemic steroid therapy is not advised. Intralesional triamcinolone has been useful in the treatment of localized periocular hemangioma, but should likely be best reserved for extraconal lesions and be performed by an experienced ophthalmologist given the attendant risks of central retinal artery occlusion.

Proliferating hemangiomas that are inadequately responsive to systemic corticosteroid may benefit from the use of vincristine. The use of interferon-alfa, although quite effective for arresting growth in proliferating hemangiomas, has been less favored due to its potential for transient and persistent neurologic complications among young infants receiving this agent.

Ulcerated hemangiomas are best managed with appropriate wound care. Topical antibiotics such as bacitracin, mupirocin, or metronidazole gel are used in conjunction with a nonadherent dressing such as petrolatum gauze or Telfa. For recalcitrant lesions, a 10–14-day course of an oral antibiotic such as cephalexin, pulsed-dye laser therapy, or becaplermin gel can all offer additional benefit at additional cost.

The use of vascular lasers is also especially useful for treating postinvolution residual telangiectasia. Early use of the pulsed-dye laser for proliferating hemangiomas has been less effective. While some cosmetic improvement may be gained by using the pulsed-dye laser in early IH lesions, this must weighed against the potential for atrophy and dyspigmentation that may result from this modality.

Rapidly Involuting Congenital Hemangioma (RICH; Congenital Nonprogressive Hemangioma)

Key Points

- Resembles IH
- Present at birth or noted intrauterine
- Rapid involution by 1–2 years of age
- Predilection for ulceration
- Glut-1-negative

RICH lesions resemble IHs given their vascular appearance and occurrence during infancy. However, in contrast to IH, RICH lesions are present fully formed at birth and may be detected prenatally on ultrasound scans. Moreover, they involute more rapidly than IH, as RICH lesions often reach maximal involution by 1–2 years of age. Because of this rapid involution, they are also more likely to ulcerate and may require appropriate wound care, antibiotic therapy, or pulsed-dye laser treatment when they do so. Otherwise, no specific intervention is needed in most cases since these undergo spontaneous and rapid involution. In cases where an atypical lesion is biopsied for tissue analysis, RICH lesions can also be differentiated from IH because RICH does not stain positively for the glucose transporter molecule Glut-1, whereas IH lesions do.

Noninvoluting Congenital Hemangioma (NICH)

Key Points

- Resembles IH, but has superficial telangiectatic appearance
- Present at birth
- Lack of involution; instead, gradual proliferation into childhood, adolescence, or adulthood
- Typically requires surgical intervention
- Glut-1-negative

NICH lesions likewise resemble IHs. Characteristic overlying telangiectatic changes are often observed on the surface of NICH tumors. Like RICH lesions, NICH is typically noted at birth. However, these vascular lesions show slow and gradual proliferation even into later childhood. As a result, they often require eventual surgical resection. NICH tumors are also Glut-1-negative, which helps to differentiate them from IHs. Curiously, RICH lesions and NICH lesions are not mutually exclusive, as RICH lesions may involute only to show signs of proliferation later along with histology indistinguishable from that seen with NICH.

Pyogenic Granuloma (Lobular Capillary Hemangioma)

Key Points

- Tendency for frequent bleeding
- Associated with minor trauma or at sites prone to trauma
- Band-Aid sign
- Infrequent spontaneous resolution, so minor surgical intervention is often necessary

Pyogenic granuloma is a misnomer for this benign, acquired vascular tumor since it is neither pyogenic nor granulomatous. The term lobular capillary hemangioma is more appropriate, although many clinicians continue to refer to these lesions as pyogenic granulomas out of long-standing tradition. These lesions typically present on the face or extremities as small, glossy, friable papules that may grow into larger nodules and tend to occur at sites of minor trauma. The tendency for these vascular tumors to bleed is a hallmark finding, and the maceration or eczematous change around them from frequent bandage changes is referred to as the "Band-Aid sign" (Figure 5-15).

Pyogenic granulomas occasionally but infrequently resolve spontaneously. However, they tend to engender significant distress among parents. Although the amount of associated bleeding is often minimal, the tendency for these lesions to bleed and stain clothing and bedding is disconcerting to patients and parents alike.

Treatment with cryotherapy or silver nitrate sticks is effective in a minority of cases. Local anesthesia followed by simple curettage is a highly effective technique that results in good cosmetic outcomes. Shave technique with or without concomitant pulsed-dye laser therapy can also be effective. Following removal, use of topical aluminum chloride hexahydrate or electrocautery provides local hemostasis.

Vascular Malformations

Spider Angioma (Spider Telangiectasia)

Key Points

- Benign telangiectasias, frequently seen on face or distal upper extremities
- Contrasted with matte telangiectasias seen in hereditary hemorrhagic telangiectasis (HHT) and capillary malformation with arteriovenous malformation syndrome
- Responsive to pulsed-dye laser when treatment desired

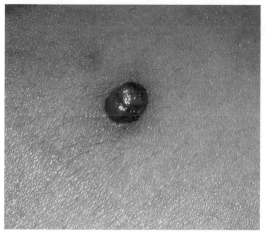

Figure 5-15 Pyogenic granuloma

Spider angiomas or spider telangiectasias are frequently observed in school-age children on the cheeks, nose, or dorsal hands and forearms (Figure 5-16). These are benign lesions that may spontaneously involute although many will persist for several years before resolving. They rarely bleed and are generally asymptomatic.

They can be distinguished from the matte-type telangiectasias classically associated with HHT which tend to lack an angiomatous papular center, and the lesions of HHT are often found on the nasal or oral mucosa, and may also be seen on palms as well as other anatomic sites.

For those desiring more rapid resolution of cosmetically distressing spider telangiectases, often one or two treatments with the pulsed-dye laser provide a satisfactory outcome.

Port-wine Stain (Capillary Malformation, Nevus Flammeus)

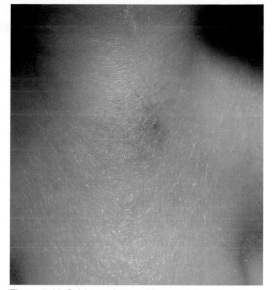

Figure 5-16 Spider angioma, with central papule and peripheral arborizing vessels

Key Points

- Port-wine stains are present from birth
- Facial lesions in the first trigeminal branch may be associated with Sturge–Weber syndrome
- Children with port-wine stains as part of Sturge–Weber require lifelong ophthalmologic follow-up
- Port-wine stains can occur as part of many syndromes with extracutaneous manifestations

Port-wine stains are common capillary malformations that present at birth and occur in approximately 0.3–0.5% of newborns. These vascular birthmarks appear as areas of blanchable, macular erythema that share the color of port wine. Nevus flammeus lesions are often localized, but may occur in what appear to be dermatomal configurations. Although many lesions remain stable for many years, some port-wine stains become less blanchable, undergo hypertrophy, and may develop small angiomatous papules or pyogenic granulomas. Segmental port-wine stains located along the first trigeminal dermatome have been associated with leptomeningeal angiomatosis, glaucoma risk, seizures, and mental retardation as part of Sturge–Weber syndrome, also known as encephalotrigeminal angiomatosis (Figure 5-17). Risk factors for Sturge–Weber syndrome include more extensive multidermatomal involvement and bilateral port-wine stains of the first trigeminal branch. Although glaucoma risk is highest during infancy, patients with capillary malformations in the first trigeminal distribution require lifelong ophthalmologic follow-up. In patients who manifest port-wine stains in the first trigeminal distribution, neuroimaging should be performed for patients with neurologic issues and considered to provide anticipatory guidance to parents regarding their child's condition. While both PHACES syndrome and Sturge–Weber syndrome involve segmental vascular lesions on the face as well as a number of extracutaneous manifestations, they can be differentiated on clinical grounds and on results of imaging studies (Table 5-3). Treatment of facial port-wine stains can be managed with the pulsed-dye or other vascular laser which can frequently lighten the birthmark. Better results can be obtained from earlier intervention with the laser.

Geographic capillary malformations of the lower extremity in association with varicosities and hypertrophy of underlying bone and soft tissues is characteristic of Klippel–Trenaunay–Weber syndrome. Patients with this condition often have combined malformations including abnormalities

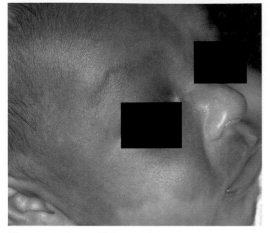

Figure 5-17 Sturge–Weber syndrome

Table 5-3 Differentiating PHACES from Sturge–Weber syndrome

System	PHACES	Sturge–Weber
Skin	Facial segmental hemangioma	Facial trigeminal port-wine stain (capillary malformation)
CNS	Posterior fossa malformation; intracranial vascular involvement	Leptomeningeal vascular malformation; seizures and mental retardation
Ocular	Microphthalmos, optic nerve hypoplasia or atrophy, cataracts, coloboma	Glaucoma
Cardiac	Coarctation of the aorta; PDA, ASD, VSD	None
Other	Midline sternal or supraumbilical defects	None

ASD, atrial septal defect; CNS, central nervous system; PDA, patent ductus arteriosus; PHACES, posterior fossa brain malformations, facial hemangiomas, arterial anomalies, coarctation of the aorta and cardiac abnormalities, structural eye malformations, and sternal clefting or supraumbilical raphe; VSD, ventral septal defect.

of lymphatics and venous circulation as well. Those affected are predisposed to lower-extremity pain, skin infections, deep venous thrombosis, and pulmonary embolism. Patients benefit from supportive stockings, prompt treatment of infections, anticoagulation when appropriate, and diuretics to manage associated edema.

Capillary malformations can also be associated with other syndromes, including but not limited to: Proteus syndrome (capillary malformation with hamartomas), phakomatosis pigmentovascularis syndromes (capillary malformation with other nevi), capillary malformation with arteriovenous malformation syndrome and Parkes–Weber syndrome (capillary malformation with arteriovenous malformation). Occasionally, port-wine stains may also occur as a post-traumatic sequela.

Lymphangioma Circumscriptum (Microcystic Lymphatic Malformation)

Key Points

* Microcystic lymphatic malformation (MLM)
* Commonly mistaken for molluscum contagiosum
* Deep underlying structure results in recurrences even after laser or surgical intervention

Lymphangioma circumscriptum is a form of MLM. Affected patients present with clusters of small translucent clear or blood-filled vesicles. They are often described as resembling "frog spawn" (Figure 5-18). Not infrequently, MLM lesions are mistaken for molluscum contagiosum lesions. Their presence from birth, long-standing duration, and persistence at one site will often help distinguish them from molluscum lesions. While only a small area may appear affected on the surface of the skin, these lesions often have

deep, complex networks of abnormal lymphatic vasculature. MLM is often asymptomatic, but if extensive, can be associated with lymphedema or pain. Patients with these symptoms may benefit from use of elastic support stockings if the lesions are present on an extremity.

Superficial vesicles, particularly heme-filled lymphangioma lesions, may respond to pulsed-dye laser therapy. Other devices, such as the Nd:YAG and the CO_2 laser, may provide longer-lasting but still temporary improvement. However, vesicles will inevitably reappear. Surgical debulking should be reserved for highly symptomatic patients since the surgery may result in disfigurement and recurrences even after extensive surgical debulking.

Venous Malformation (Venous or Cavernous Angioma or Hemangioma)

Key Points

* Slow-flow vascular malformation involving ecstatic venous structures
* Predisposition to phleboliths, thrombosis, pain
* May involve underlying bone and soft tissue
* Elastic compression, sclerotherapy, and surgical intervention can be considered in symptomatic patients

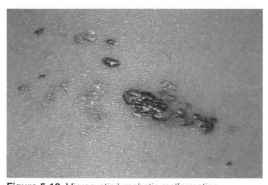

Figure 5-18 Microcystic lymphatic malformation (lymphangioma circumscriptum) with both clear and blood-filled vesicles

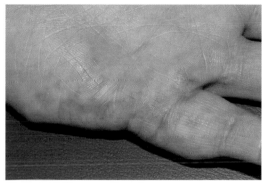

Figure 5-19 Venous malformation

Venous malformations, as the term suggests, indicate a slow-flow vascular malformation characterized by abnormal and dilated venous structures in the skin or other organs. These lesions typically present at birth as collections of bluish, compressible papules and nodules (Figure 5-19). If the venous malformation is located on an extremity, raising the extremity above the heart will result in decompression and flattening of the lesion. Exercise, increased temperature, and gravity will tend to increase the size of the lesion. Diagnostic confirmation can be made clinically in association with appropriate imaging studies such as Doppler ultrasound, MRI and angiography, and CT. Because these lesions can also affect soft tissue and bone, imaging studies are recommended to determine the extent of disease.

Differential diagnostic considerations include IH, arteriovenous malformation, glomuvenous malformation, as well as evaluation for syndromic associations such as with Klippel–Trenaunay–Weber and Parkes–Weber syndromes, which both include venous malformation as part of their clinical spectrum.

Principal clinical concerns with venous malformations include their slow flow which may predispose to phleboliths, venous thrombosis, localized intravascular coagulation, and pain. Treatment involves appropriate use of elastic stockings, and selective use of interventional radiologic techniques such as sclerotherapy, and surgical debulking or resection.

Further reading

Batta K, Goodyear HM, Moss C, et al. Randomised controlled study of early pulsed-dye laser treatment of uncomplicated childhood haemangiomas: results of a 1-year analysis. Lancet 2002;360:521–527.

Enjolras O, Wassef M, Mazoyer E, et al. Infants with Kasabach–Merritt syndrome do not have "true" hemangiomas. J Pediatr 1997;130:631–640.

Enjolras O, Ciabrini D, Mazoyer E, et al. Extensive pure venous malformations in the upper or lower limb: a review of 27 cases. J Am Acad Dermatol 1997;36:219–225.

Frieden IJ, Haggstrom AN, Drolet BA, et al. Infantile hemangiomas: current knowledge future directions. Proceedings of a research workshop on infantile hemangiomas, April 7–9, 2005, Bethesda, Maryland, USA. Pediatr Dermatol 2005;22:383–406.

Girard C, Bigorre M, Guillot B, et al. PELVIS syndrome. Arch Dermatol 2006;142:884–888.

Kasabach HH, Merritt KK. Capillary hemangioma with extensive purpura: report of a case. Am J Dis Child 1940;59:1063–1070.

Knight PJ, Raimer SB. Superficial bumps in children: what, when and why? Pediatrics 1983;72:147–153.

Metry DW, Dowd CF, Barkovich AJ, et al. The many faces of PHACE syndrome. J Pediatr 2001;139:117–123.

Mulliken JB, Glowacki J. Hemangiomas and vascular malformations in infants and children: a classification based on endothelial characteristics. Plast Reconstr Surg 1982;69:412–422.

Mulliken JB, Fishman SJ, Burrows PE. Vascular anomalies. Curr Probl Surg 2000;37:517–584.

North PE, Waner M, Buckmiller L, et al. Vascular tumors of infancy and childhood: beyond capillary hemangioma. Cardiovasc Pathol 2006;15:303–317.

Sarkar M, Mulliken JB, Kozakewich HP, et al. Thrombocytopenic coagulopathy (Kasabach–Merritt phenomenon) is associated with kaposiform hemangioendothelioma and not with common infantile hemangioma. Plast Reconstr Surg 1997;100:1377–1386.

Stockman A, Boralevi F, Taieb A, et al. SACRAL syndrome: spinal dysraphism, anogenital, cutaneous, renal and urologic anomalies, associated with an angioma of lumbosacral localization. Dermatol (Basel) 2007;214:40–45.

Tallman B, Tan OT, Morelli JG, et al. Location of port-wine stains and the likelihood of ophthalmic and/or central nervous system complications. Pediatrics 1991;87:323–327.

Drug eruptions and inflammatory eruptions of the skin

6

Howard B. Pride

Urticaria

Key Points

- Most often from infections, medications, sometimes food
- Generally acute and self-resolving
- Antihistamines

Urticaria (hives) is an extremely common condition in children. Published incidences of 10–20% probably underestimate its frequency, as most children with self-limited, brief bouts of urticaria will not seek medical attention. For the most part, it is a minor nuisance that requires little in the way of diagnostic acumen or treatment. Six weeks' duration arbitrarily distinguishes chronic from acute urticaria.

Clinical presentation

Hives are characterized by erythematous, edematous papules and plaques. As the lesion becomes annular, it develops a pale center (wheal) and brighter red periphery (flare). Individual plaques expand and fuse with other lesions, creating bizarre, polycyclic patterns (Figure 6-1). Young children and infants tend to have expansive and unusual lesions, rarely with bulla formation. Lesions evolve and transform almost before one's eyes and it is not unusual for parents to exclaim how different the lesions appeared just moments before the practitioner's exam. Outlining individual plaques with a marker can dramatically illustrate this phenomenon. The evanescence of the hives is one of its most distinctive features and can be a very helpful historical point when the child has no lesions at the time of the evaluation. Light bruising may sometimes linger after lesions resolve, especially in infants.

Dermatographism (literally meaning writing on the skin) is the development of a linear wheal and flare at the site of stroking the skin (Figure 6-2). The child's own scratching may induce linear hives. Demonstrating dermatographism may be a clue to the diagnosis of hives when a patient has no lesions at the time of the evaluation. The other physical urticarias are listed in Box 6-1.

A serum sickness-like reaction can be seen after treatment with antibiotics. This is a classic side-effect of cefaclor but its infrequent use makes amoxicillin the most common current precipitant. Large serpiginous and polycyclic urticarial plaques with conspicuous bruising are characteristic (Figure 6-3). Arthralgias and fever are common associations.

Angioedema refers to deep dermal or subcutaneous hives that generally involve the face, mucous membranes, and extremities. It may accompany regular urticaria or occur on its own. In a small minority of cases, it is a manifestation of autosomal-dominant hereditary angioedema, which is associated with repeated attacks accompanied by abdominal pain and airway edema. Anaphylaxis refers to angioedema or hives accompanied by profound tissue edema leading to airway compromise, abdominal symptoms, hypotension, and possibly shock, occurring minutes after a sting, ingestion, or medication. Stable hives do not progress to anaphylaxis, as is commonly dreaded by parents.

Papular urticaria is a confusing term used for bug bites. Lesions consist of erythematous edematous papules that are fixed and long-lasting and are best thought of as urticarial rather than a true variant of urticaria. They may be grouped in threes – the so-called breakfast, lunch, and dinner (Figure 6-4) – and tend to cluster in the most exposed areas of the arms, legs, and head. A central punctum may be noted with magnification. Some may form vesicles and bullae. Since lesions tend to occur 1–2 days following the bite, cause and effect may not be immediately obvious. Most often, the patient is the only one in the family who is overtly affected, a puzzling and hard-to-believe feature for parents. Fleas are the most common cause but bed bugs are making a comeback.

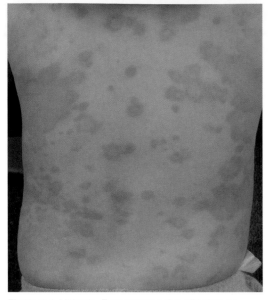

Figure 6-1 Urticaria. Evanescent, polycyclic plaques

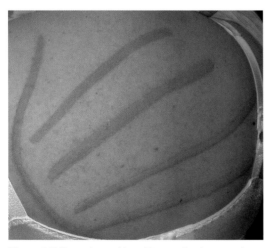

Figure 6-2 Dermatographism. Linear urticaria appearing after stroking the skin

> BOX 6-1
>
> **The physical urticarias**
>
> Pressure urticaria – from carrying a heavy object or from tight-fitting clothes
>
> Cold urticaria – from exposure to cold air or water
>
> Aquagenic urticaria – from contact with water or sweat
>
> Cholinergic urticaria – smaller papules from heat or exercise
>
> Solar urticaria – from ultraviolet light exposure

task at best, with the majority of cases having no identifiable trigger. Common viral infections account for the majority of identifiable causes, with medications, especially antibiotics, close behind. Foods, particularly nuts, dairy products, seafood, and berries, are possible causes but this is hard to prove without provocation testing. Virtually any underlying medical condition can be blamed for hives but occult infections and connective tissue diseases stand out. A very thorough history with a complete review of systems and a good physical exam are the most useful diagnostic tools. Laboratory tests not suggested by signs or symptoms are almost always unhelpful. Radioallergosorbent test or prick testing will likely add to the confusion rather than help clarify a cause. A food and activity diary kept by the parents may be helpful with chronic urticaria.

Hereditary angioedema is a serious condition and a specific diagnosis needs to be made in cases of complicated or repeated angioedema. Low levels of C4 and decreased activity of C1 esterase inhibitor will be detected on laboratory work-up. Hereditary angioedema is an autoinflammatory syndrome with recurrent bouts of severe angioedema in the absence of hives.

> PEARL
>
> The presence of hives virtually excludes a diagnosis of hereditary angioedema.

Diagnosis

Urticaria is usually an easy clinical diagnosis, recognized by patients and parents before they ever see a physician. Erythema multiforme (EM) and other figurate erythemas, excluding erythema marginatum, are distinguished by their lack of evanescence. Autoimmune blistering conditions may present with urticaria before becoming overtly bullous. Biopsy may be needed in atypical urticaria.

The greatest challenge comes in diagnosing the underlying cause for the hives, an elusive

Papular urticaria poses more of a diagnostic challenge. Biopsy in this setting may be helpful, especially when parents will not accept the diagnosis. Folliculitis, prurigo nodularis, pityriasis lichenoides, lymphomatoid papulosis, guttate psoriasis, and Gianotti–Crosti syndrome may enter the differential diagnosis.

Pathogenesis

Hives result from the release of inflammatory mediators, particularly histamine, from mast cells through an immunologic immunoglobulin

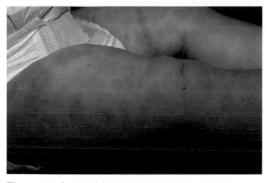

Figure 6-3 Serum sickness-like reaction. Large serpiginous and polycyclic plaques with conspicuous bruising

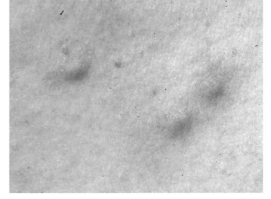

Figure 6-4 Bug bites. Erythematous edematous papules with characteristic groups of three

(Ig) E-mediated process or by nonimmunologic mechanisms. Prostaglandins, leukotrienes, and serotonin are other inflammatory mediators released by mast cells.

Papular urticaria is a delayed hypersensitivity reaction caused by fleas, mosquitoes, black flies, chiggers, bedbugs, and other biting insects.

Treatment

Asymptomatic hives do not require treatment and simply waiting for self-resolution is a very reasonable approach. Any suspected underlying condition should be treated or removed, and all unnecessary medications should be stopped.

Antihistamines are the mainstay of therapy, with diphenhydramine or hydroxyzine at 1 mg/kg per dose up to 4 times daily being a good first-line approach. More severe or persistent hives can be treated with the combination of a nonsedating antihistamine such as cetirizine or loratadine in the morning and a sedating antihistamine at bedtime or at times of breakthrough hives. Doxepin is a good bedtime substitute if this regimen fails. Cyproheptadine can be added for better serotonin blocking as well as for its antihistamine properties. H_2-blockers such as cimetidine or ranitidine are sometimes helpful adjuncts but are not very useful by themselves. Leukotriene inhibitors such as montelukast and empiric antibiotics for occult infection may be considered but are not part of standard therapy for most children. Once a patient has been hive-free for a week, the frequency of antihistamine use can be tapered.

Papular urticaria can be treated with class 1 or 2 topical steroids. Prevention with appropriately dosed N,N-diethyl-meta-toluamide (DEET)-containing repellents and environmental control are important measures. Educating and reassuring the parents are vital to the successful management of this frustrating disorder.

Drug Eruptions

Key Points

• Diffuse symmetric morbilliform erythema
• Topical steroids and oral antihistamines for treatment

Drug eruptions are commonly encountered in pediatrics, with exanthematous rashes from antibiotics and anticonvulsants accounting for the majority. Any drug, whether prescription or nonprescription, associated with any rash needs to be viewed with suspicion. The offending agent may have already been stopped or may be a drug that has been taken previously without reaction. A thorough history is needed to explore all medications, including vitamins, supplements, herbal remedies, ophthalmologic preparations, inhalers, and topical agents as parents may not consider these products as drugs. Time of ingestion and associated illnesses such as a viral syndrome or activities such as sun exposure must be queried. Some compulsivity is needed in exploring texts or computer-based references since no clinician will have an exhaustive knowledge of all possible drug eruptions. Only the most common or important eruptions will be discussed here.

Clinical presentation

Most drug eruptions will be exanthematous, indistinguishable from a typical viral exanthem. Morbilliform and maculopapular are adjectives frequently applied to the rash that usually begins 1–2 weeks after ingestion, initially on the trunk and spreading centrifugally. The distribution is diffuse and symmetric, suggesting a systemic process (Figure 6-5). Pruritus and low-grade fever may accompany the rash. Mucous membranes are not involved. The rash fades with a brownish discoloration and scaling desquamation.

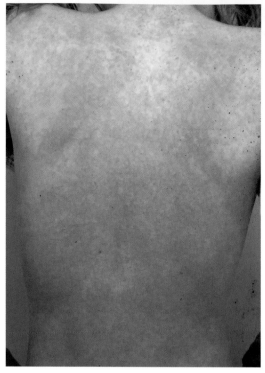

Figure 6-5 Drug eruption. Nonspecific, diffuse and symmetric, morbilliform eruption

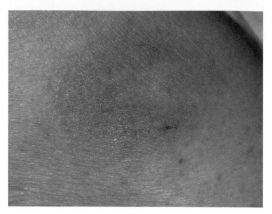

Figure 6-6 Fixed drug eruption. Well-circumscribed erythematous to dusky-brown plaque

Fixed drug eruption refers to a well-circumscribed erythematous to dusky-brown plaque that occurs in the same location each time an offending medication is taken (Figure 6-6). Bullae and crusting may develop. The face, trunk, and the genitalia are common locations. Sulfa antibiotics are the classic precipitants but others, such as acetaminophen, tetracyclines, and ibuprofen, may be responsible (Box 6-2). The eruption begins 1–2 weeks after the initial exposure but will recur rapidly after subsequent ingestions. The plaque may increase in size and new sites may develop with time. Resolution is slow and hyperpigmentation may last several weeks.

Drug reaction with eosinophilia and systemic symptoms (DRESS) is a serious reaction with 10% mortality, most commonly beginning 1–6 weeks after the initiation of anticonvulsant or sulfa antibiotic therapy. Fever and lymphadenopathy precede the eruption, which consists of facial erythema and edema with subsequent generalization ranging from a morbilliform rash to full-blown toxic epidermal necrolysis (TEN). The liver is the most frequently involved internal organ, but the kidneys, central nervous system, lungs, heart, and thyroid may be affected. Onset of clinical hypothyroidism is often delayed.

Acute generalized exanthematous pustulosis (AGEP) is a rare eruption most commonly associated with beta-lactam antibiotics. It is not always preceded by drug ingestions, suggesting a possible viral role. Diffuse erythematous, nonfollicular, pinpoint, sterile pustules associated with fever are characteristic (Figure 6-7). A marked desquamation accompanies resolution.

Diagnosis

An exanthematous drug eruption cannot reliably be distinguished from a viral exanthem and biopsy is not helpful. Reintroduction of the drug after resolution of the eruption may be diagnostic but is not routinely done. The diagnosis of fixed drug eruption may require a biopsy, particularly if there is no obvious implicated medication. Facial edema, morbilliform rash with follicular prominence, elevated liver transaminases, atypical lymphocytosis and marked eosinophilia associated with the rash suggest DRESS. AGEP may look like an infectious folliculitis or pustular psoriasis. Bacterial culture and biopsy are helpful.

Pathogenesis

The exact pathogenesis for most drug eruptions is unknown. Exanthematous reactions may be enhanced by or dependent upon concomitant viral infections, the classic example being amoxicillin and Epstein–Barr virus. Abnormal drug metabolism has been suggested in DRESS and an autosomal-recessive inheritance pattern has been seen.

Treatment

Discontinuation of the suspected medication is obviously the treatment of choice for a drug eruption, but, surprisingly, minor exanthematous eruptions may self-resolve even with continued use of the medication. In critical situations where a medication is necessary and the rash is fairly insignificant, it may be appropriate to "treat through" the eruption. High fevers, systemic abnormalities, erythroderma, or mucous

Medications that may cause fixed drug eruption

Acetaminophen

Acetylsalicylic acid

Barbiturates

Carbamazepine

Chlorohydrate

Ciprofloxacin

Codeine

Diphenhydramine

Erythromycin

Ketoconazole

Metronidazole

Nonsteroidal anti-inflammatory drugs

Nystatin

Oral contraceptives

Penicillins

Phenolphthalein

Sulfonamides

Tetracyclines

Trimethoprim

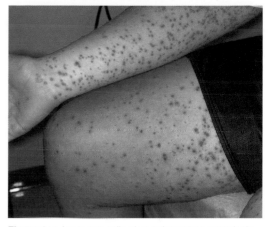

Figure 6-7 Acute generalized exanthematous pustulosis. Diffuse erythematous, nonfollicular, pinpoint, sterile pustules

membrane involvement should lead to immediate drug discontinuation. Topical steroids and oral antihistamines offer some modest relief of pruritus. Bland emollients are recommended for the desquamation phase.

DRESS is a serious reaction that may require hospitalization. Systemic steroids are generally recommended for all but the mildest of cases, with a slow taper over 2–3 weeks. AGEP can usually be managed with mid-potency topical steroids but significant reactions may warrant the use of prednisone.

Erythema Multiforme

Key Points

- Symmetrical targetoid lesions on the arms, legs, hands, and feet
- Oral lesions without other mucous membrane involvement
- Driven by herpes simplex infection
- Self-resolution

There is substantial controversy surrounding the definition, pathogenesis, and treatment of EM, Stevens–Johnson syndrome (SJS), and TEN. The literature is full of misdiagnoses, contradictory statements, and raging arguments over whether the entities are distinct or part of a clinical

spectrum. The text below attempts to present a polarized view of each entity, steering clear of the many controversial shades of gray that muddy an understanding of these important conditions.

Clinical presentation

EM is a mostly herpes simplex-induced eruption characterized by the abrupt onset of symmetrical papules and plaques that are most often seen on the arms, legs, hands, and feet. The trunk, face, and neck may be involved. Individual lesions consist of dull red, edematous plaques. Many lesions will have a central gray papule or vesicle giving the distinctive target lesion (Figure 6-8). A central red papule gives a third zone to the target in some lesions. Koebner phenomenon may be demonstrated by induction of EM lesion in areas of trauma. Lesions may be preceded by low-grade fever and malaise but usually there is no prodrome. There may have been an overt outbreak of a cold sore 1–2 weeks prior, but this is variable.

Oral lesions may be seen in up to half of affected children (Figure 6-9). Vesicles are followed by aphthous-like ulcerations on the lips, tongue, and buccal mucosa. The gums are not involved, as is the case with herpes simplex virus (HSV) infection. Mild to moderate pain is common but the severe crusting seen in SJS is not seen and no other mucous membranes are involved. Healing of mouth and skin takes place over 2–3 weeks.

Diagnosis

EM can usually be diagnosed clinically. A biopsy may be helpful in atypical cases. Many of the older reports of supposed EM actually depict giant urticaria, and this can be differentiated by its evanescence. Bug bites, vasculitis, and immunobullous diseases may look like EM.

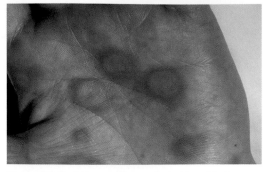

Figure 6-8 Erythema multiforme. Typical target lesions on the palms

Primary HSV infection may look like EM if the mouth dominates the clinic picture. Culture will be negative in EM. Aphthous ulcers or an immunobullous disease may enter the differential diagnosis of mouth lesions.

Pathogenesis

The majority of cases of EM represent a host response to HSV, almost always type 1 but rarely type 2. Many times, parents and patients are unaware that they are infected, but detection of HSV antibodies and the finding of HSV DNA by polymerase chain reaction in lesions of EM strongly support its role in pathogenesis. Epstein–Barr virus, cytomegalovirus, and Orf have been much less commonly implicated.

Treatment

Asymptomatic lesions do not need to be treated. Burning and itching can be relieved with oral antihistamines. Prednisone treatment runs the risk of prolonging episodes and shortening the interval between outbreaks. However, a short 2–5-day burst of prednisone can help reduce the discomfort of significant mouth lesions.

Frequent recurrences can be treated prophylactically with acyclovir 20 mg/kg per day. Valacyclovir and famciclovir are alternatives for older children. There is no reason to treat with antiviral agents in a periodic fashion since HSV infection will precede the outbreak of EM by many days.

Stevens–Johnson Syndrome

Key Points

- Extensive oral lesions with at least one other mucous membrane involved
- Some skin denudation but usually only 10% surface area or less
- Caused mostly by drugs, some by *Mycoplasma*
- Supportive care in the hospital
- Prednisone use controversial

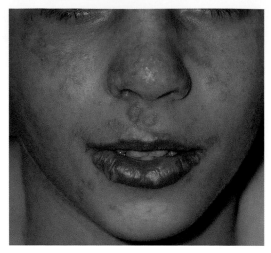

Figure 6-9 Erythema multiforme. Vesicles and bullae on the lips accompanied by typical skin lesions

Clinical presentation

Unlike EM, SJS is preceded by a 1–2-week prodrome of fever, malaise, cough, sore throat, diarrhea, and other systemic symptoms. Mucosal involvement tends to precede skin lesions and dominates the clinical picture, as opposed to TEN where skin denudation dominates. The mouth is invariably involved, with large areas of painful necrosis, ulceration, crusting and pseudomembrane formation (Figure 6-10). Esophageal and tracheal mucosa may be affected. Purulent conjunctivitis (Figure 6-11) and photophobia with associated corneal ulcerations, keratitis, and uveitis are characteristic features of ocular involvement, and there is substantial risk of permanent sequelae. Vaginal, urethral, anal, and nasal mucous membranes are less frequently involved. There should be at least two affected mucous membranes to make the diagnosis of SJS.

Skin lesions develop 1–3 days after the start of mouth lesions. Typically, dusky erythema develops on the upper trunk, neck, and face. Areas of edema give a targetoid appearance reminiscent of EM but distinctive nonetheless. Some epidermal detachment may occur, leaving painful, red, denuded skin; light pressure induces shearing. Total involved surface area will usually be 10% or less. Healing tends to leave extensive, long-lasting hyperpigmentation.

Diagnosis

Kawasaki disease is the main condition in the differential diagnosis. The mucous membrane involvement in Kawasaki disease is much less erosive, exudative, and denuded. EM is usually easy to differentiate from SJS and should not have more than one mucous membrane involved. The immunobullous diseases, particularly the rare paraneoplastic pemphigus, require biopsy

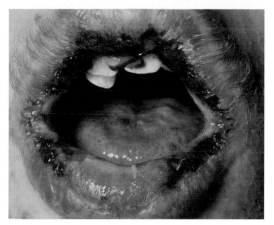

Figure 6-10 Stevens–Johnson syndrome. Painful necrosis, ulceration, crusting, and pseudomembrane formation of the mouth

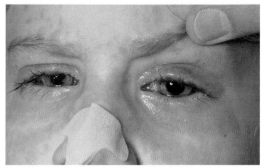

Figure 6-11 Stevens–Johnson syndrome. Purulent conjunctivitis

for definitive differential diagnosis. Perilesional normal skin or mucosa is needed to perform immunofluorescent studies. Staphylococcal scalded-skin syndrome (SSSS) with limited cutaneous involvement may look like SJS.

Pathogenesis

Most cases of SJS are precipitated by medications, particularly sulfa-based antibiotics, anticonvulsants, and nonsteroidal anti-inflammatory drugs (NSAIDs). The eruption occurs within the first several weeks of medication exposure. Some cases are the result of an underlying infection, particularly *Mycoplasma pneumoniae*.

Treatment

Most children with SJS are very ill and need hospitalization in all but the very mildest cases. An intensive care unit or burn unit may be needed depending on the extent of medical and cutaneous complications. Extensive and painful mouth involvement may prevent adequate oral hydration and intravenous fluids are needed. A topical anesthetic solution may help with mouth pain and facilitate appropriate oral hygiene. Pulmonary toilet needs to be maintained, and antibiotics effective against *M. pneumoniae* should be started for those with respiratory symptoms while awaiting titers. Ophthalmologic consultation is needed and usually antibiotic drops are instituted.

There are varying opinions regarding the use of systemic steroids in SJS. There are patients who have quite dramatic improvement in their mouth lesions if given a quick 5–8-day burst of steroids early in the course of SJS. Prolonged courses are not indicated and are apt to compound complications. Intravenous immunoglobulin (IVIG) for 3 days may be effective, but has been used to treat extensive skin necrosis in the TEN range of severity. Even in the setting of TEN, data regarding efficacy are mixed.

Toxic Epidermal Necrolysis

Key Points

- Severe and extensive skin denudation
- Caused by medications
- Supportive care in intensive care unit or burn unit
- Data are mixed regarding corticosteroids, but preponderance of evidence suggests they increase risk of sepsis
- Data are mixed regarding IVIG

Clinical presentation

The clinical picture of TEN is very similar to SJS in terms of prodrome and timing of presentation. The main differentiating feature is the more massive extent of cutaneous involvement (Figures 6-12 and 6-13) with at least 30% of body surface area being affected. Dusky erythema gives way to massive denudation, leaving behind tender, glistening, and crusted erosions. Mucous membrane involvement, although present, is not the dominant feature as in SJS.

Diagnosis

The differential diagnosis of TEN includes, in addition to those mentioned for SJS, SSSS. The young age, lack of drug exposure, typical facies, and more superficial shearing of skin are features that suggest SSSS. Microscopic evaluation of denuded skin or a biopsy specimen will distinguish the intraepidermal split of SSSS from the subepidermal split of TEN.

Pathogenesis

TEN is caused exclusively by medications, with antibiotics, anticonvulsants, and NSAIDs heading the list. *Mycoplasma* is not associated with TEN, a confounding factor in the theory that SJS and TEN are part of a continuum. There may be a genetic susceptibility to TEN, and the pathogenesis

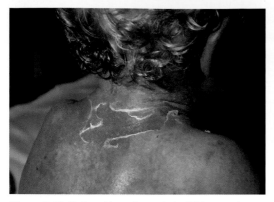

Figure 6-12 Toxic epidermal necrolysis. Widespread erythema and epidermal shearing

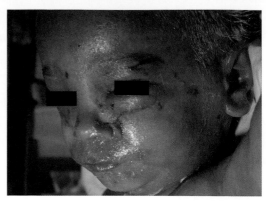

Figure 6-13 Toxic epidermal necrolysis. Extensive facial erythema in addition to mucous membrane involvement

involves activation of the death receptor Fas and its ligand, FasL.

Treatment

TEN must be managed in a tertiary care intensive care unit experienced in the care of extensive skin loss or a burn center. The care is similar as for SJS, with emphasis on meticulous wound care. Data are mixed regarding both systemic corticosteroids and IVIG. Most current evidence suggests that corticosteroids increase the likelihood of septic death, especially if used for longer than 2–3 days. Studies suggesting a benefit from IVIG have generally used a dose of at least 3 g/kg.

Vasculitis/Henoch–Schönlein Purpura

- Palpable purpura on buttocks and lower extremities
- Joint, kidney, gastrointestinal involvement
- Leukocytoclastic vasculitis with IgA on immunofluorescence

Vasculitis refers to a variety of diverse conditions characterized by inflammation of blood vessels. Nomenclature and categorization are confusing. Most of the larger-vessel vasculitides except for Kawasaki disease (Chapter 12) are very rare in childhood so vasculitis in this text will refer narrowly to postcapillary venule vasculitis (classic palpable purpura) to keep the discussion simple. Synonyms such as anaphylactoid purpura, allergic purpura, and leukocytoclastic vasculitis will be avoided for clarity.

PEARL

The mnemonic CRITICAL (cryoglobulins, rheumatologic disorders, infections, especially *Streptococcus* and hepatitis, toxins, inflammatory bowel disease, complement deficiency, allergy/ drug reaction, lymphoproliferative disorders) is helpful in remembering these causes and directing possible work-up.

Henoch–Schönlein purpura (HSP) is the most common cause of vasculitis in children and will be the focus of this discussion.

Clinical presentation

Palpable purpura of the legs and buttocks is the hallmark of HSP (Figures 6-14 and 6-15). Involvement of the joints, gastrointestinal system, and kidneys rounds out the tetrad. Fever, malaise, or nondescript flu-like symptoms may precede the initial early lesions of lower-extremity urticarial macules and papules. Nonblanching, mottled macular or palpable purpuric patches rapidly evolve and, although they may appear anywhere, they are classically located on the buttocks, thighs, and legs in a dependent manner. Lesions may coalesce into large plaques and individual lesions may form hemorrhagic vesicles, bullae, crusts, and ulcers. Healing occurs with long-lasting hyperpigmentation.

Joint pain is the most common systemic symptom, usually affecting the knees and ankles, although any joint may be involved. True arthritis may be present. Gastrointestinal involvement is manifest by colicky abdominal pain, vomiting, hematemesis, and hematochezia. Intussusception may occur. Renal involvement occurs in about a third of children with HSP, mostly presenting as isolated hematuria or proteinuria. Long-term renal impairment occurs in fewer than 2% but may be as high as 20% in those who present with nephritis or nephrosis. Much less commonly affected are the central nervous system and lungs. Scrotal involvement may lead to swelling and pain, with or without purpura.

Resolution of HSP is expected in 4–6 weeks, although parents should be warned of the possibility (perhaps likelihood) of a recurrence in the next several months. Since renal impairment may follow resolution of the cutaneous outbreak, periodic monitoring of urine and blood pressure should be done up until about 6 months after the acute eruption.

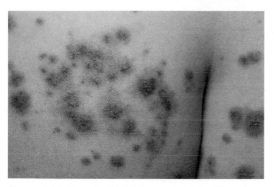

Figure 6-14 Henoch–Schönlein purpura. Palpable purpura on the buttock

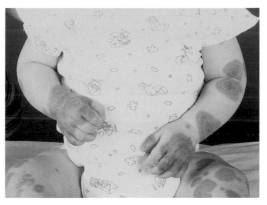

Figure 6-16 Acute hemorrhagic edema. Targetoid purpura and edema of the extremities

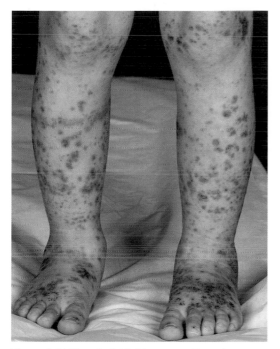

Figure 6-15 Henoch–Schönlein purpura. Extensive lower-extremity involvement

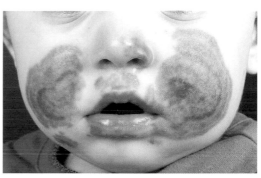

Figure 6-17 Acute hemorrhagic edema. Prominent facial involvement

Acute hemorrhagic edema (AHE) is a unique vasculitis of young children aged 4–24 months. There is sudden onset of fever with marked tender, symmetric edema and large, expanding purpura of the hands, feet, and face (Figures 6-16 and 6-17). Centrifugal spread leads to large targetoid purpura, quite distinct from the smaller palpable purpura of HSP. The physical appearance is impressive but the children look otherwise well, and internal organ involvement is very rare. Resolution without recurrence occurs in 1–3 weeks.

Diagnosis

The clinical appearance of HSP and AHE is quite distinctive and diagnosis can usually be made by physical examination findings alone. Biopsy will demonstrate small-vessel vasculitis in both conditions and immunofluorescence will show deposits of IgA in most cases of HSP, but a minority of AHE. Coagulopathy with purpura, sepsis, particularly from meningococcemia, EM, bug bites, urticaria, and child abuse may be considered in the differential diagnosis.

Internal organ involvement should be monitored with periodic stool guaiac, blood pressure, and urinalysis. Since *Streptococcus* is a purported etiologic agent, a throat culture or ASO titer may be checked. A much broader work-up may be considered for vasculitis unassociated with HSP, targeting the possible causes listed above in the CRITICAL mnemonic. A medication reaction is the most likely cause in that setting. In general, a laboratory witch hunt is not indicated.

Pathogenesis

Vasculitis is caused by immune complex deposition within the walls of small venules, leading to complement activation and neutrophil chemotaxis. Neutrophil phagocytosis and degranulation result in leakage of red blood cells and fibrin deposition within the postcapillary venules.

The inciting event in HSP is not known. Several infectious agents have been implicated, including *Streptococci*, *Bartonella*, and many viruses.

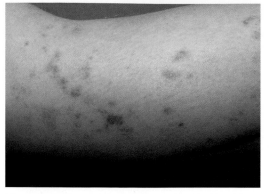

Figure 6-18 Pigmented purpuric eruption. Nonblanching, nonpalpable petechiae on the lower extremity

Table 6-1 Variants of pigmented purpuric eruption	
Variant	**Clinical characteristic**
Schamberg disease	Cayenne pepper spots
	Usually on one or both shins
Eczematoid-like purpura of Doucas and Kapetanakis	Severely pruritic
Purpura annularis telangiectodes (Majocchi disease)	Annular patches with a periphery of telangiectasia, generally found on the legs
Lichen aureus	Distinctive, rust-colored, grouped lichenoid papules that coalesce into sharply marginated plaques
Pigmented purpuric lichenoid dermatosis of Gougerot and Blum	Lichenoid papules on the legs, turn brown with time

Treatment

Uncomplicated cases of HSP or AHE do not need to be treated. Mild arthralgias can be treated with NSAIDs. Extensive, painful skin lesions, severe joint pains, and abdominal symptoms can be relieved with a course of prednisone. Steroid-sparing anti-inflammatory agents such as dapsone, colchicine, antimalarials, and tetracycline antibiotics are rarely needed.

Pigmented Purpuric Eruptions

Key Points

- Nonpalpable petechiae
- Chronic but self-limited

Clinical presentation

The pigmented purpuric eruptions (PPE) are a group of related conditions characterized by nonpalpable, pinpoint petechiae on a brownish/yellow base (Figure 6-18) clinically and lymphocytic capillaritis, leakage of red blood cells and hemosiderin pathologically. Five variants are described, although their similarities in course and prognosis favor lumping over splitting (Table 6-1).

Schamberg disease is the most common of the variants. It consists of multiple red-brown patches sprinkled with petechiae or hemosiderin, classically described as cayenne pepper spots. One or both shins are usually involved but it may be seen anywhere. The Majocchi variant is annular (ring lesions) and telangiectatic. The Gougerot–Blum variant is lichenoid. Initially, it resembles lichen planus, but the lesions become brown over time as hemosiderin accumulates. The Doucas and Kapetanakis variant is eczematous (spongiotic). *Lichen aureus* (Figure 6-19) consist of a single grouping of rust-colored macules. It results from a single incompetent valve resulting in localized increased vascular pressure.

All of the forms of PPE run chronic courses but may resolve spontaneously after many months to years. The cosmetic appearance is the only disturbing feature for most patients and itch is mild except for the Doucas and Kapetanakis variant.

Diagnosis

The PPEs are quite distinctive and usually the diagnosis can be made clinically. Biopsy will confirm the diagnosis in confusing cases. The differential diagnosis includes petechiae from platelet dysfunction or thrombocytopenia, bruising, suction purpura, vasculitis, and drug eruptions, particularly fixed drug eruption. Early mycosis fungoides (cutaneous T-cell lymphoma) can have a similar appearance.

Pathogenesis

The etiology of PPE is unknown. A minority of cases can be linked to a medication but most have no identifiable cause.

Treatment

Topical steroids offer minimal improvement, except in the eczematous variant. Antihistamines may improve pruritus in a few patients. Anecdotal reports have shown some improvement with vitamin C and bioflavonoids.

Aphthous Ulcers

Key Points

- Recurrent, painful gray to white oral ulcerations with a red halo
- Major and minor variety
- Usually idiopathic but some disease associations
- Respond to topical steroid gels
- Common triggers include walnuts and fresh pineapple
- Some severe cases may require colchicine or thalidomide

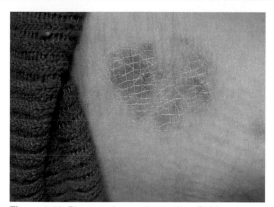

Figure 6-19 Pigmented purpuric eruption. Golden plaque characteristic of *Lichen aureus*

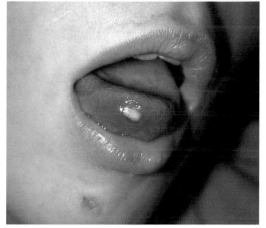

Figure 6-20 Aphthous ulcers. Round ulceration with a red halo on the tip of the tongue

Clinical presentation

Aphthous ulcers (canker sores) affect nearly 25% of the population and are more common in women, Caucasians, nonsmokers, and those of higher socioeconomic status. They are recurrent, painful, round-to-oval oral ulcerations with a gray to white center and red halo (Figures 6-20 and 6-21). Most start in childhood and many burn out in the third or fourth decade.

Aphthae can be divided into minor and major aphthous ulcers, with about 80% of those with recurrent aphthous stomatitis having the minor variety. They are 2–8 mm in size, most commonly occurring on the labial or buccal mucosae, the floor of the mouth, and the ventral surface of the tongue. They may be preceded by a tingling sensation. Healing takes place over 10–14 days. Major aphthae (periadenitis mucosa necrotica recurrens) may be 10 mm or more in size and are more painful. They are more likely to involve the dorsal surface of the tongue and hard palate and last longer than minor aphthae. Scarring may result. Although they are less common, the patients will be more likely to seek medical attention. A third, uncommon variety is called herpetiform ulceration because aphthae begin as multiple pinpoint ulcers that mimic HSV infection.

Diagnosis

Aphthae are so common that most individuals recognize the diagnosis immediately. EM can be distinguished by its associated skin lesions and HSV infection will have a positive culture. Herpangina and hand, foot, and mouth disease will have associated systemic symptoms and tend to occur in epidemic but not recurrent fashion. Cytomegalovirus and Epstein–Barr virus may rarely be the cause of mouth ulcers. Erosive lichen planus and immunobullous diseases are not as well localized as aphthae and are very rare in children.

A number of medical conditions have aphthous ulcers as part of their clinical presentation and are listed in Box 6-3. A thorough review of systems will usually rule out these processes and no laboratory work-up is needed for the typical patient with aphthae. The presence of genital ulcers suggests Behçet syndrome or inflammatory bowel disease, although major aphthosis involving the genital mucosa has been described. A complete blood count with differential is a simple test to help exclude cyclic neutropenia, iron, vitamin B12 or folate deficiency, and leukemia, although more specific tests should be ordered if these are serious considerations based on history and physical exam.

Pathogenesis

The vast majority of recurrent aphthous ulcers occur as part of an idiopathic process. Triggers may include mechanical trauma such as from sharp-edged chips, stress, hormonal changes, and food reactions (especially to walnuts and fresh pineapple). Many individuals have a positive family history of aphthae, suggesting a genetic link.

Treatment

The mainstay of treatment is avoiding trauma, particularly foods with rigid, sharp edges. Any suspected triggers, including foods and NSAIDs, should be stopped. Acetaminophen or an over-the-counter topical anesthetic (UlcerEase, Anbesol, Cepastat, Orabase Maximum Strength) will provide temporary symptomatic relief. Ulcers can be sealed with 2-octyl cyanoacrylate (Orabase Soothe-N-Seal).

Topical steroids, usually in a gel formulation, can be placed directly on the ulcers. Fluocinolone or clobetasol gels are frequently used. Steroids can be mixed in an oral paste (Orabase) but some find these formulations cumbersome to use. A steroid

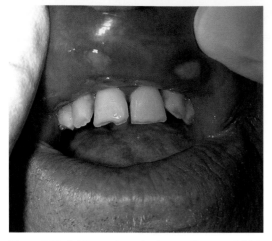

Figure 6-21 Aphthous ulcers. Lesions on the upper labial mucosa

BOX 6-3

Conditions associated with aphthous ulcers

Periodic fever syndromes – PFAPA (periodic fever, aphthous ulcers, pharyngitis, adenitis)

    TRAPS (TNF-receptor-associated periodic fevers), Muckle–Wells syndrome

Immunosuppression – particularly cyclic neutropenia and HIV

Behçet syndrome (bipolar aphthosis)

Reactive arthritis (Reiter syndrome)

Systemic lupus erythematosus

Sweet syndrome

Leukemia

Gluten-sensitive enteropathy

Inflammatory bowel disease

Deficiency of iron, folate, or vitamin B_{12}

Medications, including NSAIDs and beta-blockers

HIV, human immunodeficiency virus; NSAIDs, nonsteroidal anti-inflammatory drugs; TNF, tumor necrosis factor.

inhaler designed for use in asthma can be employed to spray steroid solution on to the oral mucosa. Systemic absorption and the development of oral candidiasis are possible concerns with steroid use. Amlexanox paste (Aphthasol) is a topical, nonsteroid antiinflammatory treatment found to demonstrate some improvement in aphthae.

Various mixtures and concoctions have been advocated, generally with various proportions of diphenhydramine, tetracycline, and antacids such as Maalox. One example of an effective mixture that can be used as a swish and spit is hydrocortisone powder 120 mg, sorbitol solution 60 ml, nystatin oral suspension 60 ml, tetracycline 3 g and diphenhydramine elixir qsad 480 ml. Of course, children should be older than 8 years of age if tetracycline is used.

Major aphthae may need more aggressive treatment if pain is debilitating and prolonged. Systemic steroids may be administered with reasonable results but chronic use is not appropriate. Dapsone, colchicine, and thalidomide may be considered for very difficult cases. Silver nitrate sticks can be used to destroy the base of a very painful ulcer. It is a painful procedure that may require some anesthesia, but resultant posttreatment pain relief is immediate.

Annular Erythemas

The annular or gyrate erythemas are an unrelated group of disorders linked by their physical exam finding of circular or polycyclic, blanching erythema. The full differential diagnosis for this group is listed in Box 6-4. Most of the entities are mentioned elsewhere in the text or are too uncommon in pediatrics to mention further, but a few entities deserve some brief discussion.

Erythema annulare centrifugum (EAC) is a persistent, chronic eruption, generally appearing on the trunk and thighs. Asymptomatic or mildly pruritic erythematous papules expand into annular or polycyclic rings over many days, eventually reaching a size of 10 cm or more. The scale, when present, is characteristically on the trailing end of the eruption (Figures 6-22 and 6-23). A potassium hydroxide scraping will rule out tinea corporis, the main entity in the differential diagnosis, but a biopsy may need to be done to make a correct diagnosis.

Like urticaria, EAC is a reaction pattern to some outside stimulus although, most often, one is never found. Medications, foods, and fungal infections head the list but mollusca, other infections, or any systemic illness can act as a trigger. Treatment with topical steroids and oral antihistamines is generally ineffective. Systemic steroids will help but are not appropriate for long-term use. The process tends to burn out over months to years.

Erythema marginatum occurs in up to 10% of patients with streptococcal-induced rheumatic fever. The other associations include carditis, arthritis, and, rarely, Sydenham's chorea. Evanescent, nonpruritic, urticarial macules and papules form on the trunk and proximal extremities, expanding into large plaques with pale or dusky centers and polycyclic borders. They occur most commonly late in the day, usually with fever, and last only hours. Eventual fading may leave a faint chicken wire appearance that is accentuated with warming. Diagnosis is based on piecing together the entire clinical picture, but sometimes biopsy will be helpful, if only to exclude other annular erythemas.

Annular erythemas

Erythema annulare centrifugum

Erythema gyratum repens

Erythema chronicum migrans

Erythema multiforme

Erythema marginatum

Urticaria

Urticarial vasculitis

Urticarial bullous pemphigoid

Tinea corporis

Psoriasis

Herald patch of pityriasis rosea

Subacute cutaneous lupus erythematosus

Neonatal lupus erythematosus

Juvenile idiopathic arthritis (juvenile rheumatoid arthritis)

Necrolytic migratory erythema

Granuloma annulare

Elastosis perforans serpiginosa

Borderline leprosy

Carriers of chronic granulomatous disease

Annular erythema of infancy

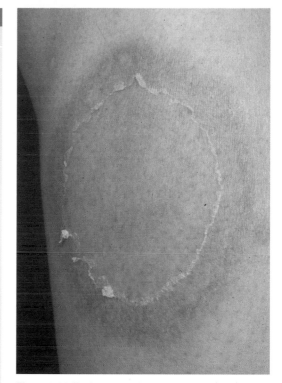

Figure 6-23 Erythema annulare centrifugum. Annular patch with characteristic trailing scale

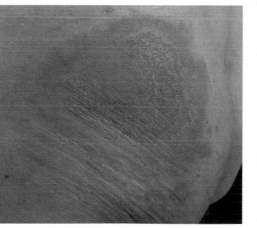

Figure 6-22 Erythema annulare centrifugum. Note the trailing scale within the annular plaque

The systemic variety of *juvenile idiopathic arthritis* (juvenile rheumatoid arthritis) is associated with a very transient eruption corresponding to periods of spiking fevers. Wheal-like, nonpruritic papules develop mostly on the trunk but also on the extremities and face. They may coalesce into larger plaques with serpiginous, annular borders. Heat or trauma may stimulate or accentuate the rash.

Sun Eruptions

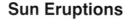

The sun eruptions (Box 6-5) or photodermatoses are a confusing group of ultraviolet light-induced disorders. Aside from run-of-the-mill sunburn, *polymorphous light eruption* (PMLE) is the most frequently encountered photoeruption – patients often refer to it as "sun poisoning." It is most common among young, light-skinned girls and occurs in up to 20% of the population. Lesions usually develop after intense sun exposure such as during a vacation or after the first significant sun exposures of the spring. Urticarial papules or vesicles coalesce into larger plaques on the sun-exposed areas of the face, neck, arms, forearms, and hands 1–4 days after ultraviolet light exposure (Figure 6-24). Itch may be intense. Self-resolution occurs in 1–2 weeks.

No treatment is necessary but some symptomatic relief may be obtained with topical or systemic steroids and oral antihistamines. Protective clothing and broad-spectrum sunscreens, containing ingredients such as titanium dioxide, zinc oxide, or combinations including avobenzone or mexoryl, are advisable. Generally the skin becomes less sensitive as the summer progresses ("hardening") so long-term treatment is not needed. Severe, repetitive bouts can be treated with oral antimalarial medicines such as hydroxychloroquine or with beta-carotene.

Conditions associated with photosensitivity

Exogenous agents (photoallergic or phototoxic)

Drugs – antibiotics, diuretics, anti-inflammatory agents

Topical agents – sunscreens, tars, perfumes

Plant material (phytophotodermatitis)

Tattoo pigment – cadmium

Porphyrias

Porphyria cutanea tarda

Pseudoporphyria cutanea tarda – naproxen or other NSAIDs

Erythropoietic protoporphyria – sun-induced pain with little rash

Congenital erythropoietic porphyria

Genodermatoses

Xeroderma pigmentosa

Bloom syndrome

Cockayne syndrome

Rothmund–Thomson syndrome

Trichothiodystrophy

Hartnup disease

Connective tissue disease

Lupus erythematosus

Dermatomyositis

Viral exanthem
Idiopathic photodermatoses

Polymorphous light eruption

Juvenile spring eruption

Actinic prurigo

Hydroa vacciniforme

Solar urticaria

NSAID, nonsteroidal anti-inflammatory drug.

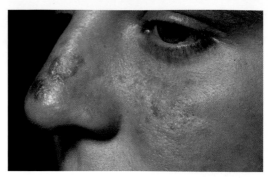

Figure 6-24 Polymorphous light eruption. Urticarial papules or vesicles on sun-exposed skin

commonly on the face but also on exposed areas of the arms and legs. With time, the eruption will spread to covered areas but is less severe. The skin does not "harden" with continued ultraviolet light exposure as it does in PMLE, and the rash continues through the summer, waning somewhat during the winter. Cheilitis and conjunctivitis may be associated findings. The process may abate in about 5 years in the childhood variety. Treatment is much the same as PMLE.

The correct diagnosis of a photosensitivity disorder may be very obvious by the clinical setting and work-up may be delayed while waiting to see the degree of chronicity and response to simple treatments. Nonessential medications or topical agents should be stopped. Skin biopsy, antinuclear antibody, SSA, SSB and serum porphyrin levels should be checked in children with chronic or undiagnosed presentations. Phototesting or photopatch testing can be considered in confusing, unrelenting photodermatoses.

Further reading

Chave TA, Mortimer NJ, Sladden MJ, et al. Toxic epidermal necrolysis: current evidence, practical management and future directions. Br J Dermatol 2005;153:241–253.

Fesq H, Ring J, Abeck D. Management of polymorphous light eruption: clinical course, pathogenesis, diagnosis and intervention. Am J Clin Dermatol 2003;4:399–406.

Gonzalez E, Gonzalez S. Drug photosensitivity, idiopathic photodermatoses, and sunscreens. J Am Acad Dermatol 1996;35:871–885.

Hernandez RG, Cohen BA. Insect bite-induced hypersensitivity and the SCRATCH principles: a new approach to papular urticaria. Pediatrics 2006;118:e189–e196.

Meadows KP, Egan CA, Vanderhooft S. Acute generalized exanthematous pustulosis (AGEP), an uncommon condition in children: case report and review of the literature. Pediatr Dermatol 2000;17:399–402.

Juvenile spring eruption may be a variant of PMLE that occurs more in young boys 5–12 years of age. Red papules and vesicles occur characteristically on the helices of the ears but may be on the dorsal hands or forearms. Episodes last for about a week and recur the following spring. Treatment is the same as for PMLE.

Actinic prurigo is most commonly seen in Native American populations but has been described worldwide. Most cases begin prior to 20 years of age but it may begin later in Canadian Inuit populations. Boys outnumber girls by a ratio of 3:1. The rash consists of intensely pruritic, excoriated papules, vesicles, and nodules, most

Metry DW, Jung P, Levy ML. Use of intravenous immunoglobulin in children with Stevens–Johnson syndrome and toxic epidermal necrolysis: seven cases and review of the literature. Pediatrics 2003;112:1430–1436.

Morelli JG, Tay YK, Rogers M, et al. Fixed drug eruptions in children. J Pediatr 1999;134:365–367.

Narchi H. Risk of long term renal impairment and duration of follow up recommended for Henoch–Schönlein purpura; a systematic review. Arch Dis Child 2005;90:916–920.

Sackesen C, Sekerel BE, Orhan F, et al. The etiology of different forms of urticaria in childhood. Pediatr Dermatol 2004;21:102–108.

Scully C. Aphthous ulceration. N Engl J Med 2006;355:165–172.

Tas S, Simonart T. Management of drug rash with eosinophilia and systemic symptoms (DRESS syndrome): an update. Dermatology 2003;206:353–356.

Tristani-Firouzi P, Meadows KP, Vanderfooft S. Pigmented purpuric eruptions of childhood: a series of cases and review of literature. Pediatr Dermatol 2001;18:299–304.

Weston WL, Badgett JT. Urticaria. Pediatr Rev 1998;19:240–244.

Yashar SS, Lim HW. Classification and evaluation of photodermatoses. Dermatol Ther 2003;16:1–7.

Pigmentary disorders: white spots, brown spots, and other dyschromias

7

Howard B. Pride

Disorders of Hypopigmenation and Depigmentation

Hypopigmentation disorders make up a varied group of conditions, from pityriasis alba to sarcoidosis and leprosy. A complete differential diagnosis appears in Box 7-1, and the most common conditions will be discussed. Most of these diagnoses are established clinically, and important differentiating features on history and physical examination include:

- Is the condition diffuse (e.g., albinism) or localized (e.g., vitiligo)?
- Is the condition hypopigmented (e.g., pityriasis alba, postinflammatory) or depigmented (e.g., vitiligo)?
- Is there surface scale (e.g., tinea versicolor, pityriasis alba) or no surface change (e.g., vitiligo)?
- Is the condition congenital (e.g., piebaldism) or acquired (e.g., vitiligo)?
- Is there underlying atrophy or induration (e.g., striae, lichen sclerosus, morphea)?

There is significant overlap in some of these differentiating features, making an algorithmic approach nearly impossible, but answering the above questions and a general knowledge of the most common entities will usually lead to the correct diagnosis.

Vitiligo

Key Points

- Symmetric patches without pigmentation
- Rarely associated with autoimmune conditions
- Treatment with topical steroids, immunomodulators, and narrow-band ultraviolet (UV) B

Clinical presentation

Vitiligo is a condition of acquired depigmentation (loss of pigment as opposed to decrease in pigment) resulting from the immunologic destruction of epidermal melanocytes. About 50% of cases begin during childhood and adolescence, and all races are equally involved. Girls slightly outnumber boys. The prevalence is about 1% in the general population.

Lesions of vitiligo are stark white macules and patches with geographic shapes. Occasionally, there will be an intermediate zone of hypopigmentation, the so-called trichrome vitiligo. The most common pattern is the generalized form where patches characteristically occur symmetrically on exposed areas such as the face, neck, and hands (Figure 7-1). Skin folds and bony prominences such as the knees and elbows are also common locations (Figure 7-2). Involved areas tend to be dynamic with subtle expansion and, sometimes, repigmentation that can be hard to appreciate without serial photographs. When repigmentation does occur, islands of follicular repigmentation or darkening along the marginal areas are often noted first. White hairs (poliosis) may be seen within the patches and may even involve eyebrows and lashes (Figure 7-3). Lesions may appear in areas of skin trauma (Koebner phenomenon).

Other variants include segmental vitiligo, which refers to involvement of asymmetric, unilateral patches with a seemingly dermatomal distribution. The acrofacial facial distribution is mostly periocular and perioral. The mucosal variety and universal (total body) vitiligo are rare variants. Halo nevi (Figure 7-4), melanocytic nevi with a rim of depigmentation, are often seen in patients with vitiligo, and the finding of a halo nevus should prompt a thorough examination for vitiligo in other areas.

Children are usually well in every other respect. There is some association with other autoimmune conditions (akin to alopecia areata) so the evaluation should include a search for signs or symptoms of thyroid disease, juvenile diabetes, connective tissue disease, pernicious anemia, alopecia areata, psoriasis, myasthenia gravis, and ulcerative colitis. In the absence of signs and symptoms, routine laboratory testing is not recommended, but families should be counseled to watch for signs or symptoms such as polydipsia and polyuria.

BOX 7-1

Differential diagnosis of hypopigmentation

Diffuse hypopigmentation

Albinism and variants

Phenylketonuria

Patchy hypopigmentation

Vitiligo

Pityriasis alba

Postinflammatory hypopigmentation

Tinea versicolor

Ash leaf spots of tuberous sclerosis

Nevus depigmentosus

Nevus anemicus

Striae

Lichen sclerosus

Morphea (late)

Mosaic (whorled) hypopigmentation

Piebaldism

Waardenburg syndrome

Early hemangioma

Incontinentia pigmenti (late fourth stage)

Sarcoidosis

Cutaneous T-cell lymphoma

Leprosy

Pinta and yaws

Diagnosis

Acquired, symmetric depigmentation is usually easily diagnosed as vitiligo. A Woods light will aid in accentuating patches in very light-skinned children. Pityriasis alba and postinflammatory hypopigmentation do not have a total absence of pigment, do not accentuate well with a Woods light, and pityriasis alba demonstrates fine overlying scale. Genital vitiligo in females may be difficult to distinguish from lichen sclerosus. The lack of induration, atrophy, bruising, and itch/pain suggest vitiligo, but a biopsy may be needed in difficult cases. Nevus depigmentosus is hypopigmented, generally appears during infancy, and tends to be more static than vitiligo. Ash leaf macules of tuberous sclerosis are hypopigmented

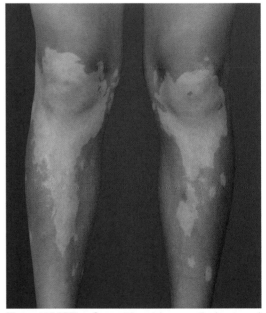

Figure 7-2 Vitiligo. Symmetric patches over the knees and shins

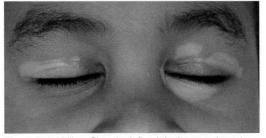

Figure 7-1 Vitiligo. Sharply defined depigmented patches on the eyelids

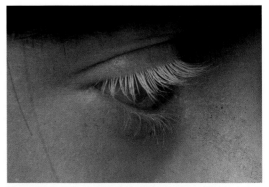

Figure 7-3 Vitiligo. White hair (poliosis) from vitiligo

rather than depigmented, but in the absence of other tuberous sclerosis findings may be mistaken for vitiligo. Tinea versicolor tends to be more truncal than acral, is hypopigmented, has a fine powdery scale, and will give a positive potassium hydroxide evaluation. Piebaldism presents on axial areas with nonpigmented skin (no melanocytes were ever present) that resembles vitiligo. The white skin of piebaldism is of congenital onset whereas vitiligo very rarely occurs at birth.

Pathophysiology

Vitiligo results from the acquired absence of epidermal melanocytes. The exact cause is not known, but there is evidence that it is an autoimmune phenomenon involving both humoral and cell-mediated immunity. There is an increased incidence among family members and a clustering among certain human leukocyte antigen types, suggesting a genetic component.

Treatment

Vitiligo can be an emotionally devastating condition and a sympathetic, patient, listening ear is needed. Reassurance that the condition is harmless should be coupled with a sensible treatment plan and some optimism for possible resultant repigmentation.

For those patients and parents who choose not to treat the condition, diligent sun protection and sunscreen use will be necessary to protect depigmented areas from chronic actinic damage. Some children may opt for camouflage makeup or use sunless tanning agents which can effectively mask the depigmented areas adequately and improve a child's social functioning with peers.

Topical anti-inflammatory agents are the most commonly prescribed medicines. Results are best with superpotent topical steroids, which will require periods of nontreatment to avoid atrophy. One week on and one week off or just treating on weekends are examples. Topical steroids should be used with caution, if at all, around the eyes where there may be some risk of inducing cataracts or glaucoma. Tacrolimus and pimecrolimus can be used solely or in conjunction with topical steroids. Repigmented areas will appear as brown dots spreading centrifugally from hair follicles (Figure 7-5).

UV light is a two-edged sword. It may induce repigmentation but will also accentuate normally pigmented skin, making the vitiliginous areas stand out in greater contrast, and will sunburn the white skin. Cautious natural sunlight exposure can be encouraged. Psoralen (topically or orally) plus UVA (PUVA) has been replaced by narrow-band UVB therapy as the treatment of choice for moderate to severe vitiligo. It appears to be safe in children and is reasonably effective. Localized, recalcitrant patches can be treated with the excimer laser, which emits light in a very similar wavelength to the narrow-band UVB light box (308 nm versus 311 nm). It is not as readily available as narrow-band UVB in most areas and is impractical for treatment of large surface areas. Topical calcipotriene (Dovonex) augments all forms of UV light therapy.

Depigmentation of normal skin is an extreme and permanent approach to normalizing appearance. High concentrations of hydroquinone (Benoquin) are used to bleach unaffected skin to match the vitiliginous skin. It should only be considered in those with very extensive, chronic, stable involvement and those who fully understand the permanence of this approach. This option is almost always reserved for adults who are fully able to give consent.

Localized areas that have failed all other therapies may respond to surgical grafting. This should only be performed by an experienced practitioner and will be poorly tolerated by very young children. It has proven to be safe, but scarring is a possible result.

It is important to be sensitive to the emotional needs of patients and families. Referral to the National Vitiligo Foundation (www.nvfi.org) is helpful for chronically involved patients.

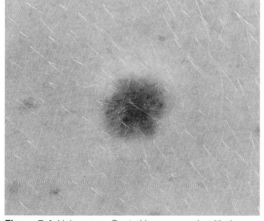

Figure 7-4 Halo nevus. Central brown papule with rim (halo) of depigmentation

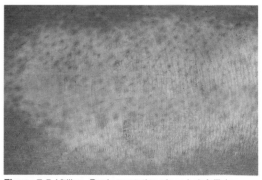

Figure 7-5 Vitiligo. Repigmentation along hair follicles giving a dotted appearance

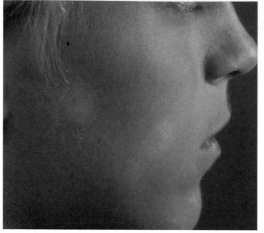

Figure 7-6 Pityriasis alba. Ill-defined hypopigmented macules on the cheek

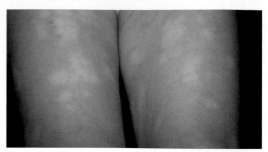

Figure 7-7 Postinflammatory hypopigmentation. White patches on the thighs of a darkly pigmented child with active atopic dermatitis

Pityriasis Alba/ Postinflammatory Hypopigmentation

Key Points

- Ill-defined hypopigmentation
- Treatment with low-potency topical steroids or topical immunomodulators

Clinical presentation

Pityriasis alba is an extremely common condition in children 3–16 years of age consisting of ill-defined, 1–3-cm circular or oval patches, sometimes with a fine scale. Cheeks (Figure 7-6) are the classic location, but the rest of the face, neck, arms, and trunk may be involved. Patches may itch slightly but usually patients' primary concern is the cosmetic appearance and the fear that they may have vitiligo. Many children with pityriasis alba have associated atopic dermatitis but this is variable.

Postinflammatory hypopigmentation has a very similar appearance to pityriasis alba and there may be some overlap between the two. Hypopigmented patches may appear anywhere on the body and occur after any inflammatory skin condition, including atopic dermatitis, psoriasis, bullous diseases, injuries such as burns, and many others. It will be noted more regularly in dark-skinned individuals (Figure 7-7) and may go totally unnoticed in pale Caucasians during the winter.

Diagnosis

Both conditions tend to be fairly obvious clinically, and the differential diagnosis is much the same as for vitiligo. Woods light examination may make the patches a little easier to see but will not give the stark contrast seen with vitiligo. Persistent hypopigmentation, lasting many months, should be biopsied to rule out cutaneous T-cell lymphoma (mycosis fungoides), although this is quite uncommon in children.

Pathophysiology

The pathophysiology is not known. Pityriasis alba may simply be a unique clinical manifestation of dermatitis. Inflammatory conditions of the skin may damage keratinocytes, making them temporarily unable to accept pigment-containing melanosomes from melanocytes.

Treatment

Low-potency topical steroids and topical immuno-modulators (tacrolimus and pimecrolimus) are the mainstays of therapy. Frequent application of emollients and avoidance of harsh soaps may also be helpful. If the primary cause of the pigmentary change causing postinflammatory hypopigmentation has completely resolved, time will result in restoration of color. Repigmentation takes several weeks.

Striae (Striae Distensae, Striae Atrophicae)

Key Points

- White or red linear atrophy perpendicular to skin tension lines
- Very common in teenagers
- Associated with obesity, weight lifting, Cushing syndrome, Marfan syndrome, steroid use, anorexia nervosa

Clinical presentation

Striae are linear, atrophic lesions located perpendicular to skin tension lines. They may be several centimeters long with color progression from red to purple to white as they mature. They tend to occur on the thighs, buttocks, and breasts of girls and the thighs and low back of boys during puberty (Figure 7-8). They are common in the general adolescent population, affecting at least 1 in 3 girls and 1 in 7 boys.

Less commonly, striae may be seen in states of endogenous or exogenous corticosteroid excess. They are large and widely distributed in Cushing syndrome and will be accompanied by other stigmata such as growth retardation, hypertension, truncal obesity, weakness, fatigue, telangiectasia, hirsutism, acne, bruising, hyperpigmentation, and acanthosis nigricans. Topical steroids, particularly superpotent steroids under occlusion, can lead to striae. Striae on tall, lanky individuals with long spindly fingers suggest Marfan syndrome. The appearance of striae in females far below ideal body weight suggests anorexia nervosa.

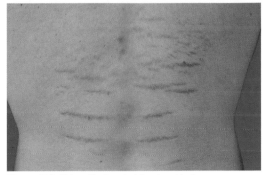

Figure 7-8 Striae. Red and white atrophic lines perpendicular to skin tension lines on the back of a teenage boy

Diagnosis

Striae are an easy clinical diagnosis, although teenagers and parents are often amazed by this diagnostic conclusion. Cushing disease should be suspected if the above signs or symptoms are present, but a work-up does not need to be done for the average teenager with stretch marks. Striae have been mistaken for whip marks and child abuse.

Pathophysiology

Striae are seldom seen before puberty, even with corticosteroid use, suggesting that there is a hormonal component. Genetics probably plays a role since there is a familial predisposition. Inflammatory-induced collagen and elastin damage followed by scar-like healing is an interesting hypothesis for striae formation.

Treatment

No treatment is very effective. Topical tretinoin 0.1% cream has offered some modest improvement but can be irritating. Pulsed-dye laser set at low fluences in lightly pigmented individuals may be helpful. Typical teenage striae tend to improve over time, naturally fading from pink to flesh-colored, and generally disappear without treatment.

Lichen Sclerosus

Key Points

- Cigarette paper wrinkling, hypopigmentation, atrophy in a figure-of-eight pattern of the perivulvar and perianal area
- Must differentiate from child abuse
- Treat with high-potency topical steroid

Clinical presentation

Lichen sclerosus (previously known as lichen sclerosus et atrophicus or LSA) is predominantly a condition of the female vulvar and perianal areas. Girls outnumber boys by about 10:1 and the genital region is involved about 90% of the time. Prevalence is about 0.1–0.2% but may be higher due to underdiagnosis.

Soreness and itching in the vulvar area are the most common presenting symptoms. Dysuria is common, and pain with defecation may lead to constipation. Boys may develop phimosis and urinary obstruction. About 10% of cases are asymptomatic. Extragenital lesions occur most commonly on the neck, trunk, shoulders, and arms and are usually asymptomatic. A relapsing and remitting course is characteristic and there is no correlation between the extent of skin lesions and the severity of symptoms.

Examination characteristically shows hypopigmentation and atrophy ("cigarette paper wrinkling") in a sharply defined figure-of-eight or hourglass pattern around the perivulvar and perianal areas, although early lesions will be more sclerotic or indurated. Erythema, hyperkeratotic scaling, fissures, telangiectasia, purpura (Figure 7-9), and scarring are often present and there may be fusion of the labia. Phimosis may be the only physical sign in boys. Extragenital skin shows guttate macules and patches with fine wrinkling (Figure 7-10).

Improvement with the onset of puberty is common but total spontaneous resolution is probably not as universal as once thought, occurring in only 7–25% of individuals.

Diagnosis

A biopsy is diagnostic but is best avoided in young children in whom a clinical diagnosis can usually be made. Vitiligo is the most difficult differential diagnosis, especially if there are no patches elsewhere. The symptomatic nature of the eruption and associated atrophy strongly suggest lichen sclerosus. Because it may present with purpura and pain, child abuse has been misdiagnosed in girls with lichen sclerosus, sometimes with disastrous consequences. Atopic dermatitis, psoriasis, seborrheic dermatitis,

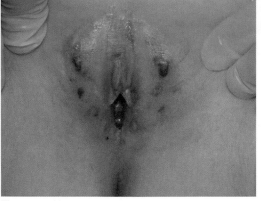

Figure 7-9 Lichen sclerosus. Hypopigmentation, atrophy, erosions, and purpura on the vulvar area

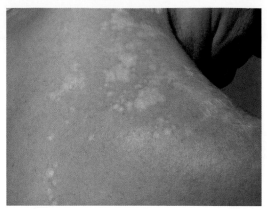

Figure 7-10 Lichen sclerosus. Guttate hypopigmented macules with "cigarette paper" wrinkling

candidiasis, perianal *Streptococcus*, and pinworms all enter into the differential diagnosis. Extragenital lichen sclerosus may look exactly like morphea, and the similarity in their histologic appearance has led some to believe that they are a spectrum of the same disease entity.

Pathophysiology

The cause of lichen sclerosus is unknown. Familial occurrence and association with certain human leukocyte antigen subtypes suggest a genetic component. A personal or family history of autoimmune diseases or presence of autoantibodies suggests that autoimmunity plays a role. The target antigen may be extracellular matrix protein 1 (ECM-1), the same protein that is abnormal in autosomal-recessive lipoid proteinosis. Infection may be an inciting event in a genetically predisposed individual.

Treatment

The response to superpotent topical steroids is very satisfying. Clobetasol propionate, usually in an ointment base, is applied twice daily for several weeks and then as needed thereafter. Surprisingly few side-effects are noted given the intertriginous location and the atrophy that is already present from the underlying condition. A lower-potency steroid or bland emollient can be used once symptoms are adequately controlled, or tacrolimus and pimecrolimus can be used as steroid-sparing agents. Topical estrogen or testosterone creams, touted in the past, are ineffective and may be systemically absorbed. Topical retinoids have shown some efficacy but irritancy limits their use.

Nevus Anemicus

Nevus anemicus is a vascular anomaly that results in a white spot on the skin. It is usually congenital and occurs in up to 1% of the normal population

and 8% of those with port-wine stains. It occurs more frequently in those with neurofibromatosis. There is a slight female predominance. Lesions consist of a well-defined, round to oval white patch, usually located on the upper trunk, neck, and upper arms (Figure 7-11). About half have multiple lesions.

Nevus anemicus results from abnormal vascular tone where blood vessels fail to dilate in response to vasodilatory stimuli. It is postulated that there is increased local hypersensitivity of the α-adrenergic receptor sites of the cutaneous blood vessels to catecholamines. This leads to vasoconstriction and the resultant pallor. The diagnosis can be confirmed by blanching the surrounding skin with a glass slide (diascopy) and noting that the border between white and normal skin disappears. No treatment is available or necessary.

Genetic Pigmentary Loss

Focal or diffuse pigmentation loss is a phenotype for a number of genetic conditions. The entities mentioned below are by no means comprehensive.

Oculocutaneous albinism (OCA) refers to a group of disorders characterized by diffusely decreased or absent pigmentation of the skin, hair, and eyes resulting from abnormal melanin synthesis (Figure 7-12). There is a significantly increased risk of sunburn and skin cancer as well as social stigmatism. Nystagmus, photophobia, decreased acuity, strabismus, and blue/grey/yellow iris color are seen in variable degrees depending on the type of OCA. Almost all are inherited in an autosomal-recessive fashion.

OCA1A is the classic form of albinism and results from the total absence of the enzyme tyrosinase. Variants of OCA1 have decreased levels of tyrosinase and are more mildly affected. OCA2 is the most common variety and results from mutations in the pink-eyed dilution protein

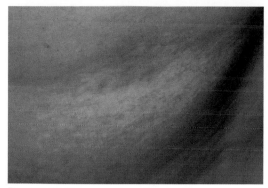

Figure 7-11 Nevus anemicus. Geographic hypopigmented patch that will match the color of the surrounding skin when blanched with a microscope slide (diascopy)

(P-protein). It occurs in about 1:15 000 of those with African skin, resulting in cream-colored to pink skin with multiple nevi and blue/yellow irides. OCA3 is characterized by reddish hair and red/brown skin. It results from a mutation in the tyrosinase-related protein 1 gene. OCA4 is phenotypically like OCA2 but is caused by an abnormality in the membrane-associated transporter protein gene.

Piebaldism is an autosomal-dominant condition caused by mutations in the c-kit proto-oncogene resulting in abnormal melanocyte embryogenesis and migration, leading to nonpigmented rather than depigmented areas. Geographic nonpigmented patches are noted on the mid-face, neck, and trunk and around the elbows and knees. Hyperpigmented islands within the depigmented areas or at the borders of nonpigmented areas may be seen. A white forelock is characteristic (Figure 7-13). Affected individuals are otherwise well, whereas children with *Waardenburg syndrome* have a similar pattern of nonpigmentation associated with deafness, a broad nasal root, irides of different color (heterochromia irides), widely spaced eyes (dystopia canthorum), or Hirschsprung disease.

Mosaic pigment abnormality (linear and whorled nevoid hypo-/hypermelanosis) is the generic name given to whorls of hypo- or hyperpigmentation following the lines of Blaschko (Figure 7-14 and 7-15). A sharp midline demarcation usually exists to the streaky pigment abnormality, which may be congenital or acquired in the first several years of life. The disorder is probably polygenic and results from a harmless postzygotic mutation in, as yet, unknown genes. It is sometimes seen in children of mixed racial parents. Children are most often otherwise well but various orthopedic, ophthalmologic, dental, and neurologic abnormalities are occasionally seen. These abnormalities in association with hypopigmentation are sometimes grouped into the entity known as hypomelanosis of Ito.

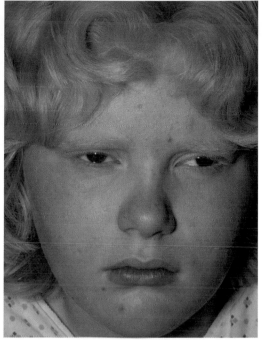

Figure 7-12 Albinism. Mildly affected girl with very light skin and hair pigment

Disorders of Hyperpigmentation

The disorders of hyperpigmentation involve another broad and varied differential diagnosis (Box 7-2). The most common entities are discussed below.

Café Au Lait Macules (CALM)

Key Points
• Uniform, brown macules or patches
• Very common to have one or two
• Multiple lesions suggest neurofibromatosis

Clinical presentation

CALM are sharply marginated, discrete, round, oval or geographic, uniformly pigmented macules (Figure 7-16). Color varies from light to dark brown. They can range in size from several millimeters to many centimeters. They are commonly located on the buttock of newborns but usually occur on the trunk of older children.

One or two CALM are quite common in the general population, somewhat more so for darkly skinned individuals. They are present in roughly 1% of newborns, 25% of children 1 month to 5 years of age, and 25–35% of school-aged children. Prevalence decreases in adults.

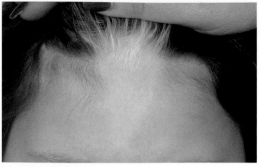

Figure 7-13 Piebaldism. Characteristic white forelock

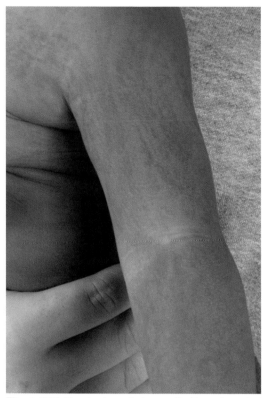

Figure 7-14 Mosaic pigment abnormality. Hypopigmented streaks on the shoulder and arm

Differential diagnosis of hyperpigmentation

Diffuse hyperpigmentation

Addison disease

Cushing syndrome

Hypo- or hyperthyroidism

Chronic hepatitis

Hemochromatosis

Ochronosis

Chronic renal disease

Drug- or heavy-metal-induced

Metastatic malignant melanoma

Patchy hyperpigmentation

Café au lait macule

Ephelide (freckle)

Lentigo

Becker nevus/congenital smooth-muscle hamartoma

Mongolian spot

Nevus of Ota/Ito

Junctional (flat) melanocytic nevus

Postinflammatory hyperpigmentation

Tinea versicolor

Melasma

Drug-induced

Incontinentia pigmenti (third stage)

Morphea

Urticaria pigmentosa (early)

Mosaic (whorled) hypopigmentation

Phytophotodermatitis

Erythema dyschromicum perstans (ashy dermatosis)

Reticulated hyperpigmentation

Tinea versicolor

Retained keratin (terra firma)

Erythema ab igne

Reticulated and confluent papillomatosis

Reticulated acropigmentation of Kitamura

Dowling–Degos disease

Dyskeratosis congenita

Naegeli–Franceschetti–Jadassohn syndrome

Hidrotic ectodermal dysplasia (Clouston syndrome)

Having multiple CALM is not common in the general population. Five or more, greater than 0.5 cm in size is highly suggestive of neurofibromatosis type 1 (NF-1) or autosomal-dominant familial CALM (previously NF-6), but multiple CALM can be totally unassociated with any underlying condition. Large, geographic CALM with a "coast of Maine" appearance may be associated with precocious puberty or other endocrinopathy and fibrous dysplasia of the bone indicative of McCune–Albright syndrome. Many other syndromes are purportedly associated with CALM, but aside from NF-2, none of them has a prevalence of CALM greater than the population as a whole.

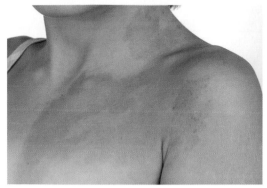

Figure 7-15 Mosaic pigment abnormality. Segmental hyperpigmentation with a sharp midline demarcation

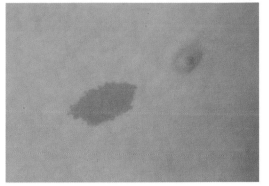

Figure 7-16 Café au lait macule. Sharply marginated, discrete, oval, geographic, uniformly pigmented patch

Diagnosis

CALM are easily diagnosed clinically. Lentigines, congenital nevi, nevus spilus, Becker nevus, and mosaic pigment abnormality enter the differential diagnosis. Pathology shows an increase in melanin without melanocytic proliferation. Giant melanosomes may be seen but are not helpful diagnostically for any particular CALM association.

Children with multiple CALM should have periodic ophthalmologic exams, close follow-up of neurodevelopmental progress, and skin exams to see if stigmata of NF-1 develop. Plain X-rays and follow-up for endocrinologic disorders are warranted for children with large segmental CALM with jagged borders suggesting McCune–Albright syndrome.

Treatment

Treatment is not necessary. Those wishing cosmetic improvement can be treated with any one of a number of pigmented lesion lasers but results are variable and recurrence is common. Cover-up makeup may be appropriate.

Freckles (Ephelides) and Lentigines

Freckles are light brown, well-circumscribed small macules found on sun-exposed skin of lightly pigmented children (Figure 7-17). They are the result of pigment release from existing melanocytes. They darken in the summer with UV light exposure and lighten or disappear in the winter. They are not associated with any syndromes but are a marker for individuals at increased risk of developing malignant melanoma.

Lentigines (singular is lentigo) are darker and bigger than freckles but smaller than CALM (Figure 7-18). They are the result of hyperplasia of melanocytes. They may be located anywhere on the body and are not affected by sunlight. They may

be an incidental finding but there are a number of syndromes associated with lentigines (Table 7-1). with which the practitioner should be aware.

Freckles and lentigines do not need to be treated but respond well to laser and, less so, light cryotherapy. Sun avoidance is important for improvement of freckles.

Morphea (Localized Scleroderma)

Key Points

- Hard, sclerotic skin
- Linear distribution most common
- Disabling disease treated with methotrexate

Clinical presentation

Morphea is an inflammatory condition, primarily of the dermis and subcutaneous fat, that leads to scar-like, bound-down, sclerotic skin. The name localized scleroderma is used synonymously with morphea but is confusing to patients and parents who will research scleroderma and discover systemic associations not encountered in morphea.

The prevalence of morphea is about 1 per 2000 in those under age 18 years, and girls outnumber boys by about 2.5:1. Mean age of onset is about 7 years, and most children are not correctly diagnosed until the disease has been present for 1–2 years. A precipitating trigger event is noted in 13% of cases. Local trauma such as an accident, bite, or injection leads the list but infections, medications, and psychological stress are sometimes mentioned.

Typical lesions of morphea begin insidiously as an asymptomatic, erythematous to violaceous patch or plaque that becomes shiny, hard, and indurated (sclerotic). As hardening progresses, the plaque becomes brown with violaceous borders. Hypopigmentation may supervene,

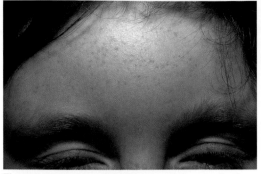

Figure 7-17 Freckles. Light brown, well-circumscribed small macules on sun-exposed skin of a red-haired child

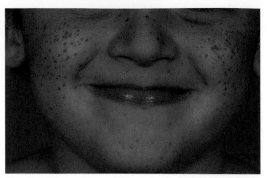

Figure 7-18 Lentigines. Multiple brown facial macules with darker color than a freckle

Table 7-1 Conditions associated with multiple lentigines

Syndrome	Location of lentigines	Gene	Other findings
Bannayan–Ruvalcaba	Penis	PTEN	Microcephaly, lipomas
Centrofacial neurodysraphic lentiginosis	Central face	Unknown	Mental retardation
Peutz–Jeghers	Buccal mucosa, lips, digits	STK11	GI polyposis
LEOPARD	Neck, upper trunk, generalized	PTPN11	ECG abnormalities, hypertelorism, pulmonary stenosis, abnormal genitalia, retarded growth, deafness
Carney complex (NAME, LAMB)	Generalized	PRKAR1A	Cardiac, cutaneous, endocrine, and neural myxomatous tumors, multiple endocrine neoplasia, many cutaneous pigmented lesions

ECG, electrocardiogram; GI, gastrointestinal.

looking much like lichen sclerosus (Figure 7-19). Hair and other adnexal structures such as sweat glands completely disappear.

Various distributions and patterns have been described. *Linear morphea* is the most common variety, accounting for 65% of childhood morphea (Figure 7-20). This occurs mostly on the extremities but can be located on the trunk and face. Significant debility accompanies sclerotic plaques over joints, resulting in limited mobility and contractures, and this problematic location requires aggressive treatment. Fat, muscle, and bone can become atrophic. When linear morphea appears over the frontoparietal region of the forehead it is called *en coup de sabre* since it resembles the blow of a sword (Figure 7-21). A faint violaceous erythema precedes the sclerotic phase by several months. Central nervous symptoms including headaches and seizures and various eye abnormalities may accompany this condition. Scarring alopecia and severe facial deformity are unfortunate sequelae. The *Parry–Romberg syndrome* (progressive facial hemiatrophy) is considered to be a variant of en coup de sabre since both may appear simultaneously in a single patient. Significant muscle and fat atrophy occurs unilaterally in a trigeminal distribution (Figure 7-22). Trigeminal neuralgia, along with other central nervous system, ocular, and oral abnormalities may be seen.

Plaque morphea, the most common adult variant, accounts for about 25% of childhood cases. The trunk is the most common location but anywhere on the body can be affected with plaques of several centimeters in size (Figure 7-23). The presence of numerous large plaques in different anatomic locations is referred to as *generalized morphea*, a rare variant in childhood. Numerous small plaques are called *guttate morphea*. Many believe that *atrophoderma of Pasini and Pierini* is a variant of plaque morphea that occurs mainly on the back of young women. Atrophy, rather than induration, is the main clinical finding, resulting in a "cliff drop" at the edge of the brown-to-violaceous patch. About 15% of patients will have more than one form of morphea simultaneously.

Most variants of morphea will burn out over time, 2–3 years for plaque morphea and 3–7 years for linear morphea. At best, there will be

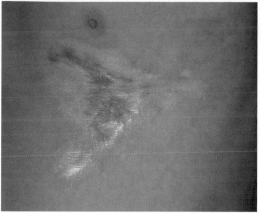

Figure 7-19 Morphea. Bound-down, indurated skin on the chest wall with hyperpigmented center and lichen sclerosus-like peripheral hypopigmentation

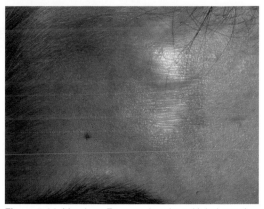

Figure 7-21 Morphea. En coup de sabre with indurated plaque extending through the lateral forehead

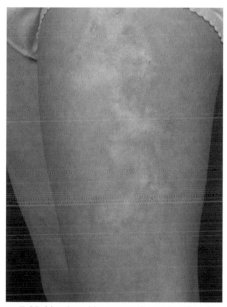

Figure 7-20 Morphea. Linear morphea extending the length of the lateral thigh

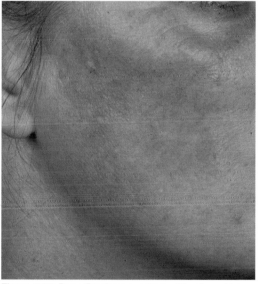

Figure 7-22 Parry–Romberg syndrome. Muscle and fat atrophy in a trigeminal distribution

mild residual hyper- or hypopigmentation, but permanent deformity, atrophy, and contracture can be disabling sequelae.

Diagnosis

Morphea is usually diagnosed clinically by its appearance and feel. Bound-down, hard, sclerotic skin with overlying hypo- or hyperpigmentation with a peripheral violaceous erythema is characteristic. A punch biopsy will confirm the diagnosis. Laboratory studies are not helpful in establishing the diagnosis. Antinuclear antibody is positive in about 40% but is not predictive of any associated complications, whereas rheumatoid

factor is positive in about 15% and correlates highly with those who have arthritis. Although the condition can be widespread, morphea does not typically progress to systemic sclerosis and parents should be reassured that this localized disease does not have the same poor prognosis as systemic sclerosis.

Morphea can be differentiated from the induration of cellulitis by its chronicity, lack of warmth and erythema, and lack of infectious symptoms. Early, nonindurated morphea may look like postinflammatory hyperpigmentation. Indurated or atrophic injection sites may have a morpheaform look. Lesions of lichen sclerosus overlap significantly in appearance with morphea and some have suggested that they are variants of the same condition. Morphea must be differentiated from progressive systemic sclerosis (scleroderma) which has Raynaud phenomenon, sclerodactyly, capillary loop abnormalities, and multiple systemic problems.

Pathophysiology

The cause of morphea is not known. There is evidence that abnormal collagen deposition results from fibroblast activation via T-cell-derived interleukin-4 and transforming growth factor-alpha. The presence of autoantibodies and the female predominance suggest an autoimmune mechanism. Twin studies do not seem to support a genetic basis, although the segmental nature of the condition suggests a possible postzygotic mutation that plants a seed of genetically susceptible cells that are triggered by some external stimulus.

Treatment

Small, nondeforming plaques of morphea do not need to be treated and will burn out over the course of years. Potent topical steroids and calcipotriene have been used successfully for mild disease. There is some evidence that oral calcitriol may be effective. Intralesional triamcinolone is a safe method of treating localized lesions. Physically or cosmetically debilitating lesions require aggressive treatment and methotrexate at doses of 0.5–1 mg/kg per week is now considered the treatment of choice. Systemic steroids, either as monthly intravenous pulses or oral prednisone, are usually added, especially for progressive disease. UVA1 phototherapy can be effective, but these photo units are not as readily available as other forms of light therapy. PUVA can be considered for those refractory to methotrexate. Patients with joint involvement should receive physical therapy to maintain full range of motion. Surgical repair or injection of fillers can be performed once the process has burnt out.

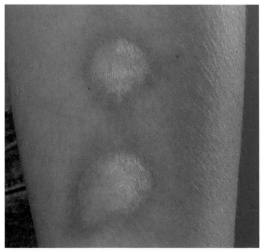

Figure 7-23 Morphea. Plaque morphea on an extremity

Becker Nevus

Key Points

- Scapula, shoulder, chest of teenage boys
- Brown, pebbly with hypertrichosis

Clinical presentation

Becker nevus classically appears in adolescence and is more common among males, although young children and females have also been reported. Sun exposure will sometimes precede its appearance. The shoulder, scapula, and chest are the most common areas of involvement but it can be seen in any body area. A tan to dark brown expanding patch, ranging from a few to several centimeters in size, eventually develops a pebbly texture (Figure 7-24). Dark hairs develop that become longer and coarser with time. The color may fade in adult years but the hypertrichosis remains. Affected individuals are otherwise well but there are reports of associated ipsilateral breast hypoplasia, arm shortening, pectus carinatum (pigeon breast), spina bifida, and scoliosis – the so-called Becker nevus syndrome.

Diagnosis

Becker nevus is most commonly mistaken for a large congenital melanocytic nevus. The acquired nature of a Becker nevus is a helpful diagnostic feature, but a biopsy will distinguish the two entities. The large plexiform neurofibromas of neurofibromatosis will have more bulk mass and a "bag of worms" feel on palpation.

Pathophysiology

The cause of a Becker nevus is unknown but it probably represents a postzygotic mutation, similar to other hamartomatous processes, and it may be part of a spectrum of congenital smooth-muscle hamartoma. The male predominance, the frequent onset during puberty, and the development of coarse terminal hairs suggest that there is a heightened sensitivity to androgenic hormones.

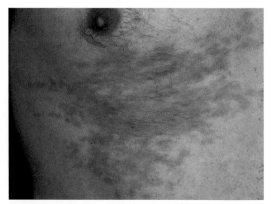

Figure 7-24 Becker nevus. Brown, pebbly patch with hypertrichosis

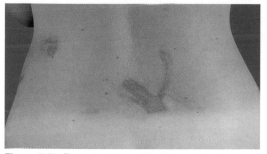

Figure 7-25 Phytophotodermatitis. Bizarre, streaky hyperpigmentation that stops at the bathing-suit line

Figure 7-26 Retained keratin (terra firma). Reticulated hyperpigmentation in the concavity of the intrascapular area

BOX 7-3

Plants that contain furocoumarins causing phytophotodermatitis

Lime

Lemon

Orange

Grapefruit

Carrot

Bergamot

Parsnips

Celery

Cow parsley

Giant hogweed

Wild rhubarb

Pigweed

Fennel

Natural grasses

Sagebrush

Goldenrod

Chrysanthemum

Ragweed

Cocklebur

Tobacco

Fig

Hot pepper

Hyacinth

Daffodil bulb

Buttercups

Shepherd's purse

Burning bush

Angelica

Treatment

Becker nevi are harmless growths that do not require treatment except for cosmetic purposes. Lasers have had variable success at removing the hyperpigmentation and recurrence is common even when laser therapy is successful. Laser can nicely remove the hair, which is a particular cosmetic concern for affected girls. Cover-up makeup, waxing, shaving, and electrolysis are other alternatives. Surgical excision is rarely appropriate and will result in very unacceptable scarring.

Phytophotodermatitis

Key Points

* Bizarre, streaky hyperpigmentation
* Furocoumarin-containing plants and sunlight

Clinical presentation

Phytophotodermatitis refers to the eruption that results from the interaction of furocoumarin-containing plant material with UV light. The phototoxic reaction first manifests with erythema in about 12–24 hours and, depending on the degree of exposure, vesiculation like a severe sunburn in 72 hours. Desquamation is followed by prolonged hyperpigmentation that takes several months to fade. The pattern of hyperpigmentation is asymmetric, streaky, and bizarre in configuration, strongly suggesting an external contact with the skin (Figure 7-25). Dribbling of juice on the skin will give a streaky, linear array, and a perfect hand print may be seen on a child's torso if the hand of a parent is coated with the furocoumarin-containing material, such as lime juice.

The most common plant offenders (Box 7-3) are from the Rutaceae family (citrus fruits) and the Apiaceae family (parsley, celery, fennel, parsnip). Limes contain five furocoumarins, with most being in the rind rather than the juicy pulp. A common history is that the family was making limeade or mixed drinks during the summer or in the tropics.

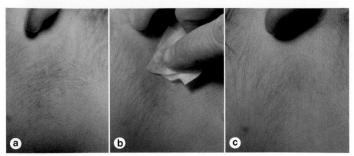

Figure 7-27 Retained keratin (terra firma). Hyperpigmentation behind the ear clears completely away with an alcohol swab

Diagnosis

The bizarre patterning will usually suggest the correct diagnosis. A scald injury or allergic contact dermatitis may enter into the differential diagnosis. The hyperpigmentation may look like a bruise but does not go through the color changes and usual life cycle of a typical bruise. Child abuse has been mistakenly diagnosed in cases of phytophotodermatitis, particularly when hand prints are seen.

Pathophysiology

UVA (wavelength 320–400 nm) irradiation combined with the plant-derived furocoumarins causes skin damage via two mechanisms. The type I reaction is independent of oxygen and forms aberrant cross-links in cellular DNA. The type II reaction results in the generation of oxygen free radicals, resulting in cell membrane damage. A heightened UV light-induced melanocyte response accounts for the prolonged hyperpigmentation.

Treatment

There is no specific treatment for phytophotodermatitis but eventually the eruption fades and disappears without scarring. Blistering is managed much the same as a sunburn with analgesics, antihistamines, and cool compresses. Prevention in the form of thorough washing after a suspected contact is the best approach.

Reticulated Pigmentary Anomalies

Retained keratin, sometimes referred to by its more whimsical name of *terra firma*, refers to asymptomatic, rough, brown, slightly hyperkeratotic patches that look like dirt. It favors concavities and is most commonly seen behind the ears (perhaps this is the origin of the question, "Did you wash behind your ears?"). It may also be seen in the central chest, intrascapular area (Figure 7-26), and brachial fossa. Parents will quite accurately insist that they cannot remove the pigmentation with cleansing, even very vigorous use of soap and water. They are usually amazed when

it wipes clean with an alcohol pad (Figure 7-27), and rubbing alcohol on a cotton ball forms the treatment of choice. Acanthosis nigricans is the main differential diagnosis, but this condition forms lower down on the neck than retained keratin and will not wipe away with alcohol.

Erythema ab igne occurs after chronic, low-level exposure to heat. Heating pads and hot-water bottles are classic causes, but fireplaces, wood-burning stoves, radiators, laptops, and several other sources of heat have been reported. Reticulated, blanching erythema eventually gives way to nonblanching hyperpigmentation (Figure 7-28). The location corresponds directly to the area of heat exposure. Cutis marmorata or cutis marmorata telangiectasia congenita may enter into the differential diagnosis but a careful history will usually clear any confusion in diagnosis. Treatment entails removing the source of heat.

Reticulated and confluent papillomatosis (of Gougerot and Carteaud) is an uncommon papulosquamous eruption, affecting mostly teenagers and young adults. About twice as many females are affected as males and there may be an increased incidence in African skin, although all races are affected. Asymptomatic, small, slightly verrucous, hyperpigmented papules coalesce into confluent plaques in the middle of the chest and back and reticulated plaques in the axillae and flanks (Figure 7-29). It can look very much like tinea versicolor, but a potassium hydroxide scraping will distinguish the two entities. Other reticulate or papulosquamous hyperpigmented conditions that enter the differential diagnosis include epidermodysplasia verruciformis, seborrheic dermatitis, dyskeratosis congenita, extensive acanthosis nigricans, and Dowling–Degos disease. A biopsy may be needed to rule out these entities.

The pathophysiology of reticulated and confluent papillomatosis is unknown, although most theories point to some abnormality in keratinization, perhaps as a nonspecific reaction to multiple stimuli such as bacterial or yeast infections of the skin. There is a perplexing array of treatment modalities that claim successful clearance of the condition, including topical and systemic retinoids, topical and systemic antifungal agents, various systemic antibacterial agents, liquid nitrogen, UV light, low-voltage radiation, calcipotriol, salicylic acid, urea, ammonium lactate, 5-fluorouracil ointment, coal tar, hydroquinone, and thyroid extract. Minocycline, with doses ranging from 50 mg daily to 100 mg twice daily, has surfaced as the treatment of choice.

Melanocytic nevi (Moles)

Key Points

- Most pediatric moles are harmless
- Halo nevi, blue nevi, scalp nevi behave harmlessly but have an unusual appearance
- Spitz nevi may be misinterpreted histopathologically as melanoma but are benign
- ABCDE criteria help clinically differentiate atypical moles and melanoma from benign moles
- Congenital moles occur in 1% of the population and are harmless
- Large and giant congenital moles are rare and potentially dangerous

Moles are seen in about 1% of newborns and are universally seen in older children and adolescents. Practitioners must be adept in correctly diagnosing

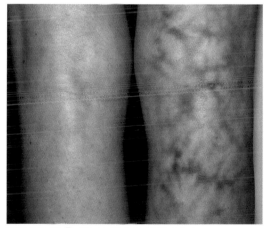

Figure 7-28 Erythema ab igne. Reticulated hyperpigmentation on the right leg where a hot-water bottle had been chronically used

and treating (or, more commonly, not treating) these lesions and must cope with daily decisions regarding removal, biopsy, observation, or simple reassurance.

The number of moles among individuals varies greatly. An increased number is seen in those with light-colored skin and hair, those with more sun exposure or sunburns, and those with a family history of large numbers of moles. More moles are seen in those with leukemia, chemotherapy, and immunosuppression for organ transplantation. The average number of moles ranges from 3–5 in preschool years to 20–30 in adolescence. Peak number is reached in the third decade, with a slow waning after 40 years of age.

Many acquired moles will traverse a life cycle of early *junctional* nevi (flat, light brown/black macules) to *compound* nevi (slightly raised with smooth or warty surface) to *intradermal* nevi (dome-shaped or pedunculated fleshy papules), although there is little to be gained by making this clinical distinction (Figure 7-30). In general, they will have good symmetry, sharp borders, uniform brown color, diameter of 6 mm or less, and will not be rapidly enlarging or changing (ABCDE rule – asymmetry, border, color, diameter, evolution) which distinguishes them from atypical nevi or malignant melanoma. Diagnosis is usually straightforward.

Treatment is seldom needed, although cosmetic concerns or intermittent trauma from rubbing may prompt removal. Shave excision after local anesthesia is simple and usually leaves a very acceptable result. Common-sense judgment is needed in the evaluation for malignant melanoma. Since the incidence of melanoma is about one in a million in prepubertal children, clinicians need not panic over minor atypical features, opting instead to follow lesions with serial exams and photography. The possibility for melanoma becomes more believable in teenage years but remains very rare so a slightly to moderately unusual mole might be followed clinically whereas the same mole might be removed more quickly in an adult. Any mole removed for any reason must be sent for pathologic review. A complete excision must be done in those removed for the possibility for melanoma.

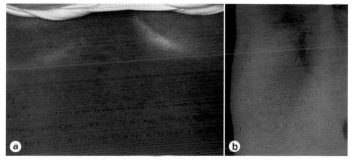

Figure 7-29 Reticulated and confluent papillomatosis (of Gougerot and Carteaud)

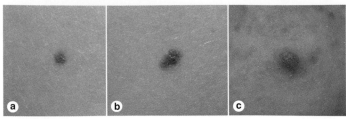

Figure 7-30 Nevi. Left to right: junctional, compound, and intradermal nevi

A few variants of melanocytic nevi deserve special mention. A *blue nevus* is a macule or papule with deep blue/black color (Figure 7-31). that can be congenital or acquired. It looks much like a graphite pencil tattoo but can also have a very ominous appearance. Its static nature is reassuring and simple observation is most often appropriate. If it is to be removed, it must be done by deep punch or elliptical excision since a shave will not approach the deep margin.

Halo nevi may be seen alone or in conjunction with vitiligo. A rim of hypo- or depigmentation is seen surrounding a pigmented macule or papule (Figure 7-4). Many halo nevi may be seen in the same patient. They are felt to represent an immunologic response to a melanocytic nevus, and the nevus will slowly resorb over the course of many years with return of the normal skin pigmentation. Regression within a melanoma must be considered in adults with this finding but halo nevi are considered a common, benign entity in childhood.

Scalp nevi tend to have a characteristic ring of hyperpigmentation at their periphery and have been referred to as "eclipse nevi" (Figure 7-32). Their larger size and the doughnut-like irregularity of the pigment tend to raise concerns among parents who may be noticing the mole for the first time after a haircut. The pathologist may interpret their histology as atypical, which can add to the confusion. They are harmless and are best left alone.

The *Spitz nevus* may be the most confusing of all the variants, as illustrated by its somewhat oxymoronic synonym of benign juvenile melanoma. The typical Spitz nevus is an innocuous-appearing, red, sharply demarcated, dome-shaped, 5–10-mm papule (Figure 7-33). Some are easily mistaken as pyogenic granulomas. Another variety of Spitz nevus has a deeply pigmented, mottled or spiculated appearance that is much more ominous in appearance and more difficult to differentiate from a malignant melanoma (Figure 7-34). When recognized clinically, they can be left alone and followed. If removed, an experienced dermatopathologist will correctly recognize the lesion as a Spitz nevus, especially in the setting of a young child, but these lesions may be mistaken histologically for malignant melanoma, prompting unnecessary concern and

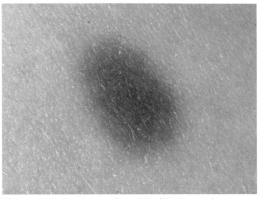

Figure 7-31 Blue nevus. Deep blue/black macule

surgical intervention. Whenever possible, any residual lesion should be completely excised to prevent future confusion and misdiagnosis should it recur at a later time.

Atypical nevi (dysplastic nevi) are another area of considerable confusion. They tend to cluster on the trunk, especially the back, but can be found in any location. Clinically they fulfill some or all of the ABCDE criteria used to assess the possibility of malignant melanoma of asymmetry, border irregularity, color variation, diameter bigger than a pencil eraser (> 6 mm), and enlargement or evolution (Figure 7-35). As such, they need to be removed if the possibility of melanoma is suspected. There are histologic criteria that must be met to be classified as an atypical nevus and the cellular atypia will be graded by the pathologist as mild, moderate, or severe. Sometimes a definite distinction from melanoma cannot be made and the clinician will need to treat the lesion as though it were a melanoma.

Clinicians struggle with what to do with a confirmed diagnosis of an atypical nevus and wonder how to explain this entity to families. At one polar end of the spectrum there is the individual studded with atypical moles (Figure 7-36). who has a strong family history of melanoma and atypical nevi. This is a patient at extraordinarily great risk, perhaps inevitability, of developing a melanoma. At the other pole is

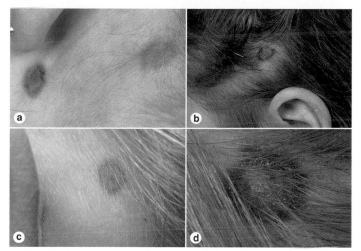

Figure 7-32 Scalp nevi. Doughnut-like ring hyperpigmentation typical of moles seen on the scalp

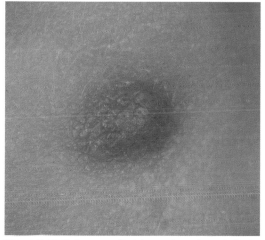

Figure 7-33 Spitz nevus. Red dome-shaped papule that was located on the earlobe

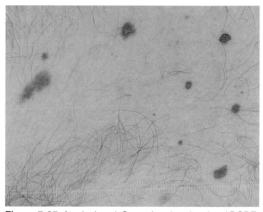

Figure 7-35 Atypical nevi. Several moles showing ABCDE criteria. Asymmetry, border irregularity, color variation, and diameter bigger than 6 mm. E is for enlarging or changing moles

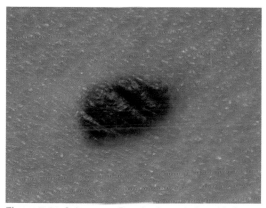

Figure 7-34 Spitz nevus. Deeply pigmented, mottled papule that is difficult to differentiate from a malignant melanoma

a patient with just one unusual mole with no family history of melanoma or atypical moles who probably has very little risk above the general population. There are countless shades of gray in between. A few points are fairly clear. An atypical mole should be completely removed because interpretation of a recurrence will be clinically and histologically difficult. At least one thorough, complete head-to-toe examination should be done and, depending on the stratification of risk factors, may be repeated on an annual basis with photographs to document the evolution of lesions. Patients must be taught self-examination skills, and very strict sun avoidance must become a lifelong practice. It should be made clear to patients that they have had neither a close brush with death nor a completely harmless lesion and that diligence without panic is required.

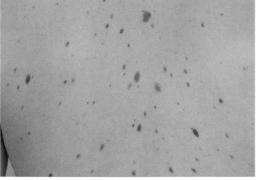

Figure 7-36 Atypical nevi. Large numbers of atypical moles in someone with familial atypical mole syndrome

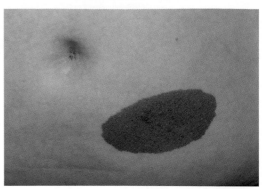

Figure 7-38 Moderate congenital nevus

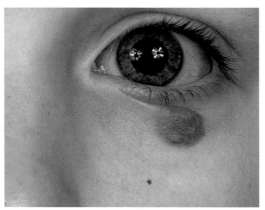

Figure 7-37 Small congenital nevus

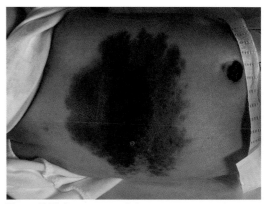

Figure 7-39 Large congenital nevus

About 1% of infants have *congenital nevi* that are present at birth or develop within the first several months of life. Most are small, less than 1.5 cm (Figure 7-37), or moderate, less than 20 cm (Figure 7-38), in size. The rules of symmetry, color, and shape are broken by almost all small and medium congenital nevi but they behave in a very harmless fashion and are cut some slack with the usual "good mole/bad mole" criteria. There may be a slightly elevated risk of malignant degeneration in adulthood compared to regular acquired nevi, perhaps simply commensurate with the increased number of melanocytes within them. Prophylactic excision to eliminate this small risk is not recommended, although some congenital nevi cause significant cosmetic disfigurement and warrant removal.

Large congenital (> 20 cm) nevi occur in 1 in 20 000 newborns, with giant congenital nevi often > 50 cm (bathing-trunk nevi) occurring far less commonly than that. These moles have substantial pigment irregularity, verrucous, convoluted surfaces, and hypertrichosis (Figure 7-39). Nodularity and ulceration may be present. These are dangerous lesions that carry significant malignant potential and, unlike small congenital

nevi, may degenerate into melanomas in the first several years of life. The risk of malignant degeneration is hotly contested but probably is about 6%, with a wide margin of error. Large lesions are often associated with smaller satellite lesions that have little risk of developing melanoma. The central nervous system may be involved – a condition called neurocutaneous melanosis. This is most common when the nevus covers the scalp, neck, or spine. It may never have any associated complications but might lead to seizures, neurologic deterioration, and central nervous system melanoma, all of which portend a very bad prognosis.

Treatment of large and giant congenital nevi is difficult at best. It is desirable to remove as much of the mole as possible but doing so without devastating scarring and poor cosmetic outcome can be difficult. Even with excision, melanoma may occur in the deep tissues or in the central nervous system so a 100% reduction of melanoma risk is impossible. Families should be referred to an experienced plastic surgeon, carefully counseled in the proven (albeit fuzzy) risks of melanoma, and then allowed to make a personal decision that they feel is best for their baby. Ongoing lifelong follow-up is necessary.

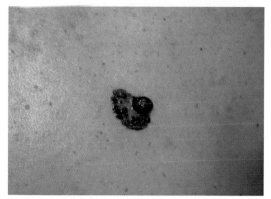

Figure 7-40 Malignant melanoma. Advanced lesion on the back

Malignant melanoma is thankfully very uncommon in the pediatric age group outside the setting of large congenital nevi. It is at least a possibility among mid to upper teen age groups. Light skin and hair, previous sun exposure and sunburns, large number of moles, presence of dysplastic moles, and family history of melanoma in a first-degree relative are all risk factors for developing melanoma. Melanomas follow the ABCDE rules that were mentioned for dysplastic nevi (Figure 7-40). and, in fact, it may be difficult clinically to tell the difference between a dysplastic nevus and a melanoma. It may develop on normal skin or within a pre-existing nevus. A biopsy specimen must be completely around and underneath the mole since prognosis and treatment are based on depth and invasiveness. An elliptical or saucerized (scoop) excision is best. Once the diagnosis is made, a wider re-excision is needed and a decision to perform sentinal lymph node analysis is made. This is best done by an experienced surgical oncologist.

Further reading

Chong WS, Klanwarin W, Giam YC. Generalized lentiginosis in two children lacking systemic associations: case report and review of the literature. Pediatr Dermatol 2004;21:139–145.

Ferrari A, Piccolo D, Fargnoli MC, et al. Does melanoma behave differently in younger children than adults? A retrospective study of 33 cases of childhood melanoma from a single institution. Pediatrics 2005;115:649–654.

Grimes PE. New insights and new therapies in vitiligo. JAMA 2005;293:730–735.

Jang H, Chang-Keun O, Cha J, et al. Six cases of confluent and reticulated papillomatosis alleviated by various antibiotics. J Am Acad Dermatol 2001; 44:652–655.

Kanzler MH. Management of large congenital melanocytic nevi: art versus science. J Am Acad Dermatol 2006;54:874–876.

Katugampola GA, Lanigan S. The clinical spectrum of naevus anaemicus and its association with port wine stains: report of 15 cases and a review of the literature. Br J Dermatol 1995;134:292–295.

Krengel S, Hauschild A, Schafer T. Melanoma risk in congenital melanocytic naevi: a systematic review. Br J Dermatol 2006;155:1–8.

Lin RL, Janniger CK. Pityriasis alba. Cutis 2005; 76:21–24.

Marghoob AA, Agero AL, Benvenuto-Andrade C, et al. Large congenital melanocytic nevi, risk of cutaneous melanoma, and prophylactic surgery. J Am Acad Dermatol 2006;54:868–870.

Silverberg NB, Travis L. Childhood vitiligo. Cutis 2006;77:370–375.

Tannous ZS. Mihm MC Jr. Sober AJ. et al. Congenital melanocytic nevi: clinical and histopathologic features, risk of melanoma, and clinical management. J Am Acad Dermatol 2005; 52:197–203.

Tasker GL, Wojnarowska F. Lichen sclerosus. Clin Exp Dermatol 2003;28:128–133.

Tollefson MM, Witman PM. En coup de sabre morphea and Parry–Romberg syndrome: a retrospective review of 54 patients. J Am Acad Dermatol 2007;56:257–263.

Uziel Y, Feldman BM, Krafchik BR, et al. Methotrexate and corticosteroid therapy for pediatric localized scleroderma. J Pediatr 2000; 136:91–95.

Val I, Almeida G. An overview of lichen sclerosus. Clin Obstet Gynecol 2005;48:808–817.

Wain EM, Smith CH. Acute severe blistering in a 24-year-old man: phytophotodermatitis, caused by contact with lime. Arch Dermatol 2006; 14: 1059–1064.

Yan AC. Smolinski KN. Melanocytic nevi: challenging clinical situations in pediatric dermatology. Adv Dermatol 2005;21:65–80.

Zulian F, Athreya BH, Laxer R, et al. Juvenile localized scleroderma: clinical and epidemiological features in 750 children. An international study. Rheumatology 2006;45:614–620.

8

Lumps and bumps

Andrea L. Zaenglein

Introduction

Recognition of lumps and bumps in the skin tends to be bipolar – the diagnosis is often either very evident or not at all clear. Important clues to diagnosis include the age of onset, color, location, firmness, overlying changes in the epidermis, and the rate of change. In the event that a clinical diagnosis cannot be made, a biopsy is usually indicated and very useful in differentiating the various possibilities. While the vast majority of lumps in the skin are benign, progressive infiltrative disorders and deadly malignancies can present as nodular lesions in the skin as well. Therefore, a solid working knowledge of lumps and bumps is vital to ensure that a proper diagnosis is made. A list of the more common lumps and bumps found in the skin is given in. Table 8-1.

Langerhans Cell Histiocytoses (LCH)

Key Points

- Persistent, petechial papules on the scalp, axillae, and groin
- Erosions in the flexures and crusted lesions on the palms
- Bone lesions common (eosinophilic granuloma)
- Diabetes insipidus may result
- Prognosis depends on the extent of vital organ involvement
- Scabies may mimic LCH clinically and histologically

Clinical presentation

The LCH are a group of disorders defined by their organs of presentation and clinical course. Both localized and severe, multiorgan variants are described. Classically the disseminated form was called Letterer–Siwe disease, while the triad of skull lesions, exophthalmos, and diabetes insipidus was known as Hand–Schuller–Christian disease. The skin is often the first organ affected in patients presenting with LCH. In some series, it is also the most common organ affected. LCH may be subtle and asymptomatic. Therefore, clinical suspicion and early recognition of the outward manifestations of LCH are vital for accurate diagnosis and prompt treatment. Skin findings include yellow to brown crusted papules, often petechial or hemorrhagic in nature, scattered in a seborrheic distribution on the scalp, creases of the axillae, and groin (Figure 8-1). As lesions coalesce, they become moist and eroded, particularly in the intertriginous areas (Figure 8-2). Oral mucosal and gingival lesions can occur and may affect dentition. Male infants are more likely to have only skin involvement. Conscientious close observation is warranted since systemic progression may occur.

Bone involvement is also common with LCH, occurring more frequently in older children and adults. Solitary lesions of LCH in the bone are called eosinophilic granuloma and typically present as bone pain or swelling. The skull is most often affected, followed by the long bones of the arms, then the flat bones of the ribs, pelvis, and vertebrae. Radiographic films show irregularly defined, single or multifocal, lytic lesions. Multiple site involvement portends a poorer prognosis. LCH can involve the mastoid bone, with extension to and obliteration of the ossicles causing subsequent deafness. Swelling and pain of the jaw may indicate mandibular involvement. When the vertebrae are affected, flattening and compression can occur.

Just about any organ can be involved with LCH. Hepatosplenomegaly is a common finding. It may be due to infiltration of Langerhans cells or obstruction from engorged regional lymph nodes, both causing biliary cirrhosis. Generalized activation of the cellular immune system, resulting in Kupffer cell hypertrophy, also results in hepatomegaly. Lung involvement typically presents with tachypnea, fever, and weight loss.

Table 8.1 Differential diagnosis of lumps and bumps	
Congenital	Encephalocele
	Dermoid cyst
	Nasal glioma
	Branchial cleft cyst
	Thyroglossal duct cyst
	Accessory tragus
Vascular	Hemangioma of infancy
	Vascular malformation (venous, AVM, lymphatic)
	Pyogenic granuloma
Inflammatory	Granuloma annulare
	Erythema nodosum
	Vasculitis
	Acne
Neoplastic	Pilomatricoma
	Juvenile xanthogranuloma
	Langerhans cell histiocytosis
	Lipoma
	Smooth-muscle hamartoma
	Dermatofibroma
	Dermatofibrosarcoma protuberans
	Recurring digital fibroma of childhood
	Infantile myofibromatosis
	Neurofibroma
	Mastocytosis
	Angiofibroma
	Syringoma
	Eccrine poroma
	Trichoepithelioma
	Nevus sebaceus
	Keratoacanthoma
	Nevus comedonicus
	Epidermal nevus
	Melanocytic nevus
	Spitz nevus
	Keloid
	Epidermoid cyst
	Steatocystoma multiplex
	Collagenoma
	Vellus hair cysts
	Osteoma cutis

Table 8.1 Differential diagnosis of lumps and bumps—cont'd	
Infectious	Wart
	Molluscum
	Nodular scabies
	Insect bite
	Cat-scratch disease
	Deep fungal infection
	Orf
	Papular urticaria
Malignant	Rhabdomyosarcoma
	Neuroblastoma
	Leukemia cutis/lymphoma
	Melanoma
	Basal cell carcinoma
	Squamous cell carcinoma
Other	Subungual exostosis

AVM, arteriovenous malformation.

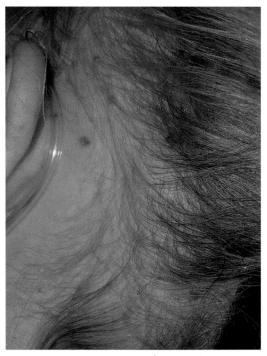

Figure 8-1 Langerhans cell histiocytosis. Classic-appearing Langerhans cell histiocytosis on the scalp of a 3-year-old girl with extensive lung involvement

A chest X-ray will show a diffuse micronodular infiltrate. Radiography can also reveal thymic enlargement. Gastrointestinal involvement may manifest as failure to thrive. Diabetes insipidus, a classic manifestation of LCH, is caused by Langerhans cell infiltration of the pituitary. Bone

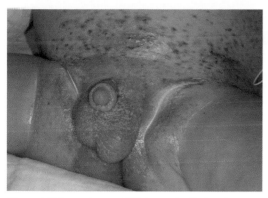

Figure 8-2 Langerhans cell histiocytosis. Red, moist persistent plaques in the groin. Note petechial hemorrhage

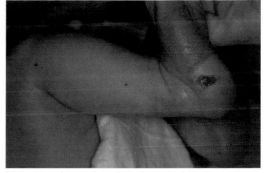

Figure 8-3 Congenital self-healing reticulohistiocytosis. Moist, exophytic nodule on the foot of a newborn

marrow dysfunction with pancytopenia portends a poor prognosis. Central nervous system involvement with intracranial hypertension, seizures, ataxia, cranial nerve defects, and dyskinesis is rare.

Congenital self-healing reticulohistiocytosis (Hashimoto–Pritzker disease) is at the benign end of the spectrum with solitary to numerous red-brown to pink papules and small nodules present in the newborn period. Some presentations may be vesicular, resembling varicella infection (Figure 8-3). The lesions resolve spontaneously over weeks to months (Figure 8-4). Systemic involvement must be ruled out, however, and an affected child should be followed closely for late progression of disease.

Diagnosis

The differential diagnosis depends on sites of involvement, but includes scabies, infantile seborrheic dermatitis, varicella or herpes infections, and the common causes of diaper dermatitis. The inflammatory disorders will typically respond to treatment whereas LCH will not. Neonates often have vesicular lesions that resemble scabies or herpetic infection, but they will not be responsive to treatment. Oil emersion examination of skin scrapings and a Tzanck smear of vesicles may aid in initial evaluation. Once suspected, however, a diagnosis of LCH should be confirmed by biopsy. The histologic infiltrate consists of CD1+, S100+ Langerhans cells with comma-shaped nuclei. Electron microscopy will reveal diagnostic tennis racquet-shaped Birbeck granules.

Pathogenesis

Langerhans cells are dendritic cells derived from the bone marrow. It is unclear what stimulates their abnormal proliferation in LCH, but infectious, genetic, immunological etiologies have all been purported.

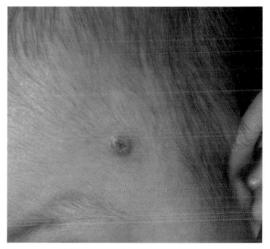

Figure 8-4 Self-healing reticulohistiocytosis (Hashimoto–Pritzker). Vesicular-appearing congenital lesion

Treatment

Treatment of LCH depends on the extent and organs involved. In pure cutaneous disease, as in congenital self-healing reticulohistiocytosis, close observation for complete resolution is all that is needed. For the solitary bone lesions of eosinophilic granuloma, surgical excision or curettage is curative, and patients with eosinophilic granuloma with bone involvement alone have the best prognosis. Systemic chemotherapy, with prednisone, etoposide, and other agents, is given in cases of LCH with organ dysfunction. Approximately 14–20% of those with multisystem disease are unresponsive to treatment and have a progressive course. The mortality rate with disseminated LCH is 50% in infants. The overall complete response rate is 85%, with 12% of patients experiencing relapse.

Juvenile Xanthogranuloma

Key Points

- Bright yellow to orange color key to diagnosis
- Spontaneously resolve over months to years
- Eye and organ involvement rare

Clinical presentation

Juvenile xanthogranuloma (JXG) may present as a single lesion or in multiples, with the most common location being the head and neck. They have a characteristic yellow to orange color that may be subtle in early lesions (Figures 8-5 and 8-6). Their size can vary, from small, micronodular 0.5 cm papules to greater than 10 cm tumors. These giant JXGs are usually present at birth and solitary (Figure 8-7). Large intramuscular lesions, localized to the trunk, are very rare. Lesions can be localized to the mucous membranes, particularly the oral cavity. JXG typically appear in early childhood, with 20% being present at birth. Males are affected more frequently than females.

While typically confined to the skin, extracutaneous involvement is well described. Ocular lesions are the most common, occurring in about 0.4% of patients, with multiple skin lesions. Children under 2 years of age with multiple lesions are more likely to have eye involvement. Spontaneous hemorrhage in the anterior chamber of the eye, or hyphema, is the most common ocular presentation of JXG. Glaucoma can also occur, and, rarely, blindness. Ocular lesions are typically treated with intralesional or systemic corticosteroids, radiation, or surgical excision based on the ophthalmologist's judgment. The infiltrative lesions of JXG have been reported in most organs, including lung, liver, spleen, testis, central nervous system, bone, kidney, and adrenal glands, although it should be emphasized that systemic involvement in JXG is very rare.

The association between multiple JXG, neurofibromatosis type 1 (NF-1), and juvenile chronic myelogenous leukemia (JCML) is a complicated one with murky statistics relating to incidences. It is known that children with NF-1 are prone to myeloid disorders, including JCML, and have a higher incidence of JXG (up to 18%). Several case reports describe the three disorders in association and suggest that children with JXG and NF-1 have a greater risk of JCML. Therefore, children with NF-1 and JXG should be observed closely for signs of leukemic disease.

Diagnosis

The diagnosis of JXG is usually made clinically based on the characteristic yellow-orange color, but a biopsy is confirmatory. Microscopic examination will reveal foamy histiocytes, foreign-body giant cells, and classic Touton giant cells (a ring of nuclei surrounded by an eosinophilic cytoplasm). Staining for CD1a and S100, used to differentiate Langerhans cells, is negative. The primary differential diagnosis of solitary JXG is a Spitz nevus since both arise abruptly on the head and neck of young children. A negative Darier's sign will rule out a mastocytoma. The other histiocytoses may also resemble JXG, especially in darker-skinned patients. Biopsy can help to differentiate these disorders.

Pathogenesis

Classified as a histocytosis, the cells of JXG are derived from dermal dendrocytes. They are considered a reactive proliferation, as opposed to a true neoplasm, but it is unclear what stimulates them. Infectious and various physical factors are implicated.

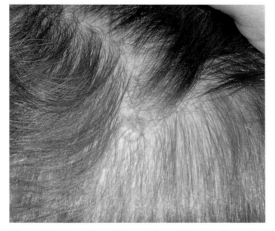

Figure 8-5 Juvenile xanthogranuloma. Typical yellow-orange juvenile xanthogranuloma on the scalp

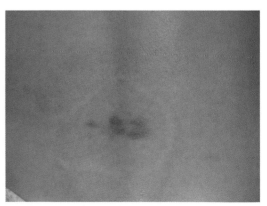

Figure 8-6 Juvenile xanthogranuloma. Grouped juvenile xanthogranuloma on the back

Treatment

Spontaneous regression occurs typically in several months to 6 years, although residual pigmentary alteration and atrophy may persist. Treatment is reserved for systemic disease and symptomatic lesions. Corticosteroids, radiation, and surgical excision are all possible therapies for select JXG.

Benign Cephalic Histiocytosis

Key Points

* Reddish-yellowish macules and thin papules on the face
* Self-resolving

Clinical presentation

Benign cephalic histiocytosis (BCH) is a non-LCH that affects young children, with the average age being 15 months. Tan to red-yellow macules and thin papules erupt on the face and head (Figures 8-8 and 8-9). Involvement of the trunk, extremities, and groin has been reported. There is some rare overlap among the histiocytoses, with reports of BCH progressing to JXG, BCH and Langerhans cell disease coexisting, and BCH coexisting with lytic bone lesions and diabetes insipidus.

Diagnosis

The lesions of BCH may resemble other histiocytic disorders, such as JXG, and LCH. A biopsy, with special stains for CD1a and S100, can help differentiate the histiocytic variants. *Generalized eruptive histiocytoma*, another non-LCH, is seen primarily in adults, but has rarely been reported in young children. Eruptive crops of yellow-brown papules in the hundreds occur symmetrically over the face, trunk, and extremities. Multiple melanocytic nevi and flat warts can also mimic BCH. Flat warts may koebnerize. Urticaria pigmentosa (UP) will exhibit a positive Darier's sign.

Pathogenesis

The cells of BCH are derived from the same dermal/interstitial dendrocyte line as JXG. It too is a proliferative disorder of unknown etiology.

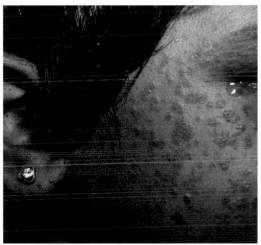

Figure 8-8 Benign cephalic histiocytosis. Lesions in a healthy 3-year-old girl

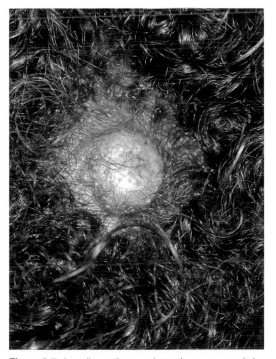

Figure 8-7 Juvenile xanthogranuloma. Large, congenital juvenile xanthogranuloma on the scalp

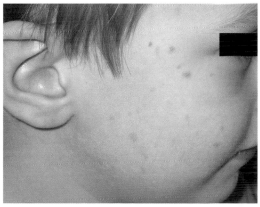

Figure 8-9 Tan, yellowish macules and papules of benign cephalic histiocytosis

Treatment

The lesions of BCH typically resolve without intervention. Atrophic scarring and hyper-pigmentation may persist.

Mast Cell Disorders

Key Points

- Reddish-tan to brown indistinct macules and papules common
- History of lesions urticating or blistering
- Resolution or marked improvement of disease by puberty

Clinical presentation

There are several distinct forms of mast cell disease defined by their clinical presentations. The most common form in childhood is urticaria pigmentosa. The lesions of UP are typically ill defined, almost fuzzy bordered macules that vary in size from a few millimeters to several centimeters (Figure 8-10). Papules and thin plaques may also be found, although nodules are uncommon. The amount of pigmentation present ranges from faint yellow-tan to dark brown (Figure 8-11). The trunk is most affected: involvement of the face, palms, and soles is rare. Pruritus is variable. Often parents will give a history of one or more of the lesions welting or blistering intermittently. As the child gets older, the blistering episodes subside.

Most cases of UP resolve by adolescence; rare cases can persist into adulthood.

A *solitary mastocytoma* is typically present at birth or early infancy. It has the same clinical appearance as a lesion of UP. Any child with five or fewer lesions is given the diagnosis of solitary mastocytoma. While classified as the second most common form, it is likely that limited cases of mast cell disease are simply underreported, as they can be misdiagnosed as a nevus, or café au lait macule. Solitary mastocytomas tend to improve at an even faster rate than those of UP, resolving without sequelae often by early to mid-childhood.

Diffuse cutaneous mastocytosis is another form of childhood mast cell disease, where the entire skin is infiltrated by mast cells. Blisters and bullae that erode and crust overlie erythema and peau d'orange (orange peel) skin (Figure 8-12). Dermatographism, also due to increased mast cell reactivity, canvasses the rest of the skin. This form is very rare and will present at birth or early infancy. As the child gets older, usually by 2–3 years of age, the blistering will improve and the skin becomes less reactive. However, the dermatographism and hyperpigmentation will often persist well into adulthood.

Telangiectasia macularis eruptiva perstans (TMEP) and systemic mastocytosis are forms of mast cell disease typically seen in adults and are rarely described in children. Small, reddish macules with subtle red telangiectatic vessels are seen with TMEP. A Darier's sign may or may not be elicited. Systemic mastocytosis is defined by extracutaneous involvement of any number of

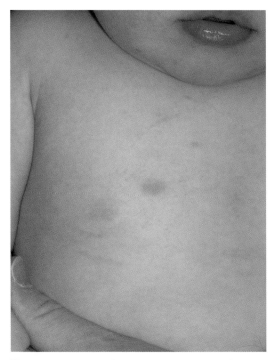

Figure 8-10 Urticaria pigmentosa. Fuzzy bordered tan patches typical of urticaria pigmentosa

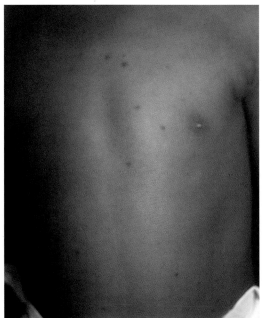

Figure 8-11 Urticaria pigmentosa. Dark brown, ill-defined papules in urticaria pigmentosa

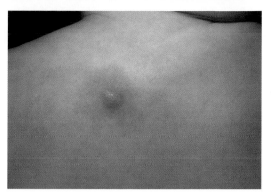

Figure 8-13 Urticaria pigmentosa. A positive Darier's sign

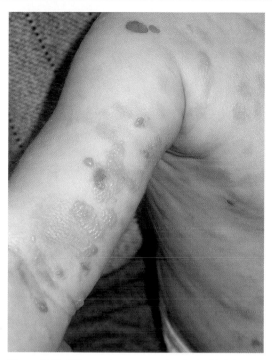

Figure 8-12 Diffuse cutaneous mastocytosis. Vesicles, bullae, and peau d'orange skin

organs, in particular the bone marrow. Overall, adult mast cell disease portends a worse prognosis than in a child.

Systemic symptoms can accompany all forms of mastocytosis, although they are very rare in cases of limited cutaneous involvement. Flushing is a fairly common event, occurring in 20–65% of patients. True hypotensive episodes are very uncommon, but it should be noted that anaphylactoid responses to bee and wasp stings may be the presenting feature of mastocytosis. Gastrointestinal cramping, pain, and diarrhea are reported in approximately 40% of children with mast cell disease. There is also an increased risk for peptic ulcer disease due to elevated histamine levels resulting in an overproduction of stomach acid. Bone pain and headache may be reported. The vast majority of children with mast cell disease have an excellent prognosis, and fatal cases are exceedingly rare.

Diagnosis

Often the diagnosis of mast cell disease can be established clinically in a patient with classic skin lesions and a positive Darier's sign. The Darier's sign is positive when a lesion welts up after rubbing it with a blunt object, like a capped pen, for 10 seconds (Figure 8-13). Adjacent skin should also be tested to differentiate dermatographism. In cases that are unclear or where confirmation is desired, a skin biopsy will reveal increased numbers of mast cells in the dermis.

The lesions of UP may resemble those of JXG or LCH, as the age of presentation and course are similar. The Darier's sign will be negative in the histiocytic disorders and histology will readily differentiate the two. Limited lesions can often look similar to café au lait macules, or melanocytic nevi. Frequently blistering lesions may be confused with another bullous disease or bullous impetigo. Diffuse cutaneous mastocytosis should be considered in any newborn with a blistering disorder.

Pathogenesis

Mutations in the c-kit proto-oncogene have been detected in some patients with mast cell disease, primarily those with systemic involvement. Children with limited cutaneous involvement do not show the same gene alterations.

Treatment

Treatment of mast cell disease depends on the severity of disease. Most children with solitary mastocytoma or UP do not require any treatment at all. Mild episodic flares of individual lesions can be managed with application of ice or topical corticosteroids. In symptomatic cases, treatment begins with an H^1-blocking oral antihistamine, such as cetirizine or hydroxyzine. H^2 antagonists may be added in refractory cases or if gastrointestinal symptoms are present. Oral cromolyn has been used with variable results for children with diarrhea. Some practitioners also provide parents with an EpiPen, although anaphylactoid reactions are exceedingly rare and unpredictable.

Children diagnosed with mast cell disease, particularly those with systemic symptoms, should be counseled to avoid any medications or foods that can cause the mass release of histamine from the mast cells. Although the list is long, very few of the potential offenders are commonly used in children. Exposure to physical triggers should also be limited. The list of mast cell degranulators is given in Table 8-2.

Table 8.2 Potential mast cell degranulators

Mechanical triggers	Rubbing, scratching, friction
	Extreme temperatures (hot or cold) Sudden changes in temperatures (jumping into a pool or hot tub)
	Exercise
Foods	Alcohol, egg whites, crayfish, lobster, chocolate, strawberries, tomatoes, citrus
Drugs	Codeine, morphine, dextromethorphan, aspirin, radiocontrast dye, quinine, scopolamine, reserpine, amphotericin B, polymyxin B, tubocurarine, NSAIDs
Venoms	Snakebites, bee stings, jellyfish stings

NSAIDs, nonsteroidal anti-inflammatory drugs.

Pilomatricoma

Key Points

- Rock-hard, calcified nodule with bluish hue
- Typically on the face of a young child

Clinical presentation

These slow-growing, irregular-bordered, mobile nodules are situated in the deep layers of the skin. They are classically rock-hard due to their propensity to calcify and often have a bluish overlying hue (Figure 8-14). Pilomatricomas most commonly occur on face, head, and neck. There is a marked female predominance, and they frequently occur in young children. While usually nonpainful, the lesion may be tender if frequently bumped or manipulated or if located in a site of pressure. Although usually sporadic, familial cases have been reported; multiple lesions have been associated with myotonic dystrophy (Steinert disease), Gardner syndrome, Rubinstein–Taybi syndrome, and trisomy 9.

Diagnosis

A clinical diagnosis of pilomatricoma can be easily made. Two useful diagnostic signs are the "tent sign" – when the skin is stretched over the affected area, the irregular, angulated contours of the lesion are highlighted – and the "teeter-totter sign" – pressing on one end of the lesion will result in the upward movement of the other end. While much is written about radiographic imaging of pilomatricoma, its utility in diagnosis of this entity is limited.

The differential diagnosis of this growth includes epidermoid cyst, dermoid cyst, and other benign follicle-derived tumors, all lesions that are treated by excision and pathologic confirmation of the diagnosis. A biopsy can confirm the diagnosis, revealing the characteristic encapsulated cyst containing "shadow cells" and calcification.

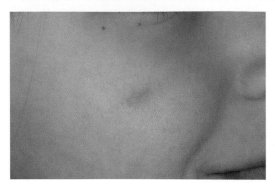

Figure 8-14 Pilomatricoma. Bluish hue of firm nodule on the cheek

Pathogenesis

Pilomatricomas are derived from the hair matrix. Defects in β-catenin have been found in some patients.

Treatment

Larger and cosmetically unacceptable lesions should be surgically excised, as they are unlikely to regress spontaneously.

Trichoepithelioma

Key Points

- Smooth-surfaced, pink to tan papule
- Most common site is the nasolabial folds
- Multiple lesions are inherited dominantly

Clinical presentation

These smooth-topped, firm, flesh to slightly tan-colored papules typically localize to the nasolabial folds, upper lip, and central forehead. Trichoepithelioma generally occurs as a sporadic, solitary lesion. However, in cases of multiple lesions, they tend to run in the family as it is an autosomal-dominant inherited condition (Figure 8-15). They may also occur concomitantly with *cylindromas* (larger, firm, pink hairless nodules on the scalp) in the Brooke–Spiegler syndrome.

Diagnosis

A clinical diagnosis of familial cases is generally straightforward. In new cases or in a child with a solitary lesion, biopsy can confirm the diagnosis. Histology shows keratin-filled cysts interspersed amongst groups of basaloid cells.

Pathogenesis

Trichoepitheliomas are benign tumors, or possible hamartomas, that are derived from the pilosebaceous unit, attempting to differentiate towards the hair follicle. The genetic defect has been mapped to chromosome 9p21.

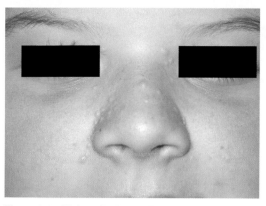

Figure 8-15 Trichoepitheliomas. Flesh-colored papules along the nasolabial folds in familial trichoepitheliomas

Treatment

A solitary trichoepithelioma can be removed by simple excision. Most patients with multiple lesions are seeking an improvement in their cosmetic appearance. Treatment modalities such as shave removal, dermabrasion, electrodesiccation, and curettage have all been employed with fairly good outcomes.

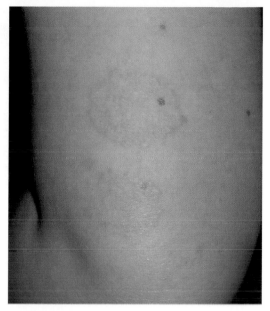

Figure 8-16 Granuloma annulare. Classic granuloma annulare showing annular nonscaling plaques on the arm

Granuloma Annulare

Key Points

- Annular, nonscaling plaques
- Common on hands and feet
- Treatment generally ineffective

Clinical presentation

Often a mimicker of ringworm, granuloma annulare (GA) is characterized by nonscaling slightly pink to tan papules that organize into annular plaques (Figure 8-16). The lesions may be solitary or multifocal, and the most common location to find GA is on the dorsal hands and feet of school-aged children. Overall, 50–75% of cases of localized GA will spontaneously resolve within 2 years. When lesions occur on the scalp, proximal extremities, shins, feet, and fingers, they often present as asymptomatic flesh-colored papules or nodules without the telltale annularity (Figure 8-17). This form of subcutaneous GA is more common in children, particularly boys, so clinical suspicion should be high for this presentation. Generalized, perforating, and macular variants of GA are uncommonly seen, particularly in children.

Diagnosis

The diagnosis is made clinically in typical cases of GA. A biopsy can confirm the diagnosis in atypical presentations, helping eliminate the more worrisome disorders in the differential diagnosis. Histopathology will show a palisading,

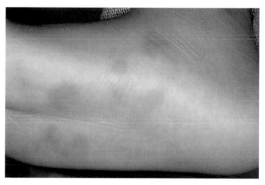

Figure 8-17 Granuloma annulare. Nodular granuloma annulare on the foot with only a hint forming an annular ring

granulomatous infiltrate with surrounding mucin. The differential diagnoses of the classic annular form of GA have been listed in Box 6-4, Chapter 6. Subcutaneous GA must be distinguished from rheumatoid nodules, in which a history of joint pain may be elicited. Knuckle pads are symmetrically distributed pink plaques confined to the skin overlying the finger joints. For nodular lesions on the shins, associated pain and erythema will define erythema nodosum.

Pathogenesis

The etiology of GA is unknown. It has been suggested that it occurs in response to a vasculitis or preceding trauma, or is perhaps a delayed-type hypersensitivity reaction. GA has followed zoster and human immunodeficiency virus (HIV) infection, suggesting an infectious trigger. A weak association with diabetes mellitus, particularly with generalized forms, has been shown.

Treatment

Untreated GA will run its course, resolving spontaneously, in several months to years. Topical or intralesional corticosteroids are often used in the treatment of GA; their effect is often unsatisfactory. In severe, generalized cases, systemic therapies, including isotretinoin, colchicine, and dapsone, have been used with variable results.

Developmental Defects

Clinical presentation

All cranial lesions, especially those located along the midline or embryological fusion planes, should raise concern for a developmental defect. The "hair collar" sign, a tuft of long, coarse, and dark hair surrounding a congenital lesion on the scalp, often heralds cranial defects (Figure 8-18). When the hair collar is seen, imaging studies should be done expeditiously and definitely before considering a biopsy. An *encephalocele* results from herniation of components of the central nervous system through the skull. Typically they are translucent to flesh-colored, bluish nodules. Most encephaloceles are found along the midline but occur along suture lines as well. Hypertelorism and structural facial or brain abnormalities can be associated. Because of their intracranial extension, these lesions will swell in size with crying or straining due to an increase in intracranial pressure. When an outpouching of meninges and cerebrospinal fluid occurs, it is called a *meningocele*. A *meningoencephalocele* is composed of brain tissue, meninges, and cerebrospinal fluid. In contrast, *heterotopic brain tissue* is defined by the presence of brain matter outside the central nervous system, without an underlying connection. This uncommon defect may occur anywhere on the head or neck. Figure 8-19 illustrates the anatomic location of many developmental anomalies of the head and neck.

Aplasia cutis congenita (ACC) is a congenital absence of skin and is seen more commonly than an encephalocele. Generally presenting with a red, oozing plaque, ACC will heal with scar (Figure 8-20). A membranous variant has a thin, shiny layer overlying the defect. ACC is most commonly located on the scalp but can affect limbs and other sites as well. While most are isolated findings, multiple associations

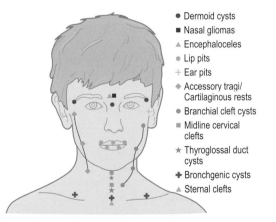

- ● Dermoid cysts
- ■ Nasal gliomas
- ▲ Encephaloceles
- ● Lip pits
- + Ear pits
- ◆ Accessory traqi/ Cartilaginous rests
- ● Branchial cleft cysts
- ■ Midline cervical clefts
- ★ Thyroglossal duct cysts
- ✚ Bronchgenic cysts
- ▲ Sternal clefts

Figure 8-19 Anatomic location of developmental anomalies of the head and neck

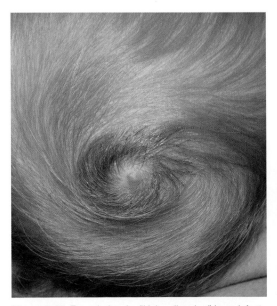

Figure 8-18 Encephalocele. "Hair collar sign" in an infant

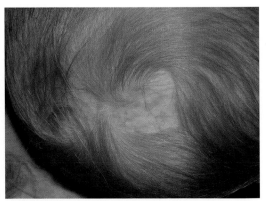

Figure 8-20 Aplasia cutis congenita

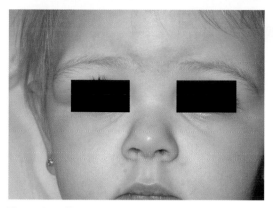

Figure 8-21 Dermoid cyst. Flesh-colored nodule in a typical location

have been reported with ACC, including methimazole use in pregnancy, other midline and limb defects, cleft lip or palate, eye abnormalities, neurological defects, epidermolysis bullosa, trisomy 13, Setleis syndrome, and Adams–Oliver syndrome.

A *dermoid cyst or sinus* occurs along embryonic fusion planes and is usually noticeable at birth. It is most commonly found along the supraorbital ridge and at the nasal root but can occur anywhere (Figure 8-21). The cysts are lined by stratified squamous epithelium and may contain appendageal elements, including hair and even teeth. Dermoid sinuses should be suspected in areas of hypertrichosis or dimpling, and infections may result. If a pit is present, intracranial extension is more likely.

Nasal gliomas are also located at the nasal root and often are coupled with hypertelorism. These flesh-colored to bluish nodules do not have an intracranial connection and thus do not vary in size with crying. Intranasal lesions may present with exophytic masses.

Accessory tragi are a relatively common finding in newborns. These flesh-colored papules occur anterior to the normal tragus, or less commonly along the cheek and neck, and may be simple or complex (Figure 8-22). They are soft and fleshy or fairly firm, depending on the presence of cartilage. Bilateral involvement occurs in about 6% of cases. Extensive defects may be associated with abnormal structural development of the ear and deafness. Several syndromes are associated with accessory tragus, the most consistent being the oculoauriculovertebral syndrome (or Goldenhar syndrome) where epibulbar dermoid cysts and vertebral defects are seen.

An overlying pit may indicate its presence but a *preauricular sinus* usually comes to the practitioner's attention when it becomes inflamed or infected. When this happens, the cutaneous extension becomes obscured by an inflamed scaling, and crusted plaque.

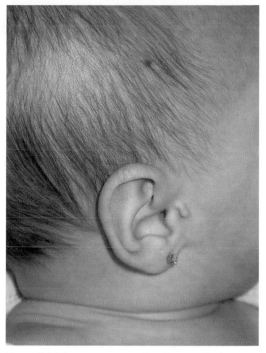

Figure 8-22 Accessory tragus. Prominent cartilaginous component

Recurrences of the tract and inflammation are common after incomplete excision. Complete excision is necessary and often difficult due to the insidious path of the sinus, often into the pharynx.

Branchial cleft defects, both cysts and sinuses, occur at the lateral cheeks, extending to the lateral neck along the margin of the sternocleidomastoid muscle. A lesion may lie quiescent until adulthood when it becomes inflamed or infected.

Midline lesions on the neck can result from the development of thyroid or bronchial structures. A *thyroglossal duct cyst* or sinus occurs midline in the location of the thyroid gland. The defect will move up and down with swallowing. Abnormal development of the thyroid may have also occurred during development so accurate knowledge of the individual's anatomy is necessary prior to excision so as not to remove an ectopic thyroid. In contrast, a *bronchogenic cyst* occurs lower down in the midline sternal notch. They are usually present at birth and are stable in location. The differential diagnosis includes a *congenital cartilaginous rest of the neck* (wattle) that appears as a firm, exophytic, flesh-colored tag at the midline to lateral neck.

Accessory nipples, also called supernumerary nipples or polythelia, occur along the central milk lines of the chest and abdomen. Rarely, they are found at the poles of the milk line on the face, neck, shoulder, groin, or thighs. Accessory nipples look like atretic versions of fully developed nipples with tan or brown to pink papules and, sometimes, central dimpling or inversion. Underlying breast tissue is generally minimal.

A variety of lesions overlying the lumbosacral region, including lipoma, hemangioma, and faun tail, may represent the cutaneous manifestation of spinal dysraphism. Multiple lesions should raise even greater suspicion. It is vital to recognize these associations and do an appropriate work-up. An approach to the evaluation and management of lumbosacral lesions is listed in Table 8-3.

Diagnosis

A computed tomography or magnetic resonance imaging (MRI) scan should be done prior to biopsy or excision to rule out intracranial extension and bony defects in all midline or atypical lesions. Ultrasound may be useful in distinguishing an infantile hemangioma or lipoma from a cranial defect or dermoid cyst but is not adequate to evaluate bony structures. Transillumination will occur with encephaloceles and may be a useful tool in establishing an initial diagnosis. Nevus sebaceus may resemble aplasia cutis, as both are congenital and without hair. A nevus sebaceus usually has an orangish, pebbly surface. Knowledge of embryological development and the typical location of neck defects will help differentiate these entities. Histologic evaluation of biopsy or excisional tissue is diagnostic for each of these entities.

Pathogenesis

Dermoid cysts and sinus occur at the fusion planes of ectodermal and neuroectodermal tissue. Accessory tragus results from defects in the first branchial arch development.

Treatment

Any congenital defect with the potential for intracranial extension should be managed by a pediatric neurosurgeon for excision and repair of the defect. Both dermoid cysts and sinuses should be surgically excised. While radiographic imaging prior to excision is not necessary in dermoid cysts located at the lateral eye margin, it may be useful in establishing a correct diagnosis. Excision of accessory tragus will result in cosmetic improvement, taking special care to remove all cartilage, as incomplete removal can result in chondritis and slow healing.

Childhood Malignancies

Key Points

- Rhabdomyosarcoma can mimic vascular tumors
- "Raccoon eyes" and prolonged blanching are seen with neuroblastoma
- Biopsy atypical bluish nodules in newborns and infants

Table 8.3 Skin signs of spinal dysraphism

Risk	Skin finding (no neurological or orthopedic symptoms)	Imaging study	
		Age < 6 months	Age ≥ 6months
High	> 2 lesions of any kind		
	Any one lesion with spinal cord dysfunction	MRI	MRI
	Lipoma		
	Faun tail		
	Dermal sinus		
	Deviation of the gluteal cleft		
	Atypical dimple	Ultrasound if abnormal	MRI
	Other hamartoma	MRI	
	Aplasia cutis congenita		
	Lumbosacral capillary vascular malformation (port-wine stain)		
	Hemangioma		
	Congenital melanocytic nevus		
Low	Simple dimple	May observe, unless other symptoms present	
	Mongolian spot		

MRI, magnetic resonance imaging.

Clinical presentation

Rhabdomyosarcoma uncommonly presents in the skin but may extend to or metastasize to the skin from its primary muscle origin. Rhabdomyosarcomas are typically rapidly growing and painful with a variable clinical presentation, from small nodules to large vascular-appearing tumors. Head and neck is the most common site involved. Early recognition and treatment are essential for cure.

Neuroblastoma will be metastatic to the skin in about one-third of patients, making the skin an important clue to diagnosis. The primary site in most cases is found in the retroperitoneum. Lesions are typically reddish-blue, firm, asymptomatic nodules. When rubbed, the lesions will show a characteristic blanching with an erythematous rim due to release of catecholamines, typically lasting over 30 min. Another important clue is periorbital bruising or "raccoon eyes" that is seen with ocular metastasis.

Leukemia cutis/lymphoma cutis may rarely present in the skin of children, but should be considered in children with systemic findings suggesting malignancy or in patients with hepatosplenomegaly. Deep red to pink firm nodules are seen. Children with Down syndrome are at greater risk for hematologic malignancies.

Diagnosis

In all cases, diagnosis of a cutaneous presentation of malignancy should be confirmed and further characterized by biopsy. Either the primary or metastatic site can confirm diagnosis. Further systemic workup will then follow. The differential diagnosis of leukemia cutis, rhabdomyosarcoma, and neuroblastoma includes the blueberry muffin lesions seen with TORCH infections (*Toxoplasma*, rubella, cytomegalovirus, and herpesvirus), vascular tumors, histocytosis, mastocytosis and other malignancies, such as fibrosarcoma.

Pathogenesis

The cells in leukemia cutis are derived from the bone marrow and will be identical to the aberrant cells found in the blood. The malignant cells of neuroblastoma are of neural crest origin. Rhabdomyosarcoma arises from the striated skeletal muscle.

Treatment

Referral to a pediatric oncologist should be made as soon as malignancy is suspected. Further workup and treatments should be performed under the oncologist's direction and will depend on the type of malignancy identified.

Miscellaneous Lumps and Bumps

Congenital smooth-muscle hamartoma is a benign growth of the smooth muscle within the reticular dermis. These tend to be subtle flesh-colored dermal plaques with a slight pebbly surface. One key to diagnosis is the overlying hypertrichosis (Figure 8-23). A pseudo-Darier's sign may be elicited by stroking the lesion and noting the chicken skin-like puckering that results.

Connective tissue nevi generally present at birth or in early childhood. They are hamartomas comprising elastic or collagen fibers or both. They are flesh-colored plaques with variable surface change, from very subtle thickening to a cobblestoned, or cerebriform thickening. The "shagreen patch" of tuberous sclerosis is a type of connective tissue nevus. Collagenomas may be autosomal dominantly inherited, with eruptive lesions symmetrically distributed over the back beginning in adolescence. Elastomas, associated with the Buschke–Ollendorf syndrome, have a similar clinical appearance to a collagenoma and may be associated with the benign radiographic finding of osteopoikilosis.

Figure 8-23 Smooth-muscle hamartoma

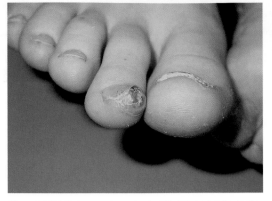

Figure 8-24 Subungual exostosis. Wart-like papule on the distal toe

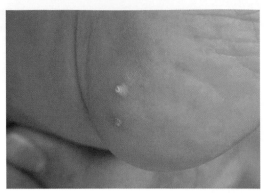

Figure 8-25 Heel stick calcification. White, firm papule on heel of infant or toddler

A *lipoma* can be present at birth or more commonly acquired later in childhood. It is a rubbery, subcutaneous nodule with normal overlying skin. It may be painful if it occurs over bony prominences but will usually be asymptomatic. Congenital lipomas overlying the lumbosacral region may herald an underlying spinal dysraphism. Radiographic imaging, either ultrasound in the newborn period or an MRI, is indicated. Several syndromes are associated with the development of lipomas, including: Bannayan–Riley–Ruvalcaba syndrome (lipoma, vascular malformation, lentigines of the penis/vulva, verrucae, and acanthosis nigricans), multiple endocrine neoplasia type 1 (MEN1: facial angiofibromas, collagenomas, café au lait macules, lipomas, confetti macules, and gingival tumors in association with parathyroid, pancreas, and pituitary tumors) and Gardner's syndrome. *Nevus lipomatosis superficialis* is characterized by superficial, soft, grouped papules generally on the buttock or thigh. The overlying skin has a wrinkled appearance. They typically occur before age 20. *Diffuse lipomatosis* is a rare disorder occurring before 2 years of age. Diffuse and infiltrative tumors of mature fat involve the trunk or extremity. Additional lipomas or hemangiomas may be associated.

Subungual exostosis most commonly affects the distal portion of the great toe. It is a painful reddish smooth papule that can resemble a wart caused by an underlying overgrowth of the bone (Figure 8-24). It can easily be diagnosed by X-ray when clinically suspected but is often discovered by accident during nail avulsion for "ingrown toenail."

Osteoma cutis is characterized by bone-hard papules to infiltrative plaques. It can occur sporadically or in association with Albright's hereditary osteodystrophy. *Progressive osseous heteroplasia* is a rare and severe form that occurs more commonly in females. *Subepidermal calcified nodule*, a rock-hard pinkish nodule, occurs on the scalp or face of children.

Calcinosis cutis presents as a rock-hard, chalky nodule. *Solitary nodular calcification* is a benign nodule found in infants and small children. It can occur secondary to heel sticks (Figure 8-25) or calcium chloride found in electrode paste.

Calcinosis universalis and calcinosis cutis circumscripta can arise idiopathically or secondary to tissue damage or connective tissue disease (scleroderma, progressive systemic sclerosis, systemic lupus erythematosus). Calcinosis universalis is more common in girls, occurring in childhood dermatomyositis.

Metastatic calcinosis cutis may result secondary to hyperphosphatemia and hypercalcemia. Symmetrically distributed lesions in the popliteal fossae, iliac crests, or posterior axillary lines are common. This form is seen in parathyroid neoplasms, hypervitaminosis D, and diseases with massive bone destruction.

Angiofibromas are reddish, firm, blanchable papules. Multiple lesions on the face may be associated with tuberous sclerosis as well as MEN-1. These lesions are rarely present at birth but appear in early childhood.

Keloids are very firm, scar-like tumors that arise within areas of trauma in susceptible individuals. African-Americans and darker-skinned persons are at highest risk for the development of keloids. In contrast to hypertrophic scars, keloids grow outside the original boundaries of the wound. Treatment is difficult. Intralesional corticosteroid injections at regular intervals and compression may help to soften and decrease a keloid.

An *epidermoid cyst* is a true cyst with a lined epithelial wall. It presents as a moderately firm, mobile flesh-colored nodule (Figure 8-26). There is often a visible pore connecting the cyst to the skin surface. The cyst contents, a whitish, cheesy smelly material, can be expressed through the pore, confirming the diagnosis. Symptomatic or larger lesions can be cured with excision of the cyst.

Figure 8-26 Epidermoid cyst. Flesh-colored mobile nodule on the back

A 4-mm punch into the center of the cyst is a simple procedure for reducing its size but is not curative. Ruptured cysts will become inflamed and tender, resembling a staphylococcal abscess, but antibiotics are of no value. Treatment entails drainage and/or injection of a steroid solution such as triamcinolone.

Further reading

Chang MW. Update on juvenile xanthogranuloma: Unusual cutaneous and systemic variants. Semin Cutan Med Surg 1999;18:195–205.

Drolet B. Birthmarks to worry about. Dermatol Clin 1998;16:447–453.

Farvolden D, Sweeney SM, Wiss K. Lumps and bumps in neonates and infants. Dermatol Ther 2005;18:104–116.

Heide R, Tank B, Oranje AP. Mastocytosis in childhood. Pediatr Dermatol. 2002;19:375–381.

Soonawala. N, Overweg-Plandsoen WCG, Brouwer OF. Early clinical signs and symptoms in occult spinal dysraphism: a retrospective case study of 47 patients. Clin Neurol Neurosurg 1999;101:11–14.

Weitzman S, Jaffe R. Uncommon histiocytic disorders: The non-Langerhans cell histiocytoses. Pediatr Blood Cancer 2005;45:256–264.

Skin conditions in newborns and infants

9

Albert C. Yan

Certain considerations must be borne in mind when evaluating and treating skin conditions in newborns and infants. A variety of skin disorders are unique to the neonatal period and present only in this age group. Subcutaneous fat necrosis (SCFN) of the newborn and sclerema neonatorum, for instance, have no corresponding adult counterparts. Moreover, because of the relative immaturity of the immune system in very young children, care must be taken to identify promptly and accurately infectious diseases presenting in the skin and to distinguish them from benign transient dermatoses of the newborn. Clinicians are frequently asked to differentiate between erythema toxicum neonatorum (ETN) and neonatal herpes simplex infection. Skin disorders that first manifest during the neonatal period may also represent harbingers of potential problems during adolescence or adulthood, as exemplified by children with infantile acne who are at risk for later more severe adolescent acne, or those with nevus sebaceous lesions or large congenital melanocytic nevi which have a low but definite risk of later malignant transformation. Finally, treatment modalities must be selected that take into account differences between infants and adults, such as the increased total body surface area relative to weight in infants. Considerations such as these inform decisions about any agents that are prescribed to infants that may place them at risk for medication toxicity.

Benign Common Conditions in Newborns and Infants

Key Points

- The newborn infant is predisposed to certain benign, transitory skin conditions that require no intervention. Recognition of these entities is important for the clinician so that unnecessary diagnostic and therapeutic interventions can be avoided:
  - ETN
  - Transient neonatal pustular melanosis (TNPM)
  - Miliaria
  - Milia
  - Sebaceous hyperplasia
  - Vernix caseosa
  - Postmaturity desquamation
  - Sucking blisters

Erythema toxicum neonatorum

ETN is a benign and transient disorder that manifests in *full-term* infants as small papules, vesicles, or occasionally pustules surrounded by a characteristic blotchy erythema (Figure 9-1). The individual lesions are typically evanescent. The rash usually appears during the first week of life and resolves within 1–2 weeks. Clusters of ETN lesions may resemble those of neonatal herpes simplex virus (HSV) infection, and scrapings of the lesions for Wright or Giemsa staining may be helpful in differentiating these diagnoses. ETN lesions demonstrate copious eosinophils on smears, as opposed to the steel gray multinucleated giant cells seen in vesicles of HSV. Erythema toxicum is a self-limited process and requires no intervention other than parental reassurance.

Transient neonatal pustular melanosis

TNPM is an idiopathic newborn eruption that often presents within the first day of life. Affected children may manifest with a widespread eruption of fragile, sterile pustules that rapidly rupture. In fact, in some children, the pustules may rupture during the birthing process, leaving behind numerous small collarettes of scale surrounding areas of hyperpigmentation (also referred to as "lentiginosis neonatorum") (Figure 9-2). Eventually, this hyperpigmentation resolves without sequelae. This condition is more commonly encountered in infants with darker skin color. Since the condition resolves spontaneously, no treatment is required.

Miliaria

Miliaria is frequently referred to as "heat rash" or "prickly heat," and is indeed observed in settings where children have been bundled tightly or may have had fevers. It is postulated that eccrine sweat ducts become occluded, possibly by resident bacterial flora, leading to papulovesicles. Miliaria crystallina results when the occlusion is superficial, manifesting as multiple tiny clear vesicles (Figure 9-3). When the occlusion is deeper, miliaria rubra, miliaria profunda, or miliaria pustulosa can result, yielding erythematous papules, erythematous nodules, or inflamed pustules, respectively (Figure 9-4). Eliminating the hot, humid environment that engendered this process by unbundling babies can help to resolve this condition more quickly. In cases where the infants are symptomatic, application of a topical antibiotic such as erythromycin or clindamycin can be considered.

Milia

Milia are small, superficial, keratin-filled cysts that can affect individuals of any age (Figure 9-5). They are often idiopathic and resolve spontaneously in newborns. In older children and adults, they are typically found at sites of prior trauma, as might be observed in burn scars or in patients with dystrophic epidermolysis bullosa, and may be more persistent. Children who suffer from allergic rhinoconjunctivitis often have multiple periocular milia, possibly from frequent rubbing

of the eyes. Some children with orofacial–digital syndromes may also present with numerous cutaneous milia, and multiple milia have been associated with Bazex syndrome.

When these keratin cysts are noted on the palate of newborns, they are referred to as Ebstein's pearls. When observed on the gingival surfaces, the term Bohn's nodules applies.

Sebaceous hyperplasia

Sebaceous hyperplasia manifests as small, yellow-white papules on the nose of newborns (Figure 9-6). It is thought to be the result of the infant's hyperandrogen state and resolves spontaneously. They can be easily mistaken for milia but are not true keratinaceous cysts.

Vernix caseosa

The vernix caseosa is a white, waxy material composed of lipids and proteins that encases the fetus at birth and provides a hydrophobic layer of protection for fetal skin while in utero. Secreted by fetal sebaceous glands at 20 weeks'

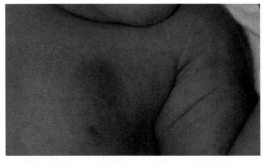

Figure 9-1 Erythema toxicum neonatorum. Note the blotchy erythema surrounding individual lesions

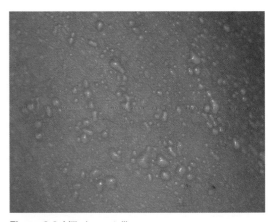

Figure 9-3 Miliaria crystallina

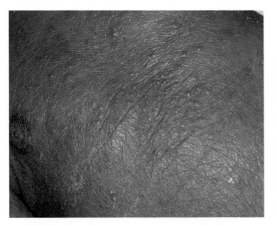

Figure 9-2 Transient neonatal pustular melanosis. As lesions fade, hyperpigmentation becomes visible

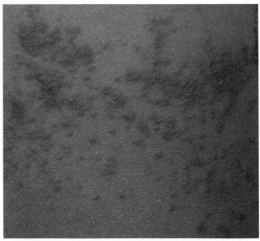

Figure 9-4 Miliaria rubra

gestation, the vernix also participates in host defense by elaborating a number of compounds, including LL-37, cystatin, uteroglobin-related protein 1 (UGRP-1), calgranulin. psoriasin, and alpha-defensins (HNP1–3), that confer broad-spectrum antimicrobial activity against bacteria and fungi. The vernix is often absent in infants born at postmaturity or greater than 42 weeks' gestation.

Postmaturity desquamation

Generalized superficial desquamation may be observed, either at birth or within the first 24–48 hours, in infants born at postmaturity or greater than 42 weeks' gestation (Figure 9-7). The desquamation resolves rapidly, typically within a week of birth.

Sucking blisters

Sucking blisters are essentially friction blisters and present as either intact blisters or erosions at sites where sucking occurs (Figure 9-8). Anatomic sites most frequently affected include the upper lip, the dorsal hands, the thumb, and the forearm areas. While blisters are often observed in the neonatal period, some may be noted at birth as a result of sucking behavior in utero.

Pigmentary Lesions in the Newborn and Infant

Key Points

* Congenital lesions of dermal melanocytosis are generally self-limited, but atypical and extensive lesions may be markers of systemic disease
* Physiologic jaundice is benign but can pose a risk:
  * Phototherapy of infants with unconjugated hyperbilirubinemia leads to "bronze-baby syndrome"
  * Infants undergoing exchange transfusion and phototherapy for unconjugated hyperbilirubinemia are at risk of developing a purpuric phototherapy-induced eruption

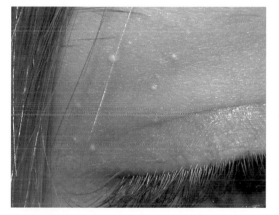

Figure 9-5 Milia

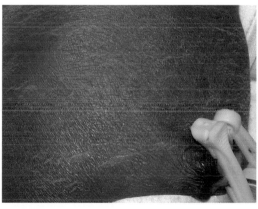

Figure 9-7 Postmaturity desquamation

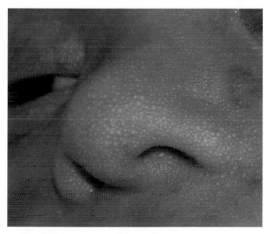

Figure 9-6 Sebaceous hyperplasia

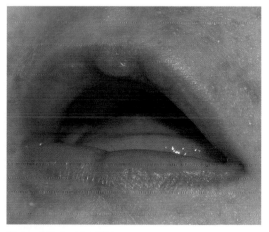

Figure 9-8 Sucking blister

Dermal melanocytosis (mongolian spots)

Dermal melanocytosis, also referred to as "mongolian spots," appear as slate-gray or bluish-gray macules and patches (Figure 9-9). These areas are more frequently observed in darker-skinned individuals and are most commonly encountered on the lower back. If the lesions resolve, they generally do so by late childhood or early adolescence. Parents can be appropriately reassured about their benign nature and likely spontaneous resolution.

Extensive and atypical dermal melanocytosis can be associated with other diseases such as mucopolysaccharidosis as well as phakomatosis pigmentovascularis (one of various syndromes in which a port-wine stain is observed in association with other skin lesions such as mongolian spots, nevus anemicus, nevus spilus, and epidermal nevi).

Nevus of Ota and nevus of Ito

Dermal melanocytosis in a periocular distribution along ophthalmic and maxillary branches of the trigeminal nerve is characteristic of nevus of Ota (Figure 9-10); when it occurs on the shoulder, the lesion is known as a nevus of Ito. In contrast to neonatal dermal melanocytosis, these do not resolve spontaneously and are likely to persist into adulthood. Both can be congenital or acquired. The clinical significance of nevus of Ota lies in its association with glaucoma, melanoma, and other syndromes such as phakomatosis pigmentovascularis. Children with this condition should be followed by a dermatologist and ophthalmologist for potential sequelae. Treatment with a laser that targets pigment – such as the q-switched Nd:YAG, ruby, or alexandrite – has been successful at lightening nevus of Ota.

Neonatal hyperpigmentation

Neonates, particularly those with darker skin, are often born with areas of accentuated pigmentation. The most common areas noted are in the periungual, scrotal, or vulvar areas. Horizontal streaks of hyperpigmentation can be observed in skin creases on the torso (Figure 9-11). These are of no clinical significance, and families can be appropriately reassured about their benign nature.

Physiologic jaundice and neonatal jaundice

Neonatal physiologic jaundice is a normal phenomenon seen in neonates typically within the first week of life. Increased circulating blood cell volume in newborns, relatively immature hepatic function, and slow initial gastrointestinal motility lead to the accumulation of unconjugated bilirubin in the blood stream.

Newborns with unconjugated hyperbilirubinemia manifest with jaundice most intensely on the face, especially around the nose. As the hyperbilirubinemia increases, the jaundice progresses in a cephalocaudal fashion.

Normal newborns may manifest mild physiologic jaundice which resolves spontaneously without sequelae. Premature infants and those with known blood group incompatibility (such as Rh or ABO incompatibility) or other

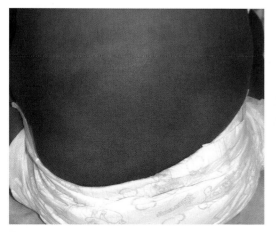

Figure 9-9 Dermal melanocytosis

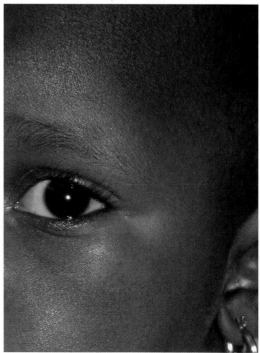

Figure 9-10 Nevus of Ota

hematologic disorder predisposing to hemolysis (such as hereditary spherocytosis, glucose-6-phosphate dehydrogenase deficiency) are at greatest risk of clinically significant unconjugated hyperbilirubinemia that may require treatment in the form of visible light phototherapy or exchange transfusion in order to avoid kernicterus.

Bronze-baby syndrome

Bronze-baby syndrome refers to the intense, gray-brown, or "bronze-like" hyperpigmentation that occurs in a subset of patients receiving visible light phototherapy for management of neonatal jaundice. Although it is classically associated with the use of phototherapy in children with conjugated hyperbilirubinemia, it also occurs in a subset of patients with unconjugated hyperbilirubinemia in association with hepatic dysfunction, particularly cholestasis. The cause of the bronze pigment is unclear, although there is evidence to suggest that biliverdin and bilifuscin-like photoproducts are involved. Phototherapy should therefore be avoided for infants with conjugated hyperbilirubinemia, and the occurrence of bronze-baby syndrome in an infant with unconjugated hyperbilirubinemia suggests the presence of coexisting hepatic dysfunction.

Purpuric phototherapy-induced eruption

A photodistributed purpuric eruption associated with visible light phototherapy has been described in children with severe hyperbilirubinemia as a result of ABO or Rh incompatibility receiving exchange transfusions. Areas that are covered by monitoring leads, diapers, or clothing are spared (Figure 9-12). It is thought that accumulation of porphyrin metabolites (such as coproporphyrin and protoporphyrin) from erythrocyte breakdown causes a transitory porphyrinemia and associated photosensitivity. Once the phototherapy is discontinued, the condition resolves spontaneously within a week.

Similar photodistributed purpuric eruptions may occur in the context of other inborn errors of porphyrin metabolism such as erythropoietic protoporphyria or congenital erythropoietic porphyria. These tend to be more severe, and may be unmasked by visible light phototherapy even without associated exchange transfusion. Screening of serum, urine, and stool porphyrin levels will indicate persistently elevated levels of porphyrins in this context.

Vascular Processes in the Newborn and Infant

Key Points

- Cutis marmorata, harlequin color change, and acrocyanosis are benign temperature-sensitive vasomotor responses that affect newborns.
- Cutis marmorata telangiectatic congenita (CMTC) is a persistent mottling of the skin that can be associated with limb length and girth discrepancies and extracutaneous manifestations.
- Umbilical granulomas can be easily treated with topical silver nitrate.
- Umbilical discharge of fluid or foul-smelling material may indicate the presence of an underlying umbilical remnant such as a patent urachus or omphalomesenteric duct remnant.

Cutis marmorata

Normal newborns may develop a "mottled" or reticulate erythema on the torso and extremities that is particularly accentuated with exposure to cold temperatures. Because of the marble-like appearance to the skin, this physiologic condition

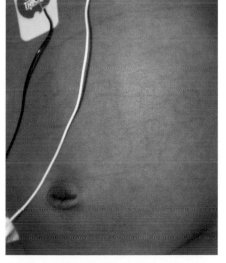

Figure 9-11 Neonatal hyperpigmentation. Note the involvement within natural skin creases

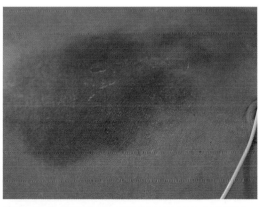

Figure 9-12 Purpuric phototherapy-associated eruption. Sparing of photoprotected areas is characteristic

is referred to as cutis marmorata. This condition is generally benign and, with maturation, cutis marmorata becomes less common as the infant is better able to maintain body temperature. Cutis marmorata may be extensive and accentuated in the trisomies and Cornelia de Lange syndrome.

Cutis marmorata telangiectatica congenita (congenital phlebectasia)

A cutis marmorata-like eruption that is present at birth in association with persistent, reticulate, violaceous erythema and areas of atrophy indicates a distinct condition known as CMTC (Figure 9-13). A "pseudoathletic" appearance is often described due to loss of subcutaneous fat when this condition is observed on affected extremities. CMTC is a unique vascular malformation in which capillary, venous, and lymphatic channels may be involved. Most children with this condition improve spontaneously over time. However, those who develop symptomatic varicosities with lower-extremity involvement may benefit from leg compression stockings. Involvement of the lower extremity has been associated with both leg length shortening and leg overgrowth, although it is more common to see a disparity in girth rather than length, as opposed to what is seen in Klippel–Trenaunay–Weber syndrome.

A variety of associated anomalies have been described, so a complete physical examination should be performed in infants affected with CMTC. Ophthalmologic and neurologic screening may be performed in those with associated findings.

CMTC-like eruptions may also be observed in the context of neonatal lupus erythematosus. Infants who manifest neonatal lupus as a result of transplacental transfer of maternal antibodies (SSA, SSB, u1RNP) may develop a reticulated, violaceous erythema with associated atrophic skin changes. Most cases of CMTC are not, however, associated with neonatal lupus, and screening of children for ANA, SSA, SSB, u1RNP should be individualized to each particular case.

Harlequin color change

As a result of neonatal vasomotor instability, some infants may manifest harlequin color change when a child is laid on its side. A clear and dramatic demarcation occurs between light or pale-colored skin on the superior half while a ruddier, redder half is noted inferiorly. Repositioning the infant will abate the phenomenon. This is a benign condition that resolves spontaneously.

Acrocyanosis

Peripheral cyanosis involving the hands and feet may occur in some infants immediately after delivery, and especially during fits of crying, as a result of peripheral vasoconstriction. This is a benign phenomenon that requires only reassurance.

However, persistent acral cyanosis in association with episodic central cyanosis in an infant may be an indicator of a cyanotic congenital heart disease, such as tetralogy of Fallot, total anomalous pulmonary venous return, truncus arteriosus, transposition of the great vessels, tricuspid atresia, and hypoplastic left heart syndrome. In these cases, a heart murmur may be detected on cardiac auscultation and an abnormal cardiac silhouette may be visible on chest radiography. Prompt consultation with a pediatric cardiologist in these cases is essential.

Umbilical granuloma

Excess granulation tissue may appear at the umbilicus following separation of the umbilical stump within the first few weeks of life. This umbilical granuloma has a glossy, red appearance and often has a friable surface (Figure 9-14). Many resolve spontaneously but treatment with intermittent applications of topical silver nitrate causes this excessive granulation tissue to regress.

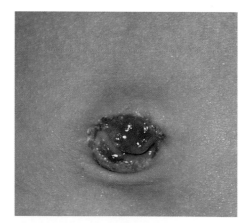

Figure 9-14 Umbilical granuloma

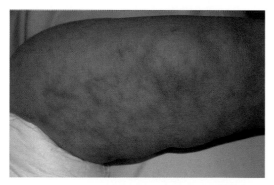

Figure 9-13 Cutis marmorata telangiectatica congenita

Umbilical remnants

If an umbilical lesion is noted that does not regress, or if an unusual discharge is noted, further evaluation may be necessary to determine whether an umbilical remnant is present. Umbilical papules or nodules seen in association with a clear or yellow discharge could indicate a patent urachus or urachal cyst, an embryologic remnant that connects the allantois to the bladder. Foul-smelling discharge from an umbilical lesion could indicate a persistent omphalomesenteric duct. Imaging studies including ultrasound, computed tomography, or magnetic resonance imaging may help confirm the diagnosis. These types of persistent umbilical remnants require pediatric surgical evaluation and intervention.

Issues of Prematurity, Labor, and Delivery

Key Points

- Caput succedaneum represents subcutaneous edema resulting from prolonged pressure in the birth canal.
- Cephalohematoma and subgaleal hematomas are more concerning because they result from birth trauma such as vacuum assistance or forceps delivery. They may be delimited by suture lines, but more severe cases can cross suture lines.
- Infants with cephalohematoma or subgaleal hematomas should be monitored for unconjugated hyperbilirubinemia as the hematomas resolve.
- Neonatal trauma to fetal or premature skin can result in persistent sequelae, such as halo scalp ring, anetoderma of prematurity, or calcinosis cutis.

Caput succedaneum

Also referred to simply as "caput," caput succedaneum occurs as a result of pressure of the fetal head against the cervix during delivery which leads to subcutaneous accumulation of serosanguineous fluid. Caput presents on the scalp as a soft, fluid-filled area with indistinct margins. Characteristically, caput does not respect suture lines, in contrast to cephalohematoma. The condition is self-limited and requires no specific intervention.

Cephalohematoma and subgaleal hematoma

Cephalohematoma refers to a painless, well-demarcated collection of blood that accumulates in the skull subperiosteum and is delimited by suture lines. This results from rupture of subperiosteal blood vessels during delivery and is sometimes accompanied by a skull fracture, especially if the hematoma crosses suture lines. The development of a cephalohematoma is often preceded by use of forceps or vacuum assistance. In contrast to the caput succedaneum, which is soft, cephalohematomas are quite firm and may actually calcify. Most cephalohematomas resolve without sequelae. Subgaleal hematomas may also result from birth trauma if bleeding occurs between the galea and the skull's periosteum.

In both cases, excessive bleeding can cause significant and symptomatic anemia, and the accumulated blood may lead to a delayed unconjugated hyperbilirubinemia.

Halo scalp ring

Halo scalp ring presents as a circular halo of alopecia that is often associated with caput succedaneum and cephalohematoma and appears to conform to a distribution suggesting pressure of the head on the cervical os. This form of alopecia is typically nonscarring and transitory, but can rarely result in permanent scarring.

Anetoderma of prematurity

Anetoderma of prematurity presents as localized areas of anetoderma that correspond to sites where trauma occurred or leads were placed. Lead placement in extremely premature infants is thought to cause pressure-induced hypoxemia in affected infants leading to loss of dermal elastic tissue and anetoderma. The affected areas appear as thinned, flaccid skin (Figure 9-15).

Calcinosis cutis

Cutaneous calcification can occur in infancy for the same reasons it does in older children and adults, and can be classified accordingly as

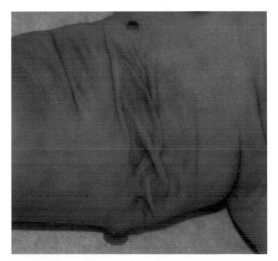

Figure 9-15 Anetoderma of prematurity

dystrophic, metastatic, idiopathic, and iatrogenic. Dystrophic calcification occurs in the setting of normal calcium and phosphate levels and develops as a result of tissue damage. This form is most commonly encountered in infants (especially premature infants) as calcified heel nodules from prior heel sticks for blood draws. These present as keratotic or verrucous papules on the lateral heel areas where prior heel sticks have occurred. Lesions may resolve spontaneously by 3 years of age, but persistent lesions may require surgical intervention if symptomatic. Metastatic calcification arises from disturbances in normal calcium and phosphate metabolism, and affected individuals typically manifest elevated calcium and phosphate levels. Metastatic cutaneous calcification in infants has been reported in individuals suffering from renal insufficiency as well as from various leukemias. Leukemic states may be associated with hypercalcemia, or may cause dystrophic calcification through tissue damage from leukemic infiltrates. Subepidermal calcified nodules of the ear are congenital lesions that represent an idiopathic form of cutaneous calcification, although some have suggested that these ear nodules may develop as a result of intrauterine tissue damage to this anatomic site. Iatrogenic calcification arises from local extravasation of calcium into the surrounding tissues. This typically occurs from infiltrated intravenous lines containing calcium chloride (or, less commonly, other forms of calcium), and this can cause significant local tissue destruction and calcinosis cutis.

Inflammatory Skin Disorders of the Newborn and Infant

Key Points

- Neonatal acne is a nonscarring process that may be caused in part by the presence of *Malassezia* species as well as transplacental transfer of maternal hormones.
- Infantile acne typically has a later onset than neonatal acne and has the potential for scarring. Appropriate topical and systemic treatment should be instituted.
- The principal concern in children with SCFN is the delayed hypercalcemia that may result as the lesions begin to resolve.
- Sclerema neonatorum is a marker for a serious neonatal illness. As the underlying process is successfully addressed, sclerema neonatorum can improve.
- Infantile acropustulosis clinically resembles scabies infestation and should be considered when the eruptions occur in a cyclical fashion.
- Diaper dermatitis can be caused by a variety of etiologies. Although most cases will improve with improvement of skin barrier function, persistent cases may indicate a serious underlying disorder.

Neonatal acne

Acneiform papules and pustules are the hallmark of neonatal acne and often involve the forehead, cheeks, chin, chest, back, and scalp (Figure 9-16). In contrast to acne vulgaris, however, comedones are notably absent. While transplacentally transferred maternal hormones may predispose infants to neonatal acne, emerging evidence suggests that a significant subset of affected infants are colonized with *Malassezia* species, and the likelihood of neonatal acne correlates with the presence of *Malassezia*. Some have therefore advocated the term "neonatal cephalic pustulosis" to describe this phenomenon. Infants typically present with neonatal acne within the first 3 months after birth, and the condition is self-limited, resolving within 1–3 months. Because the condition generally heals without scarring, no specific intervention is necessary. However, use of topical antifungals such as clotrimazole may induce more rapid remission of the condition. Use of clotrimazole, however, should be avoided in children with hyperbilirubinemia and during the first 2 weeks of life when systemic absorption of clotrimazole may interfere with normal elimination of bilirubin.

Infantile acne

Infantile acne or toddler acne can be distinguished from neonatal acne on the basis of history and physical examination. Infantile acne typically presents in children over 6 months of age, although some infants may have lesions earlier. Comedones as well as papules, pustules, and inflammatory nodules may all be present in children with infantile acne as this represents a true version of acne vulgaris, and carries a risk of permanent scarring with inflammatory lesions (Figure 9-17).

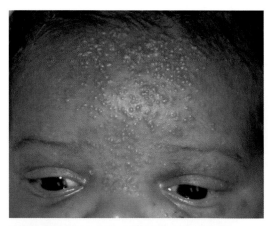

Figure 9-16 Neonatal acne. Note the lack of visible comedones

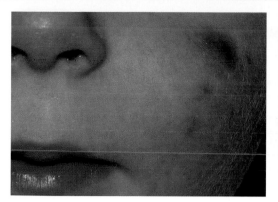

Figure 9-17 Infantile acne

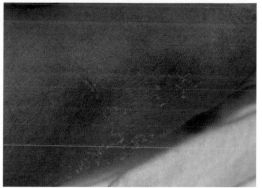

Figure 9-18 Subcutaneous fat necrosis of the newborn

Children who demonstrate findings of infantile acne should be examined closely for signs of precocious puberty, and if signs are present, consultation with an endocrinologist is recommended.

Treatment should be instituted in cases where scarring is possible or likely. A trial of topical therapy using benzoyl peroxide or topical retinoids may prove sufficient for controlling milder cases where comedones predominate. However, inflammatory cases will often require a systemic agent. Erythromycin and its derivatives (such as clarithromycin) or trimethoprim/sulfa can be used for moderate inflammatory lesions, and use of oral antibiotics may be necessary for several months until the condition subsides. Tetracycline and its related compounds must be avoided due to their ability to stain the enamel of permanent dentition. Rarely, isotretinoin is needed to control particularly severe cases.

Infantile or toddler acne has been associated with early and more severe adolescent acne.

Subcutaneous fat necrosis

SCFN manifests as firm, often erythematous papules, plaques, or nodules at sites where neonatal brown fat predominates, such as the upper back, thighs, buttocks, arms, and cheeks, although other sites can be affected (Figure 9-18). Because brown fat is higher in saturated fat and melts at a higher temperature, infants under perinatal physiologic stress may present with SCFN within the first month of life. Potential triggering stressors include: hypothermia (environmental or induced during cardiac surgery), pressure trauma (as might be seen with difficult deliveries due to macrosomia), maternal hypertension or toxemia, meconium aspiration syndrome, hypoxemia or neonatal asphyxia, familial dyslipidemia, as well as various forms of fetal distress associated with maternal diabetes mellitus, maternal cocaine use, and maternal smoking. Histologic evaluation reveals fat necrosis with needle-shaped clefts

within the adipose cells. A mixed granulomatous inflammatory infiltrate is also typically present, and areas of calcification may be observed. Some infants with SCFN may develop hypercalcemia so children with palpable lesions should be monitored, looking for signs or symptoms of hypercalcemia and a serum calcium level checked weekly until the lesions clinically resolve. If a child becomes symptomatic with hypercalcemia, calcium-wasting diuretics (e.g., furosemide) can be used to reduce serum calcium levels. Systemic corticosteroids can reduce calcium levels by interfering with vitamin D metabolism, and bisphosphonates have been used successfully in more severe cases of hypercalcemia secondary to SCFN.

Sclerema neonatorum

Sclerema neonatorum represents a phenotype associated with underlying disease rather than a specific disease entity, and has been associated with a variety of disease processes such as prematurity, sepsis, pulmonary disease (such as pneumonia), congenital heart disease, gastrointestinal diseases, and metabolic derangements such as hypoglycemia, metabolic acidosis, and hypothermia. The skin becomes indurated and waxy in appearance with decreased elasticity. Associated histologic findings include needle-like clefts within adipose cells as well as dermal edema. The process typically begins at sites where brown fat predominates – the buttocks or thighs – and then becomes more generalized as the underlying disease progresses. The skin findings parallel the progress of the underlying condition, but this is a premorbid condition that almost always ends in death.

Infantile acropustulosis

Infantile acropustulosis (or acropustulosis of infancy) is an inflammatory skin disorder that manifests during later infancy as highly pruritic crops of papules, vesicles, and especially pustules that are concentrated on the extremities

(Figure 9-19). Characteristically, episodic flares occur every 2 weeks and may last 1–2 weeks at a time, although affected infants may not completely clear between episodes. While cases of infantile acropustulosis are often idiopathic, a subset of children have a history of antecedent documented scabies infestation, indicating that these children suffer from a postscabetic pustulosis. Treatment with oral antihistamines or a low-potency topical corticosteroid such as alclometasone, desonide, or hydrocortisone 2.5% can be helpful in moderating the associated pruritus. Topical pramoxine, a topical anesthetic and antipruritic, may also be helpful. In severe symptomatic cases, dapsone has been used to treat the condition. It remits spontaneously by preschool age.

Diaper dermatitis

Irritant contact diaper dermatitis is a common consequence of diaper use. The prolonged occlusion provided by the diaper with exposure to urinary ammonia and fecal enzymes lead to conditions that favor the development of an irritant contact dermatitis. This form of diaper dermatitis is characterized by well-demarcated areas of erythema, scaling, and maceration on surfaces that contact the diaper (Figure 9-20). Sparing of the inguinal creases is common. Chronic irritant dermatitis in the diaper area can become more macerated and erosive (Jacquet's diaper dermatitis). Treatment involves more frequent diaper changes, use of superabsorbent diapers, use of barrier creams containing zinc oxide, and occasionally short-term use of a low-potency topical steroid such as hydrocortisone acetonide 1% or 2.5% cream or ointment for up to 1 week. If a presumed irritant contact dermatitis does not resolve within 1–2 weeks with appropriate

treatment, other potential diagnoses should be considered.

Allergic contact dermatitis in the diaper area is less common, but can occur in response to rubber components in diaper elastics or to dyes such as Disperse Blue. Patterned areas of dermatitis might appear where the elastic margins of the diaper come into contact with the legs. Topical medicaments used for irritant contact dermatitis may also occasionally trigger an allergic contact dermatitis, and should be suspected if the rash worsens with each application of the agent. Identification and elimination of the offending allergen will allow the dermatitis to resolve. Short-term treatment with a topical steroid for up to 1 week may be needed to accelerate the resolution of the dermatitis.

Monilial or candidal diaper dermatitis frequently evolves from a primary irritant contact diaper rash. Colonization of the rash by *Candida* species typically occurs within 72 hours and the erythema and scaling begin to involve not just contact surfaces but also intertriginous zones. Peripheral satellite papules and pustules are common (Figure 9-21). Concomitant involvement of the axillae or neck folds is sometimes noted. Use of a topical antifungal such as nystatin or clotrimazole cream twice daily for 1 week should be sufficient to clear the rash and appropriate measures should also be taken to manage any underlying irritant contact dermatitis using barrier agents, more frequent diaper changes, and more absorbent diapers. Azole antifungals should be avoided in newborns with hyperbilirubinemia due to their ability to inhibit cytochrome P450 oxidases and thereby decrease oxidation of bilirubin.

Group A streptococcal superinfection of an irritant contact diaper dermatitis can also occur. These cases are characterized by intense, fiery red intertriginous and perianal erythema and can be distinguished from moniliasis because streptococcal intertrigo is accompanied by a foul odor and typically lacks satellitosis (Figure 9-22).

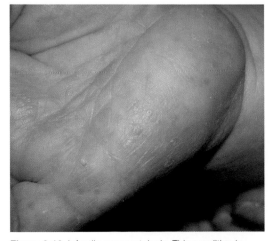

Figure 9-19 Infantile acropustulosis. This condition is frequently mistaken for scabies infestation

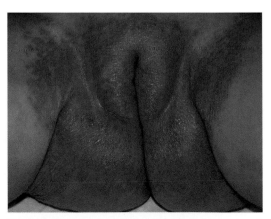

Figure 9-20 Irritant contact dermatitis. Note the sparing of the intertriginous areas

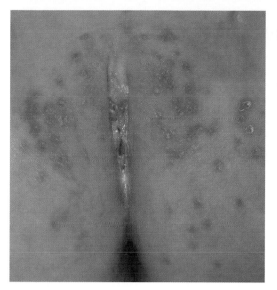

Figure 9-21 Monilial diaper dermatitis. Note the satellite lesions

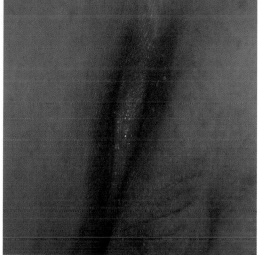

Figure 9-22 Streptococcal intertrigo

Treatment often requires prolonged therapy with an oral antibiotic such as amoxicillin in conjunction with topical therapy such as mupirocin and hydrocortisone 1% or 2.5% acetonide cream or ointment.

Seborrheic dermatitis commonly involves the diaper area and presents with a salmon-colored erythema that often includes intertriginous areas. Peripheral scaling may be present, and corroborating features of seborrheic dermatitis may be seen on the face, scalp, and other body areas. The rash is often relatively asymptomatic, so active nonintervention is reasonable. If symptomatic, short-term treatment with a low-potency topical steroid can be considered.

Infantile psoriasis in the diaper areas resembles seborrheic dermatitis and may be indistinguishable at first. Well-demarcated areas of erythema with intertriginous involvement are apparent, and children may also demonstrate other affected sites (Figure 9-23). Napkin psoriasis may precede any clinical evidence of psoriasis elsewhere on the body. Intermittent use of low-potency topical steroids or topical calcineurin inhibitors may be necessary to control the condition.

Zinc deficiency dermatitis should be considered in infants with a chronic diaper dermatitis that is well demarcated and associated with vesicles or bullae. Frequently, affected infants are being weaned from breast milk which has a greater bioavailability of zinc than formula products. Facial findings include a U-shaped dermatitis affecting the cheeks and chin while sparing the upper lip, and an acral dermatitis is typically present. Diarrhea, alopecia, photophobia, paronychia, and irritability may be present. When the zinc deficiency is the result of an autosomal-recessive zinc transporter defect, it is referred to as acrodermatitis enteropathica (Figure 9-24). Acquired zinc deficiency dermatitis may result from either decreased intake (decreased zinc content in maternal milk, anorexia nervosa in adolescents and young adults), increased losses due to malabsorption (as seen in cystic fibrosis, inflammatory bowel disease) or an associated metabolic disease (such as ornithine transcarbamylase deficiency).

Thermal burns on the buttocks or perineum should raise the suspicion of child abuse. Forced immersion injuries typically manifest with burns on contact surfaces and may demonstrate well-defined areas with splash patterns on the feet, hands, or buttocks. Sparing of the anal opening is typical, giving the appearance of a doughnut-shaped thermal burn. Unexplained burns should always be evaluated. Excessive intake of laxatives has been associated with severe, irritant burn-like diaper dermatitis of senna involvement of the anal opening and perianal area.

Langerhans cell histiocytosis should always be considered in the child with a persistent diaper dermatitis that does not respond to conventional therapy. Intertriginous erythema may be seen in conjunction with atrophic skin. Satellite lesions often have a crusted or hemorrhagic appearance. Other accompanying features include a crusted scalp dermatitis, early dental eruption, gingival hyperplasia, hepatosplenomegaly, diabetes insipidus, skeletal lesions, and pulmonary involvement.

Neonatal lupus erythematosus

Neonatal lupus erythematosus is caused by transplacental transfer of maternal antibodies to the infant. SSA, SSB, U1RNP in isolation or some combination represent the pathogenic antibodies involved. Affected infants may present with congenital heart block, thrombocytopenia, hepatitis, or skin findings of photosensitivity. The photosensitive eruption manifests as telangiectatic erythema, often encircling the eyes in a "raccoon" or "owl's-eye" pattern (Figure 9-25A). Other areas may have a psoriasiform or polycyclic appearance resembling subacute cutaneous lupus (Figure 9-25B) or a reticulate, violaceous CMTC-like appearance. The skin findings typically resolve within the first 6–12 months as the pathogenic antibody is broken down. While the skin findings, hepatitis, and thrombocytopenia resolve as the antibody disappears, the congenital heart block if present generally persists and represents the principal cause of morbidity or mortality from this disorder. In fact, neonatal lupus represents the most common cause (80%) of neonatal heart block. The heart block seen in infants with neonatal lupus is most strongly associated with SSA, less so with SSB, and not with U1RNP.

Since approximately half of all affected children have mothers who are unaware that they carry a pathogenic antibody, the mothers of affected children should be evaluated by their own physicians for evidence of an underlying connective tissue disorder. The risk of an affected mother having a child with neonatal lupus is approximately 5%. However, having had one child with neonatal lupus, the risk of a future child being affected increases to 25%.

Congenital Nevi and Anomalies of Nonmelanocytic Origin

Key Points

- Lines of Blaschko represent purported lines of cutaneous embryogenesis. Diseases which follow these lines indicate underlying genetic mosaicism.
- Most epidermal nevi are isolated phenomena; more extensive lesions can be associated with extracutaneous syndromic manifestations.

- The risk of malignant transformation of nevus sebaceus is relatively low, but children should be followed with serial skin examinations or elective excision of sebaceous nevi should be considered.
- Membranous aplasia cutis congenita (ACC) in association with a hair collar sign may indicate underlying cranial dysraphism and should undergo appropriate neuroimaging studies.

Lines of Blaschko

Lines of Blaschko refer to lines compiled and drawn by Blaschko in 1901 to indicate the cutaneous routes delineated by a variety of inherited and acquired skin disorders, such as incontinentia pigmenti, epidermal nevi, and lichen striatus (Box 9-1). These lines do not correspond to known anatomic structures, such as blood vessels or nerves, and are presumed to represent lines of cutaneous embryogenesis and indicate underlying cutaneous mosaicism. Characteristically, these lines have a swirling, arcuate pattern, forming S-like configurations, and in the midline forming V-shaped notches.

Epidermal nevus

Epidermal nevi present as linear or clustered papules and plaques that follow lines of Blaschko. They represent a class of hamartomas of ectodermal origin and, as such, epidermal nevi may possess keratinocytic, sebaceous, follicular, apocrine, and eccrine components to varying degrees. Nevi of this type are typically present at birth, or may present within the first few years of

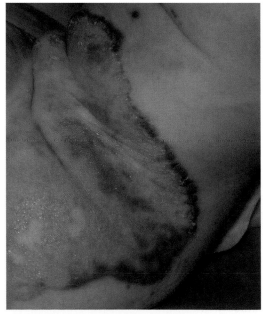

Figure 9-24 Acrodermatitis enteropathica

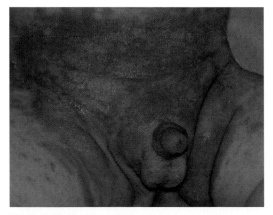

Figure 9-23 Napkin psoriasis

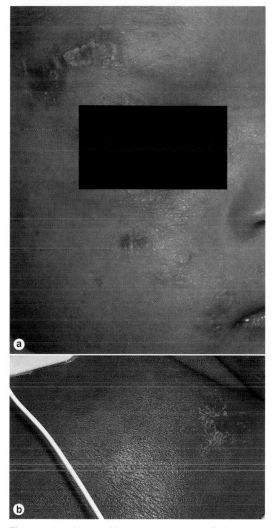

Figure 9-25a Neonatal lupus erythematosus. Periocular clustering of discoid lesions. **b** Neonatal lupus erythematosus resembling subacute cutaneous lupus erythematosus

Nevus comedonicus denotes a linear collection of keratin-plugged follicular papules that resemble comedones.

Eccrine nevi are rare hamartomas in which localized hypertrophy or hyperplasia of eccrine glands is noted. Localized hyperhidrosis is classically seen but not always present. Lesions are not typically associated with systemic manifestations.

Symptomatic lesions of ILVEN can be treated with intermittent use of topical steroids, and their appearance may be moderated by the use of topical keratolytics containing urea or ammonium lactate, topical retinoids such as tazarotene, or the vitamin D analogue, calcipotriene. Discrete lesions of epidermal nevi may be amenable to elective surgical excision, but superficial shave excisions tend to lead to recurrence. Their full extent may not be expressed until adolescence or adulthood so definitive surgical intervention may be postponed until then as regrowth at postoperative margins is possible if the entire lesion has not been removed; otherwise, additional surgery may be necessary to remove residual nevus.

Aside from symptomatic changes that might occur, epidermal nevi may also be associated with extracutaneous manifestations. While the majority of epidermal nevi are isolated phenomena, some lesions – particularly more extensive nevi – have been reported in association with neuropathologic, ophthalmologic, or musculoskeletal issues as part of a broader epidermal nevus syndrome. A skeletal survey, ophthalmologic consultation, and head magnetic resonance imaging may be indicated in appropriate cases. Hypophosphatemic rickets has been observed in the context of epidermal nevus syndromes, and epidermal nevi can be seen as part of other described syndromes such as Proteus syndrome, phakomatosis pigmentokeratotica, sebaceous nevus syndrome, pigmented hair nevus (such as Becker's nevus) syndrome, CHILD syndrome (congenital hemidysplasia with ichthyosiform erythroderma and limb defects), and nevus comedonicus syndrome.

Histopathologically, LEN show psoriasiform epidermal hyperplasia with papillomatosis, acanthosis, and hyperkeratosis. ILVEN are histologically similar with additional findings of hypogranulosis and parakeratosis alternating with hypergranulosis and orthokeratosis. In either case, epidermolytic hyperkeratosis (EHK) can be observed, and these patients should be counseled about the possibility of germline mosaicism which, if present, predisposes to having children with expression of EHK as a somatic trait. Nevus comedonicus, a developmental anomaly of the pilosebaceous apparatus, demonstrates rudimentary hair follicles with epidermal invaginations that are plugged with keratin. Eccrine nevi demonstrate increased numbers or increased size of eccrine glands.

life. Rarely, epidermal nevi manifest later during adolescence or adulthood.

Linear epidermal nevi (LEN) and *inflammatory linear verrucous epidermal nevi* (ILVEN) present as keratotic or verrucous plaques (Figure 9-26A). LEN are generally noninflammatory in appearance, asymptomatic, and favor the head and neck areas. As the name indicates, ILVEN are inflammatory, psoriasiform in appearance, often pruritic, and more commonly observed on the extremities (Figure 9-26B). ILVEN clinically and histologically resembles psoriasis, and it is interesting to note that some patients with ILVEN also complain of joint symptoms including arthralgias or arthritis. Some cases of ILVEN can spontaneously resolve, although the majority of cases tend to persist indefinitely.

Blaschkolinear lesions

X-linked

Incontinentia pigmenti

CHILD syndrome

MIDAS/MLS

Conradi–Hunerman syndrome

Focal dermal hypoplasia

Congenital or nevoid

Epidermal nevus

Sebaceous nevus

Nevus comedonicus

Linear porokeratosis

Porokeratotic eccrine ostial and dermal duct nevus

Congenital melanocytic nevi[*]

Eccrine spiradenomas[*]

Nevoid hypermelanosis

Nevus depigmentosus

Hypomelanosis of Ito

Segmental neurofibromatosis[*]

Basal cell nevus syndrome[*]

Darier's disease[*]

Hailey–Hailey disease[*]

Mosaic trisomy 7 skin pigmentary dysplasia[*]

Acquired

Drug eruptions[*]

Psoriasis[*]

Linear lichen planus[*]

Vitiligo[*]

Linear alopecia mucinosa[*]

Lupus erythematosus[*]

Linear atrophoderma (of Moulin)

Grover's disease[*]

Lichen striatus[*]

Lichen sclerosus[*]

Streptococcal exanthem[*]

[*]Some cases, but clearly not all, have a blaschkolinear distribution.

CHILD, congenital hemidysplasia with ichthyosiform erythroderma and limb defects; MIDAS, microphthalmia + dermal aplasia + sclerocornea; MLS, microphthalmia + linear skin defects.

Nevus sebaceus

Nevus sebaceus (of Jadassohn) is a type of epidermal nevus that presents as a congenital, hairless, yellow-orange plaque with a velvety

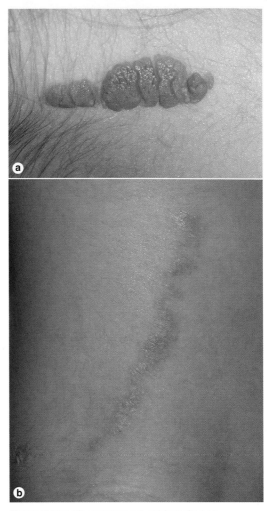

Figure 9-26a Linear verrucous epidermal nevus. **b** Inflammatory linear verrucous epidermal nevus

or cobblestoned surface and is most commonly seen on the scalp or face (Figure 9-27). Histology reveals epidermal hyperplasia with increased numbers of sebaceous glands with rudimentary or hypoplastic hair follicles.

Traditionally, nevus sebaceus has been associated with approximately a 5–15% lifetime risk of malignant transformation. Basal cell carcinoma, squamous cell carcinoma, sebaceous carcinoma, and porocarcinoma are among the malignancies that have arisen within pre-existing nevus sebaceus lesions. More recent evidence indicates that benign tumors such as trichoblastoma and syringocystadenoma papilliferum are more common and that the risk of malignant transformation has perhaps been overestimated.

Extensive lesions can be associated with nevus sebaceus syndrome. Neuropathologic changes, ocular abnormalities including ocular dermoid,

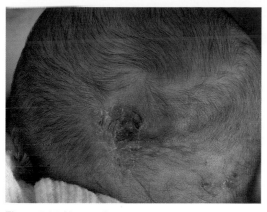

Figure 9-27 Nevus sebaceus

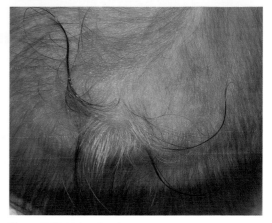

Figure 9-28 Hair collar sign

and musculoskeletal abnormalities have been reported. More rarely, hypophosphatemic rickets, renal hamartomas, and mediastinal lipomatosis have also been noted. If nevus sebaceus lesions are small, they can generally be removed without significant disfigurement. Larger lesions are likely to be noticeable and potentially carry a higher risk of malignant transformation; consultation with a plastic surgeon for elective excision can be considered. Removal at an early age will usually afford a better cosmetic outcome due to increased scalp laxity. Periodic follow-up with serial skin examinations is advised for those who decline surgical removal.

Aplasia cutis congenita and the hair collar sign

Thought to be the result of local impairment of blood flow in utero or the failure of embryonic planes to fuse properly, ACC is a disorder that manifests as the congenital absence of skin and may be associated with absence of deeper subcutaneous tissues such as fat, muscle, and bone. Lesions can be solitary or multiple and are most commonly observed on the vertex of the scalp. Two principal forms of ACC have been described: nonmembranous and membranous. Nonmembranous ACC presents with an ulcer without an overlying membrane and has irregular margins. By contrast, membranous ACC is often circular or oval and presents with a thin overlying membrane. These lesions may be associated with a collar of coarse, terminal hairs – the so-called "hair collar sign" (Figure 9-28). In its original description, the hair collar sign involved the triad of nodular membranous ACC, a collar of terminal hair, and an associated vascular stain. This hair collar is a marker for underlying cranial dysraphism, such as heterotopic brain tissue or an atretic encephalocele. Infants and children with a hair collar sign should therefore undergo

neuroimaging, but typical lesions of ACC do not need to be investigated.

Further reading

Benaron DA. Subgaleal hematoma causing hypovolemic shock during delivery after failed vacuum extraction: a case report. J Perinatol 1993; 13:228–231.

Berger PE, Heidelberger KP, Poznanski AK. Extravasation of calcium gluconate as a cause of soft tissue calcification in infancy. Am J Roentgenol 1974;121:109–116.

Bernier V, Weill FX, Hirigoyen V, et al. Skin colonization by *Malassezia* species in neonates: a prospective study and relationship with neonatal cephalic pustulosis. Arch Dermatol 2002; 138:215–218.

Commens C, Rogers M, Kan A. Heterotopic brain tissue presenting as bald cysts with a collar of hypertrophic hair. The hair collar sign. Arch Dermatol 1989;125:1253–1256.

Cribier B, Scrivener Y, Grosshans E. Tumors arising in nevus sebaceus: a study of 596 cases. J Am Acad Dermatol 2000;42:263–268.

Drolet BA, Clowry L, McTigue MK, et al. The hair collar sign: marker for cranial dysraphism. Pediatrics 1995;96:309–313.

Drolet B, Prendiville J, Golden J, et al. Membranous aplasia cutis with hair collars. Congenital absence of skin or neuroectodermal defect? Arch Dermatol 1995;131:1427–1431.

Frieden IJ. Aplasia cutis congenita: a clinical review and proposal for classification. J Am Acad Dermatol 1986;14:646–660.

Frieden IJ. The dermatologist in the newborn nursery: approach to the neonate with blisters, pustules, erosions, and ulcerations. Curr Probl Dermatol 1992;4:123–168.

Happle R. Lyonization and the lines of Blaschko. Hum Genet 1985; 70:200–206.

Harris JR, Schick B. Erythema neonatorum. Am J Dis Child 1956;92:27–33.

Hicks MJ, Levy ML, Alexander J, et al. Subcutaneous fat necrosis of the newborn and hypercalcemia: case report and review of the literature. Pediatr Dermatol 1993;10:271–276.

Mancini AJ, Frieden IJ, Paller AS. Infantile acropustulosis revisited: history of scabies and response to topical corticosteroids. Pediatr Dermatol 1998;15:337–341.

Onishi S, Itoh S, Isobe K, et al. Mechanism of development of bronze baby syndrome in neonates treated with phototherapy. Pediatrics 1982; 69:273–276.

Paller AS, Syder AJ, Chan YM, et al. Genetic and clinical mosaicism in a type of epidermal nevus. N Engl J Med 1994;331:1408–1415.

Paller AS, Eramo LR, Farrell EE, et al. Purpuric phototherapy-induced eruption in transfused neonates: relation to transient porphyrinemia. Pediatrics 1997;100:360–364.

Prendiville JS, Esterly NB. Halo scalp ring: a cause of scarring alopecia. Arch Dermatol 1987;123: 992–993.

Schneider BM, Berg RA, Kaplan AM. Aplasia cutis complicated by sagittal sinus thrombosis. Pediatrics 1980;66:948–950.

Sell EJ, Hansen RC, Struck-Pierce S. Calcified nodules on the heel: a complication of neonatal intensive care. J Pediatr 1980;96:473–475.

Tan KL, Jacob E. The bronze baby syndrome. Acta Pediatr Scand 1982; 71:409–414.

Todd DJ. Anetoderma of prematurity. Arch Dermatol 1997;133:789.

Weston WL, Morelli JG, Lee LA. The clinical spectrum of anti-Ro-positive cutaneous neonatal lupus erythematosus. J Am Acad Dermatol 1999; 40:675–681.

Wilson-Jones E, Heyl T. Naevus sebaceus: a report of 140 cases with special report of the development of secondary malignant tumours. Br J Dermatol 1970;82:99–117.

Yan AC, Wahrman J, Honig PJ. Napkin dermatitis: clinical features and differential diagnosis. In: Harper J, Oranje A, Prose N, eds. Textbook of Pediatric Dermatology, 2nd edn. Oxford: Blackwell Publishing, 2006.

Zelson C, Lee SJ, Pearl M. The incidence of skill fractures underlying cephal hematomas in newborn infants. J Pediatr 1974;85:371–373.

Genetic disorders of the skin

10

Andrea L. Zaenglein

The genetic basis for disease in the skin is varied, ranging from tumor suppressor abnormalities to enzyme defects to single-gene protein disorders. Neurofibromatosis type 1 (NF-1) and tuberous sclerosis (TS) are classic examples of genodermatoses associated with tumor suppressor defects, resulting in benign and malignant growths in the skin and various other organs. Defects in structural elements like collagen and keratin, lying above, within, and below the basement membrane zone, may result in skin fragility and blistering. Disorders of cornification, including the ichthyoses, arise from a variety of defects, for example, abnormalities in the cornified cell envelope, structural defects in keratins, and impaired desquamation. Presentations of genetic skin disease are highly variable and even within the same disorder the extent of involvement can be diverse, as evidenced by epidermolysis bullosa (EB). Two excellent resources for up-to-date reviews of numerous genetic disorders, expert recommendations for management, and available testing laboratories can be found at www.genetests.org and www.ncbi.nlm.nih.gov/omim.

Neurofibromatosis type 1

Key Points

- Greater than 6 café au lait macules (CALM)
- Lisch nodules appear after 2 years of age
- Most cases of NF-1 are diagnosed by 4 years of age
- Autosomal dominant; 50% spontaneous mutation rate
- Refer developmental delay/learning disabilities early

Clinical features

One of the classic phakomatoses, NF-1 exemplifies a tumor suppressor syndrome. The diagnosis of NF-1 is often first suspected with the appearance of multiple CALMs on the skin. These typically begin to appear in the first year or two of life and increase in numbers with subsequent years. The CALMs in NF-1 are light-tan to dark-brown in color, well-defined macules with regular borders (Figure 10-1). National Institutes of Health (NIH) criteria indicate that CALMs should be at least 0.5 cm in prepubertal children and at least 1.5 cm in children after puberty to qualify as criteria for NF-1. The other cutaneous criteria for diagnosis appear at differing times throughout development. Plexiform neurofibromas may be present at birth but may not be clinically apparent until later childhood. These tan-brown, large, ill-defined tumors can arise anywhere, may have increased hair overlying them, and are classically described as feeling like a "bag of worms" (Figure 10-2). A superficial lesion is often misdiagnosed initially as a CALM, congenital nevus, Becker's nevus, or a smooth-muscle hamartoma. Deeper plexiform neurofibromas can invade underlying soft tissue and bony structures. If pain or rapid growth is associated with these lesions, it may be a sign of malignant degeneration. Neurofibrosarcoma occurs in approximately 5% of cases, usually in adulthood, and may arise from plexiform or common neurofibromas.

Axillary freckling, originally known as Crowe's sign, appears in early childhood, usually between 3 and 5 years of age. These grouped, small, tan to brown macules can arise in the armpits or in the inguinal creases (Figure 10-3). Neurofibromas are soft, fleshy papules that begin to appear in adolescence and continue to increase in numbers throughout adulthood (Figure 10-4). They often have a pink to purplish or bluish color and can vary in size from a few millimeters to several centimeters. Commonly, they are pedunculated, mimicking skin tags. With downward pressure, neurofibromas will give way and evert within themselves. This

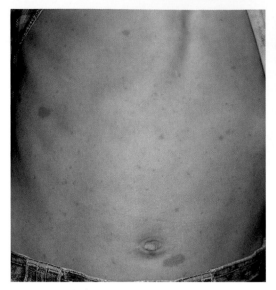

Figure 10-1 Café au lait macules. Multiple lesions on the chest

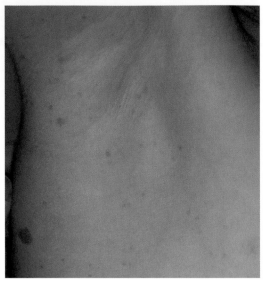

Figure 10-3 Axillary freckling. May be present in armpits and groin

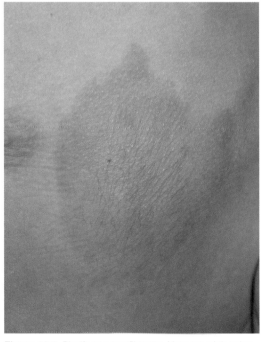

Figure 10-2 Plexiform neurofibroma. Note tan-pink color and increased terminal hair

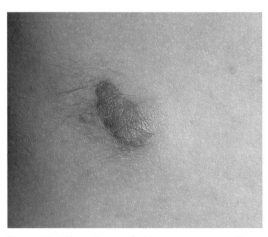

Figure 10-4 Neurofibroma. Soft tan-brown plaque with increased hair

nodules (iris hamartomas of melanocytic origin) begin to appear about the same time as axillary freckling, between 3 and 5 years of age. Lisch nodules provide diagnostic support for NF-1 but do not affect vision.

Enhanced tumorigenesis occurs with an increased incidence of pheochromocytoma, meningioma, glioma, acoustic neuroma, and optic neuroma. Of the malignancies seen in NF-1, malignant peripheral nerve sheath tumors are the most frequent, arising in about 10% of individuals. These tumors tend to occur at a younger age than the neurofibrosarcomas, and portend a poorer prognosis. Leukemias too are more common in children with NF-1, especially juvenile chronic monomyelogenous leukemia. Children with NF-1 and juvenile xanthogranuloma are reported to have an even higher risk of developing

is known as the buttonhole sign and is useful in differentiating neurofibromas from other entities such as skin tags or nevi.

The extracutaneous diagnostic criteria include the specific skeletal changes of sphenoid wing hypoplasia and pseudoarthrosis. Scoliosis and bony overgrowth are also found but are nonspecific for NF-1. Optic gliomas may arise along the tract of the optic nerve. While Lisch

leukemia. Even so, hematologic malignancies are still rare in children with NF-1. Though the overall incidence is still rare, prudent monitoring is warranted.

Hypertension is quite common in adults with NF-1 and may be essential or due to renal artery stenosis, or other vasculopathy. Pulmonic stenosis can also be seen. Moya-moya-type small-vessel cerebral vascular disease and cerebral aneurysms are more common.

While most individuals with NF-1 have normal intelligence, learning disabilities, particularly relating to language skills, occur in about 50–75%. Early intervention in children suspected of having NF-1, even if they have not met the diagnostic criteria, is essential if they are displaying any signs of developmental delay.

A specific phenotype displaying overlap between NF-1 and Noonan syndrome is seen in about 12% of individuals with NF-1. Individuals will have ocular hypertelorism, downward-slanting eyes, low-set ears, webbed neck, and pulmonic stenosis.

Diagnosis

A diagnosis of NF-1 is made by fairly strict diagnostic criteria. These are listed in Table 10-1. Having at least two or more criteria carries with it a 95% sensitivity and specificity for NF-1. It may take several years for a person with NF-1 to fully develop all of the findings necessary to make a diagnosis. In children with multiple CALM and no family history of NF-1, only about 50% will meet the NIH criteria for diagnosis by 1 year of age. By 8 years, almost all suspected children will have fulfilled the required criteria. Genetic testing is also now commercially available for NF-1 and may provide earlier detection to identify affected individuals. Therefore it is important for patients with multiple CALM to be followed regularly by a dermatologist, geneticist, ophthalmologist, and/or other clinician experienced in diagnosing the disorder.

It is important to note that several disorders have been associated with multiple CALM and must be considered until the criteria for NF-1 have been met. Other forms of NF-1 should be considered in incomplete or atypical presentations (Table 10-2). McCune–Albright syndrome is associated with large, irregular, jagged bordered CALM (coast of Maine), in contrast to the smooth regular borders of the CALM found in NF-1 (coast of California.) Polyostotic fibrous dysplasia and endocrine abnormalities are additionally seen with this syndrome. NF2 is also important to consider in a child with multiple CALM. The presence of bilateral acoustic schwannomas is diagnostic. Numerous entities have been identified as having multiple CALM, although many have an incidence that matches the general population

Table 10.1 Diagnostic criteria for neurofibromatosis type 1	
Cutaneous critera	**Extracutaneous criteria**
6 or more café au lait macules > 0.5 cm in childhood > 1.5 cm in adulthood	Optic glioma
1 plexiform neurofibroma	Skeletal changes: pseudoarthrosis or sphenoid wing hypoplasia
Axillary or inguinal freckling (Crowe's sign)	Affected first-degree relative
Lisch nodules	
2 or more neurofibromas	

Table 10.2 Types of neurofibromatosis	
Type 1	Von Recklinghausen
Type 2	Acoustic schwannomas
Type 3	Mixed
Type 4	Variant
Type 5	Segmental
Type 6	Café au lait macules only
Type 7	Late-onset
	NF NOS

NF NOS, neurofibromatosis not otherwise specified.

and the association may be weak. These are listed in Table 10-3.

Pathophysiology

NF-1 is caused by a mutation in the tumor suppressor gene, neurofibromin, located on chromosome 22. This is a very large gene, with hundreds of different disease-causing mutations. Its function is to inhibit the ubiquitous oncogene, Ras. There is a 50% spontaneous new mutation rate, meaning one-half of all persons with NF-1 do not have an affected family member.

Treatment

A multidisciplinary management of patients with NF-1 is essential. In the absence of a multispecialty NF clinic, one provider should supervise and coordinate the specialist referrals. Cosmetically unacceptable CALM can sometimes be effectively treated with an appropriate laser by an experienced laser surgeon. Surgical treatment of neurofibromas should be limited to troublesome or conspicuous lesions. Removal of all lesions is often impractical and would not likely result in the best cosmetic outcome. Experienced oncologists, neurosurgeons, or other appropriate specialists must manage any malignant tumors that arise.

Table 10.3 Disorders reportedly associated with multiple café au lait macules

Disorder	Major clinical features	Genetic defect
Neurofibromatosis type 1	CALM, neurofibromas, axillary freckling, optic gliomas, Lisch nodules	AD Neurofibromin
Neurofibromatosis type 2	CALM, bilateral acoustic neuromas, meningiomas, spinal schwannomas	AD Neurofibromin2 (Merlin)
McCune–Albright syndrome	Large irregular CALM, polyostotic fibrous dysplasia, precocious puberty and other endocrine dysfunction	Mosaicism in GNAS1
Watson syndrome	CALM, pulmonic stenosis, other findings of NF1	AD Neurofibromin (alleleic with NF1)
LEOPARD syndrome	Lentigines, electrocardiographic conduction abnormalities, ocular hypertelorism, pulmonic stenosis, abnormal genitalia, retardation of growth, and sensorineural deafness. CALM and café noir macules	AD PTPN11 (alleleic with Noonan syndrome)
Russell–Silver syndrome	IUGR with postnatal growth retardation. Triangular-shaped facies. Down-turned corners of mouth. CALM. Hypoglycemia. Camptodactyly, brachydactyly	Genetically heterogeneous. 10% with uniparental disomy chromosome 7
Fanconi anemia	Progressive bone marrow failure, short stature. Cardiac, renal, and limb malformations. CALM and hyperpigmentation	AR Defect in one of the Fanconi anemia complementation group genes
Banayan–Riley–Ruvalcaba	Macrocephaly, lipomas, hemangiomas, CALM, lentigines on penis, pseudopapilledema	AD PTEN (allelic with Cowden syndrome)
Turcot syndrome	Adenomatous colonic polyps, malignant CNS tumors, CALM, sebaceous cysts, BCC	AD APC or MLH1 or PMS2
Multiple endocrine neoplasia, type 1 (MEN1)	Peptic ulcer disease. Pituitary, parathyroid and pancreas tumors. CALM, angiofibromas, collagenomas, lipomas, gingival papules	AD MEN1
Tuberous sclerosis	Angiofibromas, connective tissue nevus, periungual fibromas, hypopigmented macules, cortical tubers, renal angiomyolipomas, subependymal giant cell astrocytoma, cardiac rhabdomyoma, lymphangiomyomatosis. Gingival fibromas, CALM	AD Tuberin TS1 Hamartin TS2
Johanson–Blizzard syndrome	Nasal alar hypoplasia, hypothyroidism, pancreatic insufficiency, and congenital deafness. GU structural abnormalities. CALM, sparse and unruly hair, transverse palmar crease, aplasia cutis	AR UBR1
Bloom syndrome	Pre- and postnatal growth deficiency, photosensitivity, recurrent infections, diabetes, chronic pulmonary disease, predisposition to cancers. CALM, dyspigmentation, hypertrichosis	AR BLM (DNA helicase)
Rubinstein–Taybi syndrome	Mental retardation, broad thumbs and toes, abnormal facies, short stature. CALM, hemangiomas, transverse palmar crease, keloids	AD CREBBP

AD, autosomal dominant; APC, antigen-presenting cell; AR, autosomal recessive; BCC, basal cell carcinoma; CALM, café au lait macules; CNS, central nervous system; GU, genitourinary; IUGR, intrauterine growth retardation.

Tuberous Sclerosis

Key Points

- Autosomal dominant; however, many cases arise spontaneously as sporadic mutations
- Hypopigmented macules from infancy
- Angiofibromas arise in childhood
- Developmental defects correlate with the severity of neurologic involvement and seizures

Clinical features

The clinical manifestations of TS appear staggered throughout childhood, with some signs not developing until adulthood. Clinical suspicion should prompt an age-appropriate work-up based on the working knowledge of when each sign typically develops. The first skin lesion to appear is a well-defined hypopigmented macule, formerly known as an ash-leaf macule (Figure 10-5). These may be present at birth or during early infancy. Multiple lesions eventually develop. Additionally, cortical tubers and cardiac rhabdomyomas develop in utero and are early-appearing diagnostic criteria. However, in the absence of seizures or cutaneous signs of TS, detection of their presence would likely be happenstance. As the child grows, angiofibromas begin to emerge. These small pink-to-red, somewhat blanchable, vascular papules appear grouped about the central face, forehead, and chin (Figure 10-6). Collagenomas, both fibrous forehead plaques and Shagreen patches, are also diagnostic and appear later in childhood (Figure 10-7). Firm, pink, smooth-topped, exophytic papules grow outward from under the proximal nail folds. These periungual fibromas were classically known as Koenen tumors, and usually develop later in adulthood (Figure 10-8).

Extracutaneous manifestations of TS involve many solid organs, including heart, kidney, lungs, eyes, and brain. Cardiac rhabdomyomas are at their largest in the neonatal period, and spontaneous regression is common. Treatment is only necessary in symptomatic cases. One of the major diagnostic findings of TS is renal angiomyolipomas, but various other renal tumors are also found, including epithelial cysts, oncocytoma, and, rarely, malignant tumors. Renal involvement appears before 10 years of age in about 80% of persons. Renal failure may result in extensive cases. In a subset of affected individuals, there is phenotypic overlap between TS and polycystic kidney disease. These patients will display classic features of TS along with cystic degeneration of the kidneys, possibly leading to renal failure. Liver and central nervous system (CNS) involvement may also occur.

Lung involvement is uncommon and a late finding, occurring primarily in females between 10

Figure 10-5 Hypopigmented macule in tuberous sclerosis

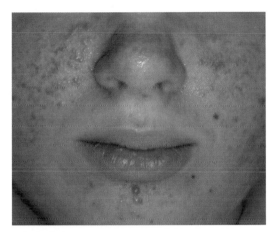

Figure 10-6 Facial angiofibromas

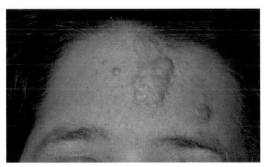

Figure 10-7 Collagenoma. Forehead plaque in woman with tuberous sclerosis

and 40 years of age. Lymphangiomyomatosis may present with shortness of breath or hemoptysis. Progressive disease may result in respiratory failure. The eyes are commonly affected, and regular ophthalmologic examination can reveal asymptomatic iris hamartomas or achromic macules.

CNS tumors are the greatest cause of morbidity in patients with TS and the degree of mental impairment can be directly correlated to the severity of CNS disease and seizure activity. Developmental delay (including pervasive

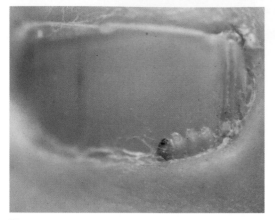

Figure 10-8 Periungual fibroma

Table 10.4 Diagnostic criteria for tuberous sclerosis*

Major	Minor
Hypomelanotic macules (ash-leaf macule)	Dental pitting
Collagenomas (Shagreen patch)	Rectal hamartomatous polyps
Facial angiofibromas (adenoma sebaceum)	Bone cysts
Periungual fibromas (Koenen tumors)	Cerebral white-matter radial migration lines
Cortical tubers	Gingival fibromas
Subependymal nodule	Retinal achromic patch
Subependymal giant cell tumor	Confetti-like hypopigmented macules on skin
Retinal hamartoma	Multiple renal cysts
Cardiac rhabdomyoma	
Renal angiomyolipoma	
Lymphangiomyomatosis	

*Must have two major criteria or one major and two minor criteria for diagnosis.

developmental disorder and autism) and mental retardation occur in up to 50% of patients with TS. In order of frequency, subependymal glial nodules, cortical tubers, and subependymal giant cell astrocytomas can occur. Premature death occurs in one-third of patients and is directly related to the degree of mental retardation and severity of seizures.

Diagnosis

A diagnosis of TS is made by established diagnostic criteria, as listed in Table 10-4. Two major criteria, or one major and two minor, must be met in order to confirm a diagnosis of TS. Therefore, a thorough cutaneous examination is necessary in patients and first-degree relatives. TS should be considered in all children with new-onset seizures. Confirmation of the diagnosis is made by magnetic resonance imaging of the brain, revealing classic tubers, by biopsy of the kidney, or by critical skin examination to detect additional criteria. Patients who do not meet these criteria, but have elements suggestive of TS, should be followed closely for future development of disease. Singular hypopigmented macules are fairly common in children.

The differential diagnosis of the hypopigmented macules includes nevus depigmentosus, nevus anemicus, postinflammatory hypopigmentation, and perhaps pityriasis alba. These entities are detailed in Chapter 7. Solitary angiofibromas, also called fibrous papules, are common in adulthood but rare in children. Multiple angiofibromas are also seen in other genetic disorders, including multiple endocrine neoplasia type 1 and Birt–Hogg–Dube syndrome. The small, reddish lesions can be confused with acne and perhaps familial trichoepitheliomas.

Pathophysiology

The TS complex results from a mutation in either of two separate genes, TSC1, encoding the protein hamartin, or TSC2, encoding tuberin. It is inherited in an autosomal-dominant manner. Approximately 50% of cases arise from a spontaneous new mutation, without an affected parent.

Treatment

Disfiguring facial or digital angiofibromas can be treated by various surgical modalities, including electrodesiccation and curettage, dermabrasion, or appropriate laser ablation. Disfiguring facial collagenomas can be surgically removed but a large scar is the inevitable outcome. A multidisciplinary approach to the other manifestations of TS should be taken, including cardiology, nephrology, neurology, ophthalmology, and oncology.

Epidermolysis Bullosa

Key Points

- Noninflammatory blistering, particularly at sites of trauma
- Variable severity depending on genetic defect
- Worse at sites of friction and trauma

Clinical features

EB is a heterogeneous group of blistering disorders, all defined by the presence of non-inflammatory vesicles and bullae. The severity of blistering will depend primarily on the type of EB and specific genetic defect. The forms of EB are detailed in Table 10-5. Within each general category there is much phenotypic variation.

The most common form of EB is *EB simplex* (EBS). Blistering in the Weber–Cockayne

Table 10.5 The types of epidermolysis bullosa

	Epidermal bullosa type	Clinical characteristics	Genetic defect
Simplex	Weber–Cockayne	Blistering predominantly on hands and feet	AD Keratins 5 and 14
	Koebner	Bullae overlying joints and at sites of trauma. Milia may be present	AD Keratins 5 and 14
	Dowling–Meara	Generalized blistering with milia common. Nails and mucosa may be involved	AD Keratins 5 and 14
	w/ Muscular dystrophy	Generalized blistering with milia and scarring. Characterized by progressive muscular weakness. Dystrophic teeth and nails. Laryngeal and urethral involvement may occur	AR Plectin
Junctional	Lethalis	Widespread sheets of bullae without scarring. Prominent facial involvement healing with granulation tissue. Significant morbidity with respiratory, gastrointestinal, and corneal disease. Hands usually spared	AR Laminin 5
	w/ Pyloric atresia	Generalized blistering of skin and mucous membranes. Gastric outlet obstruction in newborn. Urinary tract involved	AR $\alpha6\beta4$ Integrin
	Generalized atrophic benign	Widespread blistering with a high rate of squamous cell carcinoma. Dental enamel impairment and nail loss	AR Collagen XVII
	Cicatricial	Generalized blistering resulting in significant scarring with joint contractures, syndactyly	AR Laminin 5
Dystrophic	Recessive dystrophic (Hallopeau–Siemens) epidermal bullosa	Severe, generalized blistering, erosions and ulcerations. Milia and scarring. Resultant mitten deformity of hands and feet. Oral involvement and feeding problems result in failure to thrive	AR Collagen type VII
	Dominant dystrophic epidermal bullosa	Variable phenotype from very mild to more severe. Acral blistering with nail dystrophy	AD Collagen type VII

AD, autosomal dominant; AR, autosomal recessive.

subtype (EBS-WC) does not present at birth but typically later when the child starts crawling or walking, or sometimes even later. The hands, feet, and knees will be most affected (Figure 10-9). The more severe, generalized form of EBS, the Dowling–Meara subtype (EBS-DM), will present in the newborn period. Hemorrhagic blisters cluster at sites of trauma, such as the diaper area, and are more widespread. They typically heal without scarring, though nail dystrophy and milia are common (Figures 10-10 and 10-11). However, dyspigmentation may take several months to resolve. The severity of blistering usually improves over time. Palmoplantar hyperkeratosis may be the only manifestation in adulthood. While the teeth and mucous membranes are not typically affected in EBS-WC, the more extensive variants may have involvement that is severe enough to cause feeding problems. The Koebner variant typically displays an intermediate degree of blistering, more widespread than EB-WC, but not as severe as EBS-DM. In another form, EBS with mottled pigmentation, the blistering is extensive at birth

and is replaced by prominent hyperpigmentation. Eventually the dyspigmentation also improves but a palmoplantar hyperkeratosis may persist.

The *junctional EB* forms are often the most severe, and are associated with a high mortality rate. The Herlitz variant (JEB-L) is particularly severe, marked by eroded sheets of bullae at birth with prominent central facial denudation. Despite the extent, the blistering does not typically scar. Widespread mucosal and airway involvement leads to respiratory compromise, nutritional deficiency, infections, and eventual death. *Dominant dystrophic EB* (DDEB) classically presents with recurrent blistering, particularly on the hands, feet, knees, and elbows. Milia are prominent and in very mild forms may be the only manifestation seen. With recurrent blistering, scarring results; and loss of nails or dystrophic nails are very common with this presentation, especially on the toes (Figure 10-12).

Recessive dystrophic EB (Hallopeau–Siemens RDEB), in contrast, presents with a more severe phenotype. Generalized blistering of the skin and

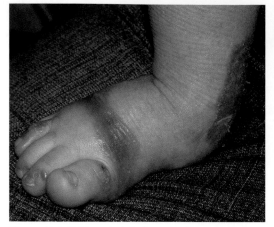

Figure 10-9 Epidermolysis bullosa simplex. Note superficial blistering on feet

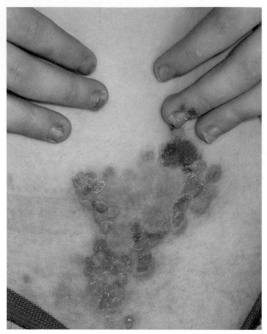

Figure 10-11 Epidermolysis bullosa simplex. Superficial blistering on the abdomen with prominent nail dystrophy

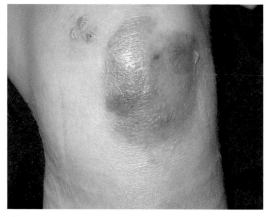

Figure 10-10 Epidermolysis bullosa simplex. Healing bulla on the knee with milia in Dowling–Meara subtype

mucous membranes relentlessly occurs starting from birth (Figure 10-13). Pseudosyndactyly, or mitten deformity, of the hands and feet will result from chronic, repeated blistering and scarring. Conjunctival and cornea involvement may cause a permanent loss of vision. Oral, tracheal, and laryngeal blistering results in profound morbidity, with feeding difficulties, failure to thrive, and growth retardation. Ankylostomia, microstomia, and esophageal webbing are common. As a result of malnutrition and increased blood loss, a persistent, severe anemia is of particular concern and often refractory to treatment, as is osteoporosis. Pulmonary and renal amyloidosis may result from years of chronic disease. A dilated cardiomyopathy has also been described in affected individuals and may result from carnitine and/or selenium deficiency. As with most chronic scarring disorders, RDEB has an increased risk of cutaneous squamous cell cancer, with the lifetime risk nearing 90%. It is an exceedingly aggressive type, frequently causing death in these physically frail individuals. Many additional

variants of RDEB (non-Hallopeau-Siemens RDEB) with variably less severe phenotypes than the classic RDEB have been described.

Diagnosis

A diagnosis of EB is suspected clinically and can be confirmed by biopsy of normal skin that has been gently abraded with a pencil eraser or similar object. Regular hematoxylin and eosin-stained sections are not helpful, and biopsies must have immunofluorescent mapping of basement membrane zone antigens or be sent for electron microscopy. Either way, a highly specialized pathology laboratory is needed. Electron microscopy can sometimes be beneficial in establishing a level of blister cleavage; however, experienced interpretation of results is needed for accuracy. In the severe forms – junctional and RDEB in particular – genetic testing should be performed as the detected genotype may give some foresight into expected phenotype. In less severe forms of EB, mutation analysis is most helpful for genetic counseling.

Pathophysiology

The specific genetic defects that cause EB are listed in Table 10-5. The forms of EBS are due to various mutations in keratins 5 or 14 found in the basal layer of the skin. The exception is EBS with muscular dystrophy, which is caused by a plectin mutation. Plectin is a major structural component of the intermediate filaments, providing

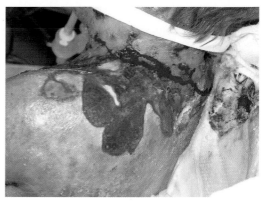

Figure 10-13 Recessive dystrophic epidermolysis bullosa (Hallopeau–Siemens). Sheets of eroded bullae with excessive granulation tissue on the neck of a 6-year-old boy

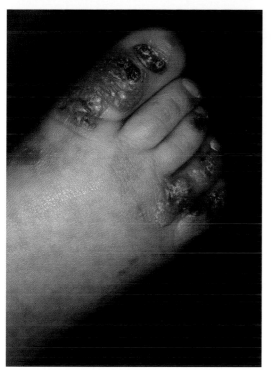

Figure 10-12 Dominant dystrophic epidermolysis bullosa. Prominent milia and loss of nails

mechanical strength to both muscle and skin. The junctional forms of EB are the result of defects in proteins within the basement membrane: laminin 5, α6β4 integrin (associated with pyloric atresia), or collagen XVII. The dystrophic forms of EB (DDEB and RDEB) are both due to defects in collagen VII, the major component of anchoring fibrils. The severity of disease depends on whether it is a homozygous or heterozygous mutation and the site of mutation within the gene.

Treatment

The mainstay of treatment of all the forms of EB is avoidance of trauma and wound care. In general, tape and other adherent bandages should not be applied directly to the skin in children with EB. Sterile incision and drainage of larger blisters can alleviate painful pressure and prevent expansion of the blisters. The roofs of the bullae should be left intact. Secondary infections are a risk and should be treated with appropriate topical or oral antibiotic therapy when they occur. In most forms, with EBS-DM being the exception, blistering is generally worse in warm weather so trying to maintain a cool environment is important. Due to the long-term risk of squamous cell carcinoma in the scarring forms of EB, nonhealing wounds should be biopsied.

For the severe forms of EB, a multidisciplinary approach should be taken, incorporating dermatology, gastroenterology, ophthalmology,

hematology, genetics, and pain management and any other relevant specialty. Since failure to thrive, chronic anemia, and feeding difficulties are common, aggressive nutrition supplementation and gastrostomy tubes may be required. Pain is often severe, especially when changing bandages, and appropriate pain control measures should be taken.

Hypohidrotic Ectodermal Dysplasia

Key Points

- Light sparse hair, decreased sweating, and absent dentition
- Characteristic facies
- Risk of hyperthermia in warm weather

Clinical features

The ectodermal dysplasias are an expansive group of disorders defined by the presence of defects in the ectodermal structures: hair, teeth, nails, and sweat glands. Nearly 200 different disorders fall under the classification of ectodermal dysplasia. There are several different classification systems based on different criteria, including the number of structures involved and the basic category of genetic defect identified.

The classic example of an ectodermal dysplasia is *hypohidrotic ectodermal dysplasia* (Christ–Siemens–Touraine syndrome). At birth, affected neonates are often red and scaly, and the condition may be confused with an ichthyosis. The skin improves over time, but remains slightly fragile. Affected individuals will have light-colored, sparse scalp and body hair. There is a marked decrease in the numbers of eccrine sweat glands resulting in ineffective sweating. Hyperthermia during warm weather or exercise is a major risk and basal body temperature should be closely monitored, especially in young children who are unaware of the warning signs. Late eruption of teeth with pronounced hypodontia, usually about 5–6 teeth, is common. The teeth that are present may be conical or misshapen (Figure 10-14). Persons with hypohidrotic ectodermal dysplasia also have a characteristic facies evident even in infancy. The findings of periorbital hyperpigmentation and depressed nasal bridge (saddle-nose deformity) are supportive features. Other clinical findings include the lack of dermal ridges and a hoarse, raspy voice. Decreased sebaceous secretions resulting in impaction of aural cerumen and nasal secretions can occur. It is important to note that, despite the defects in the ectodermal structures, the physical growth and psychological development of a person with hypohidrotic ectodermal dysplasia are completely normal.

Heterozygous female carriers of this X-linked recessive disorder will demonstrate a decreased number of sweat glands in a mosaic pattern following the lines of Blaschko. They may have mild dental abnormalities, including pegged, conical, or a few absent teeth, along with mild hypotrichosis. Due to underdeveloped milk ducts, maternal milk production may be inadequate. The defects are so mild in most female carriers that no clinically significant expression of the disorder is ever evident until an affected child is born, prompting close examination for the subtle manifestations.

Diagnosis

Hypohidrotic ectodermal dysplasia is suspected in infancy based on the physical appearance of the child and the skin changes. Delayed eruption of teeth, absence of sweating, and sparse hair will confirm the diagnosis. Once suspected, the diagnosis can be corroborated by genetic analysis if necessary. A biopsy from the palm will demonstrate a marked decrease in sweat glands but this invasive test is seldom necessary. A sweat iodide test can be used to determine the extent and distribution of functioning sweat glands in carriers of X-linked recessive hypohidrotic ectodermal dysplasia.

As stated, there are numerous ectodermal dysplasias and any combination of ectodermal appendageal defects is possible. In patients presenting with one or more abnormalities of hair, teeth, nails or sweating, other forms of ectodermal dysplasia are possible. If cleft lip or palate is present, one of the ectodermal dysplasia clefting syndromes, such as Hay–Wells or Rapp–Hodgkin syndrome, should be considered. The services of a geneticist or dysmorphologist are extremely helpful in these confusing and rare genodermatoses.

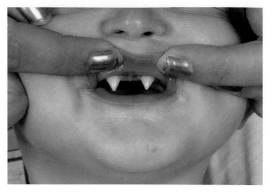

Figure 10-14 Hypohidrotic ectodermal dysplasia. Pegged and absent teeth

Pathogenesis

Although 95% of affected individuals have the X-linked recessive form, autosomal-recessive and autosomal-dominant forms exist. The autosomal-recessive form is clinically indistinguishable from the X-linked form while the AD form is generally milder in phenotypic expression. In the X-linked recessive form, a defect in ectodysplasin A (EDA), a ligand involved in the early epithelial–mesenchymal interaction that regulates ectodermal appendage formation, is responsible for the disease. In the autosomal-recessive and autosomal-dominant forms, defects in the ectodysplasin receptor (EDAR) or death domain adaptor (EDARADD) are causative.

Treatment

Monitoring for hyperthermia in hot weather is vital. Affected individuals should mist cool water on the skin to encourage evaporative loss of excess heat. Cooling vests are also commercially available. An experienced dentist should monitor dental abnormalities and treat according to the severity of abnormalities. Replacing absent or misshapen teeth with implants or dentures may be necessary to achieve adequate functional and cosmetic outcomes. Impacted earwax and nasal secretions may require regular monitoring by ear, nose, and throat specialists.

Ichthyosis Vulgaris

Key Points

* Worse in cold, winter months
* Often associated with atopic disorders
* Treat with emollients, such as petroleum ointment

Clinical features

Affecting approximately 1:250 people, ichthyosis vulgaris is the most common genetic scaling disorder and one of the most common single-gene

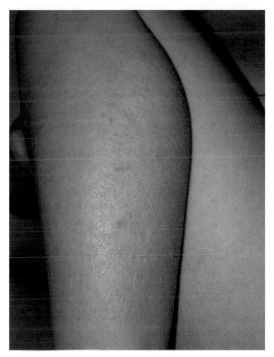

Figure 10-15 Ichthyosis vulgaris. Dry scaling of the arms in a child with atopic dermatitis

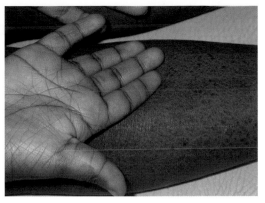

Figure 10-16 Ichthyosis vulgaris. Thick scaling on the legs with hyperlinear palms

disorders occurring in humans. The skin of a patient with ichthyosis vulgaris may appear normal during the summer months when the heat and humidity are high. As winter approaches, the large, dirty-appearing scales emerge on the lower extremities followed by the trunk and arms (Figure 10-15). Hyperlinearity of the palms and soles often accompanies the scaling skin (Figure 10-16). Classically there is flexural sparing due to higher relative humidity in those areas. Affected areas are often quite pruritic. The scaling disorder is often secondarily associated with atopic dermatitis and can occur concomitantly with keratosis pilaris.

Diagnosis

The differential diagnosis of ichthyosis vulgaris is listed in Table 10-6. In male patients without a family history of scaling skin or atopy, it is often difficult to differentiate X-linked ichthyosis clinically from ichthyosis vulgaris. In older children or patients with acquired ichthyosis, an underlying systemic illness (particularly lymphoma) should be considered. A biopsy showing a decrease in the granular layer may be beneficial in differentiating ichthyosis vulgaris from other forms of ichthyosis but is seldom necessary. Targeted mutation analysis is also available.

Pathophysiology

Ichthyosis vulgaris results from homozygous or heterozygous loss-of-function mutations in the fill agrin gene. This condition exhibits semidominant

inheritance. Therefore the severity of disease in each affected family member may vary.

Treatment

The staple treatment of all ichthyoses is hydration and moisturization. Soaking baths followed by liberal application of a thick, bland emollient such as petroleum ointment is recommended. The addition of a keratolytic agent such as lactic acid, glycolic acid, or urea, may be beneficial but may be associated with burning and irritation. Topical corticosteroids should be used judiciously in patients with prominent itch and associated atopic dermatitis.

X-linked Ichthyosis

Key Points

- Only males affected
- Fine scaling on extremities, abdomen, flexures, and neck
- Corneal opacities and undescended testes
- Contiguous gene syndrome with Kallmann syndrome and Conradi–Hünermann syndrome

Clinical features

With scaling appearing shortly after birth, boys born with X-linked ichthyosis will have fine, white-to-tan dry scales, pronounced on the legs but also represent behind the ears and on the sides of the neck, extensors of the upper arms, and characteristically across the abdomen (Figure 10-17). Thicker, darker scales cover the distal legs. As with ichthyosis vulgaris, the creases and central face are typically spared (Figure 10-18).

Extracutaneous manifestations of X-linked ichthyosis include undescended testes in 20% of affected individuals and asymptomatic corneal opacities in the majority of patients by adulthood. Additionally, prolonged labor in carrier mothers due to a placental insufficiency of steroid sulfatase

Table 10.6 The ichthyoses

Type	Clinical features	Genetic defect
Ichthyosis vulgaris	Dry, fine scaling greatest on the extremities. Spares face and flexures. Often associated with atopic dermatitis	AD Filaggrin
X-linked ichthyosis	Coarser, dirty-appearing tan-brown scales. Sides of necks and retroauricular region commonly affected. Males only. Associations include corneal opacities, undescended testes, and prolonged labor in carrier mothers. Contiguous gene syndrome with Kallmann syndrome and Conradi–Hünermann syndrome	XLR Steroid sulfatase
Epidermolytic hyperkeratosis (bullous CIE)	Blistering and erosions at birth. Progresses to generalized scaling. Hyperlinearity in the creases. Musty odor	Keratins 1 and 10
CIE	Generalized erythema with fine scaling. Often collodion at birth (> 90%)	AR ALOX12B ALOXE3 Transglutaminase
Lamellar ichthyosis	Coarse, plate-like scaling. Ectropion, eclabium. Often collodion baby	AR Transglutaminase 1 (90% of classic cases) ALOX12B ALOXE3 ICHTHYIN
Harlequin ichthyosis	Dramatic restrictive, armor-like scaling with deep fissures at birth. Extensive ectropion and eclabium. Often premature. High mortality in infancy. Later progresses to severe, generalized erythroderma and scaling along with alopecia, palmoplantar keratoderma	AR ABCA12

AD, autosomal dominant; AR, autosomal recessive; CIE, congenital ichthyosiform erythroderma; XLR, X-linked recessive.

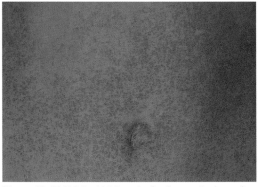

Figure 10-17 X-linked ichthyosis. Scaling on the legs of a newborn boy

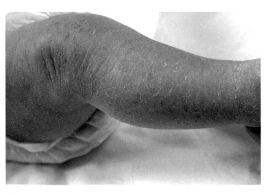

Figure 10-18 X-linked ichthyosis.

is commonly reported and not surprisingly a high percentage of these children are delivered by cesarean section. Of note, X-linked ichthyosis is part of a contiguous gene syndrome located on Xp22.3 with Kallmann syndrome (cryptorchidism, anosmia, stippled bones, and unilateral renal agenesis) and Conradi–Hünermann chondrodysplasia punctata (linear ichthyosis following the lines of Blaschko, cataracts, and short stature).

Diagnosis

Biopsy findings in X-linked ichthyosis are nonspecific. An enzymatic assay for steroid sulfatase function is diagnostic. Asymptomatic corneal opacities may be noted on ophthalmologic examination. A thorough family history will usually demonstrate generations of affected males born to female carriers, confirming the X-linked recessive nature of the condition. This will help

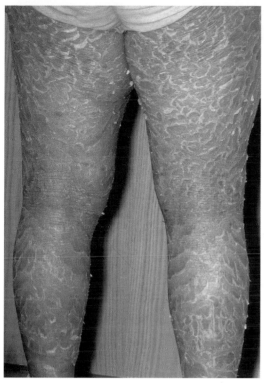

Figure 10-19 Lamellar ichthyosis. Thick plates of scale

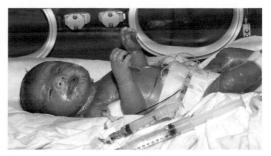

Figure 10-20 Collodion baby. Congenital membrane of scale leading to ectropion and eclabium

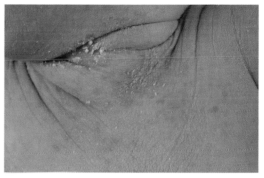

Figure 10-21 Epidermolytic hyperkeratosis. Thick, grooved, warty brown scaling

distinguish it from ichthyosis vulgaris, the most difficult entity in the differential diagnosis.

Pathophysiology

X-linked ichthyosis is due to a defect in the gene encoding the enzyme steroid sulfatase. This results in a decreased level of cholesterol in the stratum corneum, impaired desquamation, and a retention hyperkeratosis.

Treatment

Treatment focuses on moisturization and increasing desquamation. Keratolytic agents, such as ammonium lactate, urea, and retinoids, are particularly useful in increasing the rate of shedding of the retained stratum corneum. Surgical correction of cryptorchidism should be done upon detection.

Other Forms of Ichthyosis

Lamellar ichthyosis is an autosomal-recessive disorder consisting of generalized, large, plate-like scales (Figure 10-19) associated with scarring alopecia and ectropion (eversion of the eyelids). *Congenital ichthyosiform erythroderma* is another autosomal-recessive ichthyosis. Fine, white powdery scaling overlies a bright red erythema and variable degrees of ectropion. Overlaps exist with features of both lamellar ichthyosis and congenital ichthyosiform erythroderma, and several patients with

uncategorized autosomal-recessive ichthyosis have fairly mild components of each. There is also much genetic overlap amongst the autosomal-recessive ichthyosis, with defects in transglutaminase, the ALOX genes, and rarely, ICHTHYIN being reported.

Sweating is impaired in both forms, and hyperthermia can be a problem in hot weather. The condition is devastating from a cosmetic standpoint, and no treatment is very effective. Tub soaks for hydration and gentle scale removal followed by aggressive use of emollients are helpful. Systemic retinoids such as isotretinoin may help. Keratolytics are not well tolerated. The initial presentation is often that of a *collodion baby* with parchment-like, restrictive scaling and erythema (Figure 10.20). These infants need very close monitoring for temperature instability, fluid and electrolyte balance, nutritional deficiency, and secondary infection. Several of the ichthyoses present as collodion babies and the specific phenotype may not be evident for weeks.

Epidermolytic hyperkeratosis is an autosomal-dominant disorder of keratin 1 or 10. Infants present with blisters that look just like EB. Eventually blistering gives way to generalized, thick, warty, brown scaling (Figure 10.21) that spares the face. Palmoplantar keratoderma may occur. Summer heat tends to induce fissuring and blisters, and secondary *Staphylococcus aureus* infection may complicate the wounds. Emollients and systemic retinoids are moderately helpful. Bathing in dilute chlorine bleach or other antibacterial cleansing agent can reduce the characteristic, socially stigmatizing, strong odor.

Further reading

Crino PB, Nathanson KL, Henske EP. The tuberous sclerosis complex. N Engl J Med 2006;355: 1345 -1356.

Ferner RE. Neurofibromatosis 1 and neurofibromatosis 2: a twenty first century perspective. Lancet Neurol 2007;6:340–351.

Lee M, Stephenson DA. Recent developments in neurofibromatosis type 1. Curr Opin Neurol 2007; 20:135–141.

Parisi MA, Sybert VP. Molecular genetics in pediatric dermatology. Curr Opin Pediatr 2000;12:347–353.

Shwayder T. Disorders of keratinization: diagnosis and management. Am J Clin Dermatol 2004; 5:17–29.

Smith FJD. The molecular genetics of keratin disorders. Am J Clin Dermatol 2003;4:347–364.

Trent JT, Kirsner RS. Epidermolysis bullosa: identification and treatment. Adv Skin Wound Care 2003;16:84–90.

Wright TJ, Grange DK, Richter MK. Hypohidrotic ectodermal dysplasia. GeneReviews. Available at www.genetests.org. Accessed June 10, 2007.

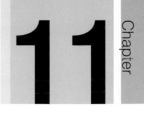

Chapter 11

Disorders of hair and nails

Howard B. Pride

Disorders of Hair

There are few chief complaints that are as emotionally charged as that of hair loss, and these visits can be some of the most challenging and time-consuming for clinicians. It is important to be very detailed in obtaining information on all aspects of the patient's past history and medication history and to do a thorough review of systems. Particular attention must be paid to other ectodermal structures such as nails and teeth and the entire skin surface needs to be observed for any associated rashes or abnormalities in sweating. It is helpful to have a diagnostic algorithm (Figure 11-1) clearly in your mind to guide history and physical exam and the clinician may find it helpful to discuss what is sought on examination with parents ahead of time so that the diagnostic conclusion at the end of the visit makes sense.

If hair follicles can be seen on close examination of the thin or hairless scalp, as will almost always be the case, then the alopecia is labeled as nonscarring and will likely be one of the entities discussed below. Scarring (Figure 11-2) is indicated by a shiny, smooth surface devoid of hair follicles. Sometimes doll's hairs, many hairs emanating from the same node, will be seen. The scarring (cicatricial) alopecias are a complicated group of rare disorders that require specialized evaluation and biopsy for diagnosis. The evaluation of tissue specimens from patches of scarring alopecia using transverse and horizontal sections requires a pathologist with experience and expertise.

Alopecia Areata

Key Points

- Distinct, smooth patches of hair loss
- Positive pull test and exclamation mark hairs
- Biopsy is diagnostic but not usually needed
- Spontaneous regrowth is the rule
- Treat with intralesional or topical steroids, minoxidil, topical contact sensitizers or anthralin

Alopecia areata is a common form of hair loss, affecting 0.1% of the population at any given time and with a lifetime risk of about 1.7%. While it affects all ages, 60% of individuals have their first bout of hair loss before the age of 20 years. Congenital occurrence has been reported. Males and females are equally affected and it is more common in children with Down syndrome.

Clinical presentation

Most children present with the sudden onset of hair loss in an isolated area or areas that is typically round or oval and completely smooth and bald (Figure 11-3). The patch may be small and hidden, and it is common for the first observation to be made by the patient's barber or hairdresser. Usually it is totally asymptomatic but some patients report itching, burning, or tenderness prior to or during the hair loss. Most often the children are otherwise totally healthy although some relate the onset of alopecia to a physically or emotionally stressful event.

On examination, a patch of alopecia areata is sharply demarcated and as smooth as a baby's bottom. It will usually be flesh-colored but may be red or pink. There may be partial regrowth or subtotal loss, and blond or gray hairs may be spared (Figure 11-4). This occurrence may lead adult patients to complain that they suddenly turned gray when in fact they suddenly lost most of their pigmented hair – the so-called "white overnight" or "gray in a day" phenomenon. Close inspection with a magnifying glass may reveal "exclamation mark" hairs: short, broken hairs that taper from a thicker distal tip to a thinner proximal shaft at the scalp (Figure 11-5). Although not totally specific, they are a finding highly suggestive of alopecia areata. A pull test should be done around the periphery of the alopecic patch and in locations around the scalp by lightly squeezing several hairs between the thumb and index finger and gently pulling away from the scalp. This should obtain a hair every 2–4 pulls in a normal individual but will obtain several hairs in a single pull in active

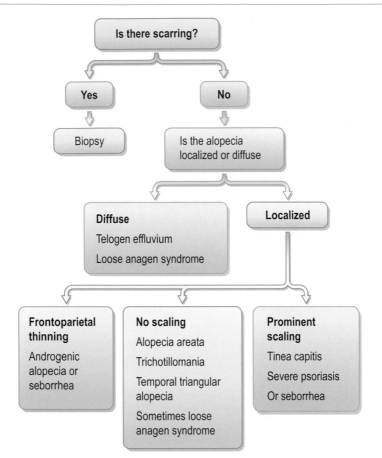

Figure 11-1 Diagnostic algorithm for hair loss

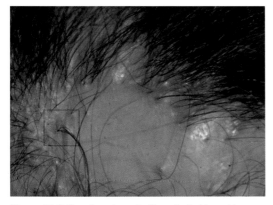

Figure 11-2 Scarring alopecia. Smooth, hairless skin devoid of any follicles. Note doll's hairs

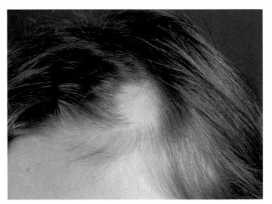

Figure 11-3 Alopecia areata. Typical smooth, sharply marginated patch of alopecia areata

areas of alopecia areata. Hairs extracted from a normal scalp demonstrate a nonpigmented club-shaped bulb. In contrast, hairs extracted from a patient with alopecia areata demonstrate a tapered fracture, resembling a pencil point.

In addition to the common patchy form of alopecia areata, other presentations of hair loss include a reticulated pattern and a diffuse pattern (particularly difficult to diagnose clinically).

Ophiasis refers to a distribution of an "inverse monk" that consists of a band of hair loss in the occipital and temporal hair margins (Figure 11-6). This carries a poor prognosis.

Inspection of the eyebrows and eyelashes may reveal spotty or total alopecia (Figure 11-7) and it is important to examine beard, trunk, and extremity hair. Categorization of alopecia is based on the extent of hair loss with alopecia areata

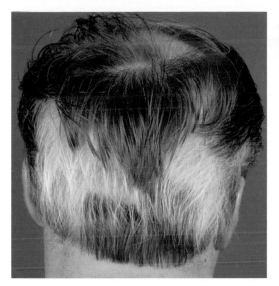

Figure 11-4 Alopecia areata. Sparing of white hairs within a patch of hair loss

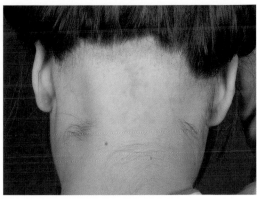

Figure 11-6 Alopecia areata. Ophiasis pattern of tempero-occipital hair loss

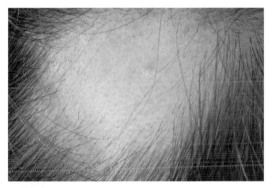

Figure 11-5 Alopecia areata. Many exclamation mark hairs

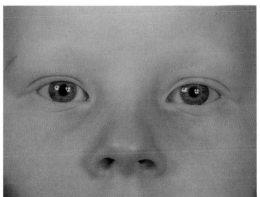

Figure 11-7 Alopecia areata. Total eyebrow and eyelash loss of alopecia universalis

being partial alopecia, alopecia totalis being total scalp alopecia and alopecia universalis being total scalp and body hair loss.

Nail changes (Figure 11-8) may be seen in up to half of children with alopecia areata, but good lighting is needed to appreciate this finding, and magnification with a hand lens can be helpful. The severity of the nail changes tends to correlate with the severity of hair loss and may precede, present concomitantly, or follow the alopecia. A few or all 20 nails may be involved. Small pits, either randomly scattered or arranged in rows, are the most characteristic finding. Rough-surfaced nails (trachyonychia), longitudinal splitting of the nail (onychorrhexis), separation or shedding of the nail (onychomadesis), and white or red spots may be seen.

Diagnosis

Classic, active alopecia areata is an easy clinical diagnosis, seldom needing laboratory studies or biopsy. The most difficult differential diagnosis

is hair pulling (trichotillomania), especially if the alopecia areata is not active at the time of examination. Compounding the confusion is the fact that some children with alopecia areata are concomitantly pulling their hair. A rough, sandpaper texture to the scalp, regrowth of hairs of different lengths, a negative pull test, absence of nail abnormalities, and bizarre patterns of hair loss suggest pulling. Isolated eyebrow and eyelash loss without any scalp hair loss is very characteristic of pulling but may occasionally be seen in alopecia areata. A 4-mm punch biopsy will generally distinguish the two entities and may need to be done in confusing cases or in circumstances where parents or patients need objective proof of the correct diagnosis to move forward with treatment.

Diffuse alopecia areata can be impossible to distinguish clinically from telogen effluvium. Biopsy will help but watchful waiting while the process resolves or declares itself is a good approach. Tinea capitis will usually be accompanied by pruritus, scaling, erythema, adenopathy, and many broken hairs. A potassium hydroxide (KOH) examination of the hairs or culture will document the infection.

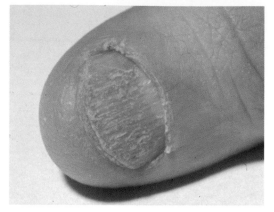

Figure 11-8 Alopecia areata. Rough, sandpapery nails

Pathogenesis

There is strong evidence that alopecia areata is an autoimmune process mediated by activated T lymphocytes with a Th1 profile. Autoantibodies to hair follicle antigens have been found in humans and in animal models and may precede hair loss, implying that they are pathogenic rather than reactive. There is a genetic component to alopecia areata but it is likely complex and polygenic. Infections, bacterial superantigens, or trauma may be inciting events that initiate the autoimmune process in a genetically susceptible host.

Patients or, more commonly, family members may have other autoimmune conditions, with thyroid disease being the most common. Other associations include vitiligo, pernicious anemia, type 1 diabetes mellitus, lupus erythematosus, rheumatoid arthritis, myasthenia gravis, and ulcerative colitis. A thorough review of systems is a sufficient screen for these entities, although many clinicians will prefer to check thyroid studies, particularly if there is a strong family history of thyroid disorders.

Treatment

No treatment is consistently effective in alopecia areata and since most children spontaneously remit in 6–12 months, simple observation is a very reasonable approach in many patients. If treatment is desired, steroids are the most commonly used agents. Intralesional injections of triamcinolone are very effective and usually well tolerated. Concentrations of 2.5–5 mg/ml are used with a maximum concentration of 10 mg/ml. About 0.1 ml/cm^2 is injected into the dermis of active alopecic areas with a maximum of 3 ml during any one session at intervals of 4–6 weeks. Some reversible atrophy may result, especially with higher concentrations or injection of too much triamcinolone into one spot. Intradermal injections are generally more effective than subcutaneous injections and are associated with a lower risk of atrophy. A topical anesthetic cream can be used prior to the injection but most children are surprised to find that the pain is not as bad as they imagined. This approach is only practical if less than 50% of the scalp is involved.

Superpotent topical steroids (for instance, clobetasol solution) are a less effective compromise for large surface areas or for young children who will not tolerate injections. Once- or twice-daily application can be done for a month and then switched to one-week-on and one-week-off application to reduce the chance of atrophy.

Topical steroids may be supplemented with other nonsteroid topical agents. Minoxidil in a 5% solution applied twice per day is reasonably effective. Systemic absorption is very low but some patients experience local irritation, dermatitis, and facial hair growth. Anthralin (Dritho-Scalp 0.5%) in a 0.25–1% cream, an immune-modulating agent that has historically been used for psoriasis, has been utilized in treating alopecia areata with some success. It is applied about 30 min prior to showering with gradually increasing contact time as tolerated. Side-effects include staining of skin and clothing, irritation, folliculitis, and lymphadenopathy. Trials with topical agents should extend for 3 months before being considered a treatment failure.

Topical immunotherapy is a novel and effective modality for treating alopecia areata, and it is particularly suited to the treatment of large surface areas and areas resistant to other topical treatments. Three contact sensitizers have been used: dinitrochlorobenzene (DNCB), squaric acid dibutyl ester (SADBE), and diphenylcyclopropenone (DPCP). DNCB has been found to be mutagenic on Ames testing and is used less often. Because these agents may also be employed in treating warts (Chapter 2), any clinic may consider having a pharmacy mix these agents to have them available for therapy. A 2% solution in acetone is used to induce sensitization and a small application can be done to the scalp or the forearm. This is repeated at 5–7-day intervals until a poison ivy-like rash is obtained. A dilute solution, usually about .001%, is then applied to the areas of alopecia once or twice per week with a cotton-tipped applicator, the intent being to perpetuate a low-grade contact dermatitis that is usually tolerable to the patient, albeit uncomfortable. Too vigorous a reaction will require less frequent application or a more dilute solution and the opposite is true of too little reaction. Care must be taken to keep the solution inside the treatment area. In various studies 20–60% of patients have responded to this regimen. Treatment should be abandoned if there is no response in 4–6 months.

Systemic steroids will stimulate growth in most patients but side-effects limit their long-term use and most children will lose the regrown hair without constant use. A burst of prednisone with a slow taper over about a month may be appropriate for explosive, extensive hair loss but should only be a stopgap measure while topical therapy is being instituted. Even though patients may note a recurrence of hair loss after discontinuation of systemic steroid therapy, frequent, repeated use of systemic steroid is not advised.

Photochemotherapy with psoralen plus ultraviolet A (PUVA) and oral cyclosporine have been reportedly effective but their side-effects are out of proportion to their therapeutic effects and cannot be routinely recommended. There is hope that the biologic agents that more specifically target a single aspect of the immune response will eventually replace these risky forms of treatment.

When confronted with the failure of topical therapy and the potential side-effects of systemic therapy, many patients and parents will very appropriately abandon treatment. Physicians should remain hopeful about the possible spontaneous regrowth of hair and offer supportive measures such as referral for wigs and providing information about the National Alopecia Areata Foundation (www.naaf.org).

Intentional Hair Pulling (Trichotillomania, Trichotillosis)

Key Points

- Preschool variety: good prognosis
- Adolescent variety: terrible prognosis
- Bizarre patterns of hair loss
- Regrowth of hair with differing lengths and negative pull test
- No treatment necessary for the preschool form
- Psychology or psychiatry evaluation for the adolescent variety

The term "trichotillomania" implies a psychiatric illness and is an unfortunate label applied to all forms of hair pulling. However, it is a name that is firmly ingrained in the medical literature and in common medical vocabulary so trichotillomania will be used here synonymously with intentional hair pulling of all varieties. Some prefer the term "trichotillosis," because it translates simply to "condition of pulling hair."

There are clearly two distinct entities that carry the label of trichotillomania. Infants and preschoolers twist and pull their hair as part of a habit or for tactile stimulation, often while they are falling asleep. It may be analogous to thumb sucking. The prognosis is good for spontaneous

resolution without intervention. School-age children and adolescents are usually pulling in reaction to various stressors and are much more likely to have associated psychological comorbidities. Some respond to simple behavior modification, but for most in this age group the prognosis is poor. The age at which these distinct presentations blend is in early grade school.

Incidence data vary widely, and studies no doubt greatly underestimate the frequency of this disorder. Roughly 10% of individuals will have practiced some form of hair pulling in their lifetime. Females outnumber males, and the average age of onset is about 12 years. There is a slight preponderance of males in the preschool variety of hair pulling.

Clinical presentation

Patients will not usually disclose that they are pulling their hair and parents infrequently witness pulling. Some parents will have some suspicion but, more often, there is denial on everyone's part. The patient may describe various sensations from the scalp but usually the process is asymptomatic.

The alopecia of trichotillomania is usually subtotal with a bizarre pattern of loss (Figure 11-9). A linear row may extend from the frontal scalp to the vertex (Figure 11-10). The margins are usually indistinct and the scalp has a rough, stubbly feel, totally unlike the smoothness of alopecia areata. Regrowth of hairs of many differing lengths is characteristic (Figure 11-11). Gentle pull test is negative. There may be excoriations and crust formation from picking. Patches may be multifocal,

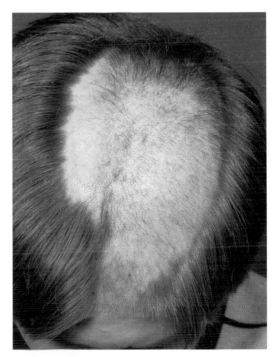

Figure 11-9 Trichotillomania. Bizarre patterning

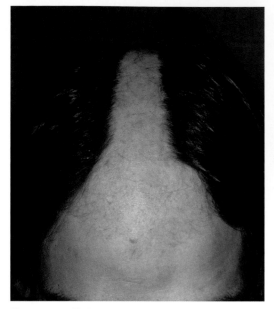

Figure 11-10 Trichotillomania. Midline row of alopecia sometimes seen in trichotillomania

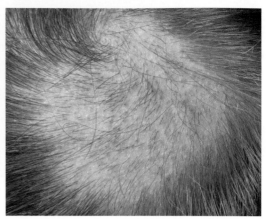

Figure 11-11 Trichotillomania. Regrowth of hairs of differing lengths

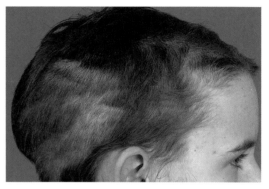

Figure 11-12 Trichotillomania. Sharply defined waves of alopecia

may spread in a wave (Figure 11-12), or may show an ever-expanding centrifugal spread from an original starting point. Some patients also exhibit trichophagia with bezoar formation. The scalp is the most common location for hair pulling, but eyebrows and lashes (Figure 11-13), beard hair, body hair, and pubic hair might be involved.

Diagnosis

Trichotillomania is usually an easy diagnosis and can often be detected even before starting the examination. Bizarre patterning and hairs of various lengths may be obvious, even from a distance. It is extremely important, though, to be thorough in the history and meticulous in the physical exam lest parents feel that you have made a snap diagnosis. Before examining the child, it can be helpful to outline the key features that will distinguish the conditions considered in the differential diagnosis and why a set of findings leads to a particular diagnosis. The hope is that parents and patients will have enough faith in the clinician's meticulousness and knowledge to accept the diagnosis, something that may be a highly unlikely conclusion to them.

Alopecia areata is the most likely condition to be confused with trichotillomania but the smooth, sharply-marginated patches of hair loss with a positive gentle pull test contrasts significantly with trichotillomania. Exclamation mark hairs and nail changes are helpful when present. Tinea capitis can be ruled out with KOH examination or culture. The moth-eaten pattern of alopecia seen with secondary syphilis may mimic trichotillomania and serologic testing should be done if there is a history that

supports this or there is an associated pityriasis rosea-like rash on the trunk and extremities.

There are times when the diagnosis may not be obvious or it is important to have objective proof to convince parents and patients that pulling is taking place. A 4-mm punch biopsy from an affected area will show multiple catagen hairs, melanin casts, and dilated follicular ostia with keratin plugs. While awaiting the biopsy results, the family can ponder the possibility of the diagnosis of trichotillomania and may be more accepting by the time they are phoned with results.

Pathogenesis

It is well established that infants with trichotillomania do so as part of a habit or soothing behavior that self-resolves. Older children are far more complex. There are some features similar to obsessive-compulsive disorder but trichotillomania is more likely a behavior seen with a heterogeneous group of psychologic disorders, including depression, bipolar disorder, anxiety, body dysmorphic disorder, and substance abuse.

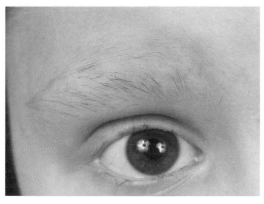

Figure 11-13 Trichotillomania. Eyebrows and eyelashes are being forcibly pulled. Note the differing lengths of regrowth

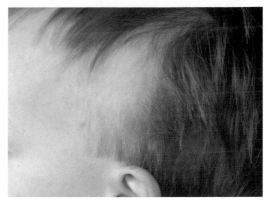

Figure 11-14 Temporal triangular alopecia. Isolated, lancet-shaped hair thinning

Treatment

Treatment of trichotillomania begins with establishing a trusting and empathic relationship with the family. The diagnosis must be presented in a nonjudgmental, nonaccusatory fashion in an unhurried setting that allows discussion and questions. Follow-up visits with extra time set aside may help. The compassion of a caring clinician has tremendous therapeutic effect.

Very young children do not need to be treated and families may simply need to be reassured about the eventual resolution of the problem. Petrolatum or other thick emollient creams may be used as aversion therapy to discourage habit twirling and pulling. A team approach is generally needed for older children. Referral to a psychologist or psychiatrist is necessary and may be facilitated by pointing out the other troubles that are invariably associated with the trichotillomania, such as school anxieties, family issues, or peer relations, which will benefit from a counselor's interception. No single intervention is consistently helpful for trichotillomania in older patients and treatments usually involve combinations of behavior modification techniques, relaxation, psychotherapy, and hypnosis. Pharmacotherapy such as the use of serotonin reuptake inhibitors may be helpful, although controlled studies are lacking and results are variable. Overall, the prognosis with any treatment is poor in the older age group.

Temporal Triangular Alopecia

Unilateral, frontotemporal, lancet-shaped or oval hair thinning (Figure 11-14) characterizes temporal triangular alopecia. About 20% of cases are bilateral. Despite the scarcity of reports, this is probably a fairly common and overlooked condition. It may be present at birth but parents generally first notice the thinning at about 2–4 years of age. Close scrutiny of old photographs demonstrates that the condition was present before becoming clinically obvious. The patch is well marginated and has a normal hair density when examined closely with a magnifying glass, but the majority of hairs are fine, vellus hairs. This observation along with the long-lasting, static nature of temporal triangular alopecia distinguishes this condition from alopecia areata. Biopsy will help confirm the diagnosis but is not necessary. Treatment with topical minoxidil should theoretically help this condition but most parents are happy with obtaining a diagnosis and reassurance.

Tinea Capitis

Dermatophyte infection of the scalp is discussed in detail in Chapter 2. Patches of alopecia are associated with pruritus, scaling, inflammation, broken hairs, and adenopathy (Figure 11-15). A KOH examination of dystrophic hairs will show innumerable fungal spores, but scale will not usually show hyphae. Culture is diagnostic but may take weeks to grow. *Trichophyton tonsurans* is the organism responsible for most cases of endemic tinea capitis seen in cities and *Microsporum canis* is obtained from infected dogs and cats. Treatment with griseofulvin oral suspension 25 mg/kg per day in two divided doses for 6–8 weeks is curative but longer courses are needed for *Microsporum*, perhaps as long as 4–5 months in some stubborn cases. Terbinafine, itraconazole, and fluconazole are alternative treatments.

Androgenetic Hair Loss

Key Points

- An underappreciated and common problem among adolescents
- May affect adolescent girls as well as boys
- Frontoparietal thinning or bitemporal recession in boys
- Christmas-tree pattern in girls
- Biopsy can help with the diagnosis
- Treat with 5% minoxidil solution in both sexes and finasteride 1 mg/day in boys only

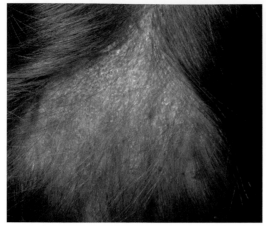

Figure 11-15 Tinea capitis. Scaling, broken hairs, and inflammation

About 15% of adolescent boys experience early male-pattern balding or androgenetic hair loss and young women can be affected too, at much greater loss of self-esteem. This can be a psychologically devastating condition that needs to be taken seriously and sympathetically by clinicians.

Clinical presentation

The onset of hair thinning is insidious, although some patients will relate a telogen effluvium-like shedding. Onset has been reported as early as 7 years of age, with mean age of onset in adolescents being about 15 years in boys and 14 years in girls. Most often there is a family history of androgenetic hair loss, although this is not invariably the case. Three patterns are noted in males: frontal scalp thinning, vertex thinning, and bitemporal recession (Figures 11-16 and 11-17). Any or all of these patterns may be observed simultaneously. Girls may be subtler. The thinning is usually over the frontal region with increased spacing between hairs and a widened central part. The pattern may resemble a Christmas tree pointing toward the vertex (Figure 11-18). The frontal hairline is usually maintained. There is decreased density and/or miniaturized, shorter, finer hairs.

Diagnosis

The history, family history, and examination will often lead to a clinical diagnosis, although differentiation from telogen effluvium and diffuse alopecia areata can be challenging. A 4-mm punch biopsy is invaluable in distinguishing these entities and can be helpful for the patient who cannot accept this unthinkable diagnosis.

Pathogenesis

Androgenetic alopecia results from the effect of normal androgen on a genetically suscep-tible hair follicle. Testosterone is converted to

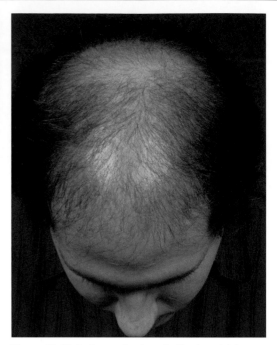

Figure 11-16 Androgenetic alopecia. Frontoparietal pattern

dihydrotestosterone (DHT) by 5α-reductase and DHT then activates the gene responsible for shortening the hair cycle and shrinking the hair follicle. Patterned hair loss is a polygenic trait inherited from either side of the family, not just the mother's side, as many believe.

Treatment

Minoxidil is a safe and reasonably effective topical agent that has stood the test of time in treating androgenic alopecia in men and women. It comes as a 2% and 5% solution, the 5% showing superior results in men, but at higher cost. Its mechanism of action is not known but the end result is to lengthen the anagen phase, resulting in longer, thicker, and more pigmented hair. As many as 50% may experience some regrowth while others may simply notice a cessation of loss. Clearly there are those who do not respond at all. Minoxidil is applied to a dry scalp twice daily, and it appears to be safe, although mild irritation and excessive facial hair growth have occasionally been reported.

Finasteride (Propecia) is an inhibitor of 5α-reductase that is taken as a 1-mg pill once daily. Results are superior to topical minoxidil, but side-effects consist of loss of libido (generally in abundance at this age), erectile dysfunction, and decreased volume of ejaculate. Women of child-bearing potential should not take finasteride because genital malformations in men could occur in male fetuses. Topical or systemic treatment needs to continue indefinitely as there is a rapid return to the genetically programmed baseline when stopped.

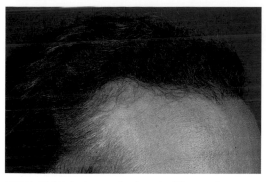

Figure 11-17 Androgenetic alopecia. Bitemporal recession pattern

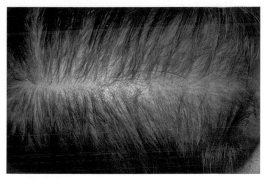

Figure 11-18 Female androgenetic alopecia. The part is widened and the thinning is most prominent anteriorly, tapering posteriorly – the so-called Christmas-tree pattern

Other Localized Alopecias

Traction alopecia is usually an obvious clinical diagnosis, seen most frequently when the hair is pulled into very tight braids (Figure 11-19). The hair loss is greatest at the outer edge of the braid where the most tension occurs. The prognosis is very good if caught before scarring occurs, but chronic, ongoing traction can lead to permanent scarring alopecia.

Postoperative pressure alopecia may occur after prolonged immobilization during and after surgical procedures and is generally seen in the setting of endotracheal intubation for open-heart surgery. Symptoms of pain, swelling, crusting, and ulceration may precede or occur concomitantly with the alopecia that comes days to weeks after the surgery. The vertex of the scalp, corresponding to the area of maximum pressure, is the most commonly affected area. Recovery occurs spontaneously in most cases but a permanent scarring alopecia may result.

The characteristic yellow-orange plaque of nevus sebaceus and the flesh-colored-to-brownish scar-like patch of aplasia cutis congenita (Chapter 9) make these two fairly common birthmarks an easy clinical diagnosis. Surgical excision is the treatment but aplasia cutis associated with a surrounding collar of long dark hair, a vascular stain, or an underlying nodule (generally with two of these three) should be imaged first to rule out heterotopic brain tissue with a central nervous system connection.

Telogen Effluvium

Key Points

- Diffuse hair loss 2–3 months after a stressor
- Clinical diagnosis
- Forcible pluck (trichogram) and biopsy are diagnostic
- If no obvious cause, look for scaling on scalp and check thyroid-stimulating hormone (TSH), iron saturation, and ferritin
- Spontaneous recovery is the rule

Clinical presentation

Telogen effluvium is a form of diffuse hair loss. Parents or patients will relate a marked increase in hairs obtained while combing and washing the hair, sometimes blocking the shower drain. Despite the impressive history, the patient may look entirely normal since about 10% of the entire scalp needs to be lost before thinning is appreciated. Gentle pull test may be positive, although not generally to the extent as seen in alopecia areata and, since patients have usually showered and groomed for their appointment, the loose hairs may have been removed prior to the physical exam. The absence of physical findings may lead clinicians to minimize the problem, an error that will quickly alienate very distressed parents.

Diagnosis

The diagnosis can usually be made by history and physical examination alone. A forcible pluck of 20–30 hairs will show greater than the usual 10% of telogen bulbs, characterized by a nonpigmented drumstick follicle without a root sheath, but this requires some experience and expertise in interpretation and is painful for the patient. A gentle pull of a hair tuft will extract 5 or more telogen hairs, and a 1-min combing will yield at least 10 telogen hairs. A 4-mm punch biopsy will demonstrate the increase in telogen hairs and help rule out the very difficult clinical diagnosis of diffuse alopecia areata, but this is only necessary in atypical cases.

Other causes of diffuse hair loss should be ruled out (Box 11-1) and a minimal work-up for diffuse hair loss should include a thorough review of systems, a complete medication history which includes all nonprescription and prescription products, and a careful examination for signs of psoriasis or seborrheic dermatitis on the scalp. Thyroid studies (TSH) and iron studies (saturation and ferritin) should be performed if no other obvious cause is found.

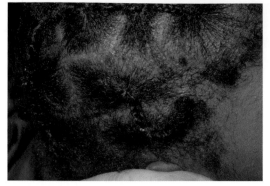

Figure 11-19 Traction alopecia. Hair pulled tightly into braids

Low ferritin is diagnostic of iron deficiency, but ferritin behaves as an acute-phase reactant, so can be paradoxically normal in some cases of iron deficiency.

Pathogenesis

The pathophysiology of telogen effluvium relates to a shift in the ratio of growing (anagen) hairs to resting (telogen) in response to some physical or severe emotional stressor such as a severe febrile illness, delivery of a baby, surgical procedure, crash diet, or death of a family member. It may take considerable probing to acquire a history of the event that probably occurred 2–4 months prior to the onset of hair loss. The conversion to a higher percentage of telogen hairs accompanying the stressor is then followed by recovery to the normal 9:1 anagen-to-telogen ratio, resulting in the resting hairs being shed by the new growing hairs. The paradox of telogen effluvium is that hair loss heralds growth and recovery, a piece of good news highly welcomed by the family.

Treatment

Recovery from telogen effluvium may take 6–12 months. In those who are predisposed to androgenetic (pattern) hair loss, the hair may never fully recover its previous fullness or texture. There is no treatment, and most parents are satisfied with reassurance as long as their concerns have been acknowledged, the child has been thoroughly examined, and the laboratory work-up is negative.

Loose-Anagen Syndrome

Key Points

- Young, blonde girls
- Scalp hair is thin and seldom needs to be cut
- Hair pulls out easily and painlessly
- Dystrophic anagen hairs are seen on trichogram
- Improves with age

BOX 11-1

Causes of diffuse hair thinning

Endocrinologic

Hyperthyroidism

Hypoparathyroidism

Hypopituitarism

Hypothyroidism

Malnutrition

Biotin deficiency

"Crash" dieting

Essential fatty acids deficiency

Iron deficiency

Protein/calorie malnutrition

Zinc deficiency

Medications (not inclusive)

Angiotensin-converting enzyme inhibitors – captopril, enalapril

Anticoagulants – warfarin, heparin

Anticonvulsants – phenytoin, valproic acid, carbamazepine

Beta-blockers

Birth control pills

Chemotherapeutic agents

Cimetidine

Lithium

Nonsteroidal anti-inflammatory drugs

Retinoids – isotretinoin, etretinate, vitamin A toxicity

Loose-anagen syndrome is characterized by easily extracted hairs and slow hair growth. It is probably far more common than the scarcity of reports would imply.

Clinical presentation

The stereotypical patient with loose-anagen syndrome is a young, blonde girl with short hair that will not grow long. Boys account for about 15% of cases but, without doubt, many are unrecognized and there is probably no significant difference between the incidence in males and females. Children with dark hair have been reported. Mean age of diagnosis is about 6 years. The scalp hair is diffusely thin and pulled clumps of hairs may give a patchy pattern of loss. The hair is often described as unmanageable, dry, lusterless, dull, matted, or sticky. Occasionally there is a positive family history; siblings and parents are often diagnosed only after the index patient has been evaluated.

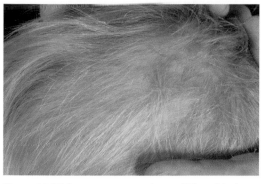

Figure 11-20 Loose-anagen syndrome. Diffuse thinning and patchy alopecia

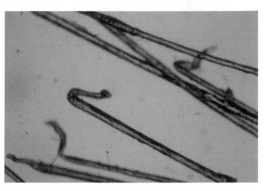

Figure 11-22 Loose-anagen hair. The bulb is bent like a fishhook and lacks an inner and outer root sheath

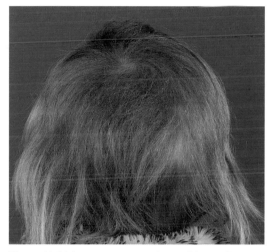

Figure 11-21 Loose-anagen syndrome. Frizzy, unkempt-looking hair at the occiput

On physical examination, the children have fine, thin hair with patchy or diffuse alopecia (Figure 11-20). Inability to comb the hair may give it an unkempt look. The hair in the occipital area of the scalp may be rough and tends not to lie flat (Figure 11-21). The forcible extraction of 20–30 hairs can be performed easily and remarkably painlessly but the shafts are neither fragile nor easily broken.

Three phenotypes have been described: children with sparse hair that does not grow long, children with diffuse or patchy unruly hair, and children with increased hair shedding. The presence of different phenotypes within the same family suggests that these clinical variations are genotypically related.

Diagnosis

The clinical picture is often enough to make the diagnosis. In particular, the absence of a pained reaction to forcible hair extraction is quite striking. The microscopic examination of the forcibly obtained hairs will show a predominance of dystrophic anagen hairs characterized by the absence of an inner and outer root sheath, distortion of the bulb that is usually bent in an obtuse angle like a fishhook (Figure 11-22) and ruffling of the cuticle, resembling a sagging leg warmer or rumpled stocking. About 60% of all children will have some loose anagen hairs so the finding is not specific, albeit very suggestive when these abnormal hairs dominate the trichogram. Biopsy is only helpful in ruling out telogen effluvium, trichotillomania, and alopecia areata.

Pathogenesis

The cause of loose-anagen syndrome is not known. It is believed to be a keratin disorder of the inner or outer root sheath that impairs adhesion. An autosomal-dominant inheritance pattern is suggested by reports of familial occurrence.

Treatment

There has been one report of improvement in some patients with minoxidil 5% solution, but most patients are not treated. The condition improves spontaneously with adolescence.

Disorders of Nails

Trachyonychia (Twenty-Nail Dystrophy)

Key Points

- Rough-surfaced nails
- May be one or all 20 nails
- Idiopathic process or associated with lichen planus, psoriasis, or alopecia areata
- Resolves over time

Trachyonychia refers to rough, dull, lusterless nails with a sandpaper-like surface (Figure 11-23). Pitting, distal chipping, longitudinal striations (onychorrhexis), and superficial splitting

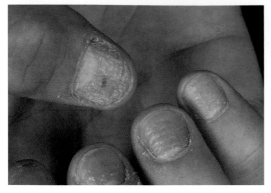

Figure 11-23 Trachyonychia (twenty-nail dystrophy). Rough, ridged nails with some pitting of the middle fingernail

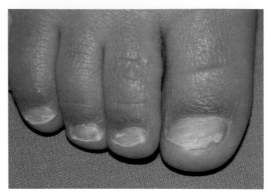

Figure 11-24 Beau's lines. Transverse groove on all toenails, most notable on the great toenail

(onychoschizia) may be seen. Any number of finger or toenails may be involved so the term "twenty-nail dystrophy" is a misnomer, albeit firmly ingrained in the medical literature. Onset is insidious, usually in a child 3–12 years of age. It is not usually symptomatic but may be a source of some embarrassment.

Trachyonychia usually occurs as an isolated finding but may be associated with lichen planus, alopecia areata, and psoriasis. A thorough examination of the skin, hair, teeth, and mucous membranes is warranted. A fungal culture or fungal staining of the nail plate will rule out the uncommon patient with onychomycosis, but no studies are routinely needed, except for a good physical examination.

Treatment for this condition is unsatisfying, although normalization of the nails over many years is the rule. Injections of triamcinolone (2.5–5 mg/ml) into the nail matrix are helpful but poorly tolerated and need to be done repetitively. Topical steroids applied to the proximal nail fold have some minimal effect and may induce atrophy of the soft tissue or premature closure of the underlying epiphysis if overused. Systemic therapy is certainly not warranted. Nail hardeners or a product with acetyl mandelic acid (DermaNail, Summers Laboratories) are sometimes helpful, and filing of the distal tips should be performed to prevent trauma to the nail.

Beau's Lines

Key Points

- Transverse groove in one or more nails
- Results from systemic illness or stressor
- Self-resolves

Transverse depressions or grooves occurring in one or more nails are called Beau's lines (Figure 11-24). They occur after temporary cessation of nail growth, characteristically after a significant illness, surgery, or trauma. It is somewhat analogous to

telogen effluvium in this respect. The time of the inciting event can be fairly well estimated by noting the location of the groove on the nail plate, knowing that the nail takes 4–6 months to grow from the proximal nail fold to the distal tip in children. No treatment is needed as the abnormal portion will grow out and disappear with time.

Ingrown Toenails

Key Points

- Foreign-body reaction to the nail piercing the lateral nail fold
- Remove a portion of the nail if conservative measures fail
- Phenol or surgical matrixectomy to prevent repetitive problems

Ingrown toenail (onychocryptosis) is a relatively common problem among teenagers, especially among those with chronic hyperhidrosis and those on isotretinoin for acne. The outside edge of the nail lacerates the lateral nail grove and enters the nail fold, inciting a foreign-body reaction and secondary infection. The inflammatory reaction results in pain, swelling, and abundant, heaped-up granulation tissue (Figure 11-25). Antibiotics against *Staphylococcus aureus*, warm soaks, and time may be enough to get patients through mild cases. Conservative procedures such as forcing a small wad of cotton under the nail, feeding dental floss under the nail, or trimming away a distal nail wedge are easy interventions that don't require anesthesia and may be effective if performed early. An advanced ingrown nail requires surgical removal. If a nail has been a repetitive problem, then matrixectomy should be performed so that the removed section of nail does not regrow. Chemical matrixectomy with phenol can be done easily and safely and is at least as successful in accomplishing permanent removal as surgical matrixectomy. A new treatment is to glue a flexible plastic strip to the nail that gently pulls up the sides of the nail as it grows out.

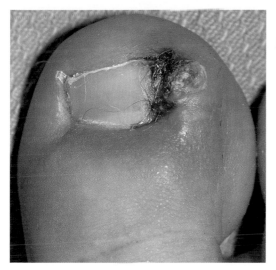

Figure 11-25 Ingrown toenail. Boggy erythema and heaped-up granulation tissue of the lateral nail fold

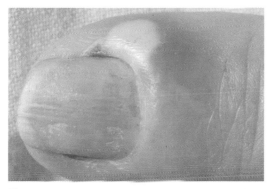

Figure 11-26 Acute paronychia. Erythema and a purulent pocket at the lateral nail fold

Paronychia

Key Points

- Acute paronychia is an infection with staphylococcal or streptococcal bacteria and needs appropriate antibiotics
- Chronic paronychia is multifactorial and responds best to topical steroids
- The inciting trauma to the nail and nail fold needs to be corrected

Paronychia, or inflammation of the soft tissue surrounding the nail unit, can be either acute or chronic. The acute form comes on quickly, leading to an exquisitely painful, red finger or toe tip. With time, a pustule will become visible but this may not be seen in the early stages (Figure 11-26). Surgical drainage with a number 11 scalpel blade will relieve some of the pressure and a culture of the lanced pustule will grow *Staphylococcus aureus*, *Streptococcus* or, much less

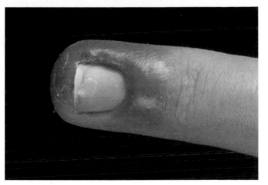

Figure 11-27 Chronic paronychia. Erythema and edema of the lateral nail folds and loss of the normal cuticle

frequently, *Pseudomonas*. Surgical drainage is the most important intervention, with antibiotics such as a cephalosporin or dicloxacillin serving an adjunctive role. In refractory cases, culture results should guide the choice of antibiotics.

Chronic paronychia is a more indolent, multifactorial process. Ongoing, low-grade irritant dermatitis, allergic contact dermatitis, trauma, manipulation of the cuticle, persistent contact with moisture such as sucking on fingers, chemical exposure, or underlying skin conditions such as eczema or psoriasis may contribute to chronic paronychia. Colonization with *Candida* species and many different bacteria contributes to the host inflammatory response. With time, the nail folds become boggy and erythematous (Figure 11-27).

The most important interventions include identifying and controlling the precipitating factors, especially limiting contact with moisture. Frequent applications of petrolatum or zinc oxide-containing emollients may act as an artificial cuticle until a new one can grow back and a thick wad of zinc oxide tends to discourage placing fingers in the mouth. Topical anticandidal agents, antibiotics, and drying agents such as thymol mixed as a 4% solution in alcohol will provide some relief but the best results are obtained with topical steroids. One- to 2-week courses of a superpotent steroid such as clobetasol, preferably in an ointment base, give results superior to anti-infective therapy. Intralesional injection of triamcinolone (2.5–5 mg/ml) is helpful in very difficult cases but is limited by pain.

Further reading

de Berker D. Childhood nail diseases. Dermatol Clin 2006;24:355–363.

Harrison S, Sinclair R. Telogen effluvium. Clin Dermatol 2002;27:389–395.

Hautmann G, Hercogova J, Lotti T. Trichotillomania. J Am Acad Dermatol 2002;46:807–821.

Madani S, Shapiro J. Alopecia areata update. J Am Acad Dermatol 2000;42:549–566.

Norris D. Alopecia areata: current state of knowledge. J Am Acad Dermatol 2004;51:S16–S17.

Price V. Androgenetic alopecia in adolescents. Cutis 2003;71:115–121.

Scheinfeld NS. Trachyonychia: a case report and review of manifestations, associations and treatments. Cutis 2003;71:299–302.

Tosti A. Loose anagen hair syndrome and loose anagen hair. Arch Dermatol 2002;138:521–522.

Tosti A, Peluso AM, Piraccini BM. Nail diseases in children. Adv Dermatol 1997;13:353–373.

Trakimas C, Sperling LC, Skelton HG, et al. Clinical and histologic findings in temporal triangular alopecia. J Am Acad Dermatol 1994;31:205–209.

Chapter 12

The skin in systemic disease

Howard B. Pride

Lupus Erythematosus

- Butterfly rash over cheeks and nose
- Discoid scaling plaques
- Annular, papulosquamous plaques in subacute lupus
- Mucous membrane lesions
- Biopsy diagnosis ± immunofluorescence
- Treat with topical steroids, oral hydroxychloroquine

Clinical presentation

Childhood systemic lupus erythematosus (SLE) occurs with a prevalence of about one case per 10 000 children per year, accounting for one-fifth of all cases. It is extremely rare under 5 years of age. SLE is most common among Native Americans and is more common and severe among those of African or Hispanic descent. Preadolescent children have a roughly equal sex ratio, but there is a distinct female predominance in postadolescent years. Children in general have a worse prognosis than adults.

Diagnostic criteria for SLE are listed in Box 12-1, and it is notable that mucocutaneous findings account for four of them. A mucocutaneous finding is present in 80–90% of childhood cases of SLE and is part of the presenting symptom complex 60–70% of the time. One of the most common and characteristic skin findings is the malar or butterfly rash. Erythema with a faint violaceous hue and scant scaling is noted on the cheeks and nose (Figure 12-1) but generally spares the nasolabial fold. Pustules, papules, and telangiectasia typical of rosacea are conspicuously absent.

Discoid lesions can be seen with negative lupus serologies and without systemic complications but will more typically be associated with SLE in children than adults. Lesions consist of

---

BOX 12-1

Diagnostic criteria for systemic lupus erythematosus*

Malar rash – butterfly distribution of mildly scaling erythema sparing the nasolabial fold and without papules, pustules, or telangiectasia

Discoid lesion – well-circumscribed, violaceous-to-erythematous plaques with adherent scale

Photosensitivity – pink, macular erythema in sun-exposed areas

Oral or nasal ulcerations

Arthritis – nonerosive, tender

Serositis – pleuritis or pericarditis

Renal disorder – proteinuria, casts

Neurologic disorder – seizures, psychosis

Hematological disorder – anemia, leukopenia (either lymphopenia or neutropenia), thrombocytopenia

Immunological disorder – anti-dsDNA, anti-Sm, antiphospholipid antibodies, false-positive test for syphilis

Positive antinuclear antibody

Hypocomplementemia – criterion added by the Pediatric Study Group of the Japanese Ministry of Health and Welfare

*Should have at least four of the criteria.

---

well-demarcated, violaceous-erythematous plaques with thick adherent scaling that plugs the follicular orifice (Figure 12-2). These follicular plugs resemble carpet tacks when attached to the removed scale. The face, scalp, and neck are the most common locations but they can be seen anywhere. Scarring, atrophy, hyperpigmentation, hypopigmentation (Figure 12-3), and alopecia may be permanent sequelae.

Subacute cutaneous lupus (SCLE) is much less common in children than adults. Scaling papules and plaques (papulosquamous lesions) develop suddenly

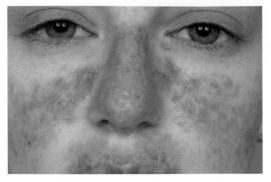

Figure 12-1 Systemic lupus erythematosus. Erythema with a faint violaceous hue noted on the cheeks and nose. Note whitening of the vermillion border of the upper lip

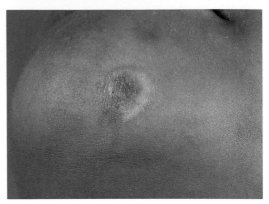

Figure 12-3 Discoid lupus. Scarring and hypopigmentation within a plaque on the chin

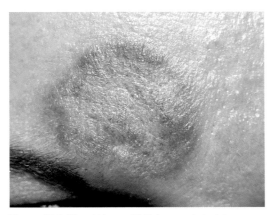

Figure 12-2 Discoid lupus. Well-demarcated, violaceous-erythematous plaque with thick adherent scaling

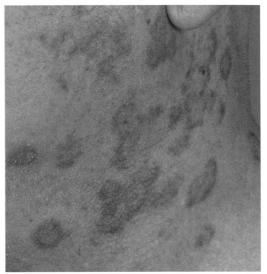

Figure 12-4 Subacute cutaneus lupus. Annular and polycyclic scaling plaques on the neck and face

on sun-exposed areas of the face (Figure 12-4), chest, back, arms, forearms, and hands. Annular and polycyclic plaques evolve from individual lesions. Resolution occurs without scarring.

Other skin findings, such as scarring and nonscarring alopecia, petechiae, nail fold telangiectasia, Raynaud's phenomenon, ice-pick digital infarcts, chilblains, livido reticularis, panniculitis (lupus profundus), urticaria, or urticarial vasculitis, are seen in SLE but are not part of the major diagnostic criteria. Mucous membranes may show oral aphthous ulcers, gingivitis, friability with hemorrhage, and vermillion border whitening (Figure 12-1).

Fever and arthralgia/arthritis are the most common systemic complaints in SLE. The arthritis is characteristically a very painful, symmetric, nondeforming polyarthritis of small and large joints. The most common systemic manifestations are renal, cardiac, neuropsychiatric, and hematologic disease.

Diagnosis

The diagnosis of SLE is based on meeting the diagnostic criteria in Box 12-1 and by obtaining confirmatory laboratory data. Skin biopsy can be very helpful and can be supplemented by direct immunofluorescence performed on lesional skin showing deposition of immunoglobulin, the so-called lupus band. Antinuclear antibody (ANA) is a highly sensitive, albeit nonspecific test for SLE, and a negative ANA all but rules out this diagnosis. The anti-ds DNA antibody is much more specific for SLE and correlates with the presence of renal disease but it is not as sensitive a test. The presence of anti-RNP antibodies is associated with a lower risk of renal disease and better prognosis. SCLE (fairly uncommon in childhood) will have positive anti-Ro and anti-La (SSA and SSB) antibodies, which tend to correlate with severe sun sensitivity. Complete blood count (CBC) with differential, erythrocyte sedimentation rate, blood urea nitrogen, creatinine, urinalysis, and complement levels should be checked in all patients.

Lupus can be a great mimicker so the differential diagnosis is wide. The facial lesions of acne/rosacea can be confused with the rash of SLE. However, papulopustules are not seen in SLE and the erythema of lupus (and dermatomyositis) tends to have a purplish hue. The acral lesions of dermatomyositis are characteristically on the knuckles whereas those of SLE are on the interphalangeal spaces. Lupus falls within the differential diagnosis of papulosquamous conditions (Chapter 2), polycyclic, annular lesions (Chapter 6), and scarring alopecias (Chapter 11). Biopsy is needed to make the correct diagnosis.

A number of medicines, particularly minocycline, can induce a lupus-like syndrome. Others include D-penicillamine, zafirlukast, isoniazid, hydralazine, procainamide, quinidine, chlorpromazine, sulfasalazine, and methyldopa.

Pathogenesis

Twin studies and family clustering suggest that SLE has some genetic (probably polygenic) predisposition for autoimmunity. This results in an attack on the cellular and nuclear structures of the body by the immune system, spurred by some environmental factor such as sex hormones, pregnancy, ultraviolet (UV) light, drugs, and/or infection.

Treatment

It is important to manage SLE with a multi-specialty team that includes a rheumatologist, nephrologists, and dermatologist. Sun avoidance is very important, and patients must be instructed to avoid peak times of sun exposure, wear protective clothing, and wear broad-spectrum sunscreens that block both UVB and UVA. Cutaneous lesions usually respond nicely to topical steroids or the nonsteroid agents tacrolimus/pimecrolimus. Generally high potencies are needed. Small or stubborn lesions can be treated with intralesional steroid injections. Hydroxychloroquine at a dose of 5 mg/kg per day is well tolerated and reasonably effective. Clofazimine, thalidomide, and retinoids are much less commonly used.

Oral prednisone is used to treat moderate to severe systemic disease, with intravenous pulses of methylprednisolone given for acute flares. Other immunosuppressive agents such as cyclophosphamide, azathioprine, mycophenolate mofetil, and methotrexate are reserved for more aggressive and unresponsive disease, particularly for lupus nephritis and central nervous system lupus.

Dermatomyositis

* Fatigue, pain, and proximal muscle weakness with elevated muscle enzymes

* Purplish papules on the knuckles, elbows, and knees
* Purplish discoloration and edema around the eyes
* Scalp dermatitis
* Treat with systemic corticosteroids

Clinical presentation

Juvenile dermatomyositis (JDM) is a rare inflammatory myopathy with about 2–4 new cases per million children per year. The mean age of onset is about 7 years, but the distribution is bimodal with peaks at 2–5 and 12–13 years of age. Girls outnumber boys by about 2:1. There is no racial predominance. Unlike adults, it is not associated with underlying malignancy.

One of the most characteristic cutaneous features of JDM is the appearance of purplish-red, slightly scaling plaques (Gottron's papules) on the extensor surfaces of the finger joints, elbows, and knees (Figure 12-5). Lesions are typically right on the knuckles (Figure 12-6), as opposed to lupus, where they tend to be in the interphalangeal spaces. Proximal nail fold erythema, capillary dilatation (Figure 12-7), capillary loop dropout, digital ulceration, and thickening of the margins of the palms with erythema (mechanic's hands) are other hand findings.

Periorbital purplish erythema, edema, and telangiectasia are found in 50–90% of affected children – the so-called heliotrope sign (Figure 12-8). This photosensitive rash may involve the nose and cheeks, prompting confusion with SLE. When present on the shoulders and upper trunk, it is referred to as the shawl sign. Scalp involvement (Figure 12-9) is common but often overlooked and consists of psoriasis or seborrhea-like scaling, atrophy, and alopecia.

Ulcerations and poikiloderma (atrophy, telangiectasia, hypopigmentation, hyperpigmentation) are late, chronic skin findings. Calcinosis

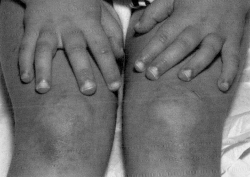
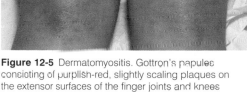

Figure 12-5 Dermatomyositis. Gottron's papules consisting of purplish-red, slightly scaling plaques on the extensor surfaces of the finger joints and knees.

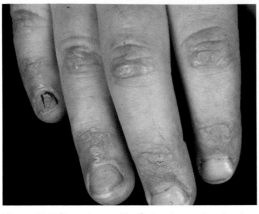

Figure 12-6 Dermatomyositis. Gottron's papules showing the typical location on the knuckles, as opposed to lupus where they are interphalangeal

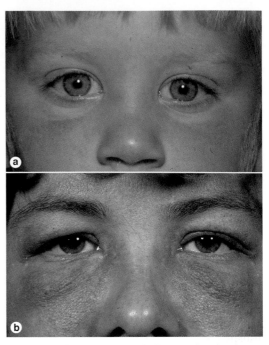

Figure 12-8 Dermatomyositis. Heliotrope sign showing purplish erythema, edema, and telangiectasia of the periorbital region and cheeks

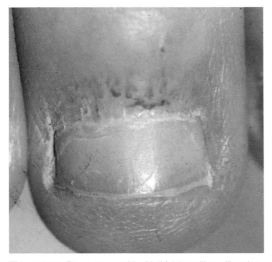

Figure 12-7 Dermatomyositis. Nail fold capillary dilatation and capillary loop dropout

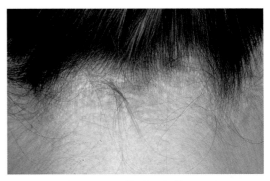

Figure 12-9 Dermatomyositis. Psoriasiform scalp dermatitis

(Figure 12-10) may develop and tends to be found on sites exposed to trauma such as the knees, elbows, and buttocks. It is highly correlated with the chronicity and severity of the disease. There is good evidence that the rapid initiation of aggressive therapy will eliminate this most vexing complication and highlights the need for establishing an early diagnosis. Other skin findings include panniculitis, lipodystrophy, acanthosis nigricans (AN), and erythroderma.

The myopathy of JDM typically involves the proximal muscles and may present as tenderness, stiffness, or weakness. Tasks such as walking up stairs, getting out of a chair, or bending to pick something up may become more difficult. Children seated on the floor can be observed bracing their hands against their legs to push themselves up from a sitting position. Myositis may be very subtle and only discovered after

laboratory work-up. It can develop after the skin signs have become well established, and rarely does not develop at all – the so-called amyopathic dermatomyositis. Other systemic problems can include fever, arthritis, gastrointestinal complaints, cardiac conduction defects, and respiratory compromise.

Diagnosis

A diagnosis of JDM can be established by the combination of the very typical rash in association with proximal muscle weakness and/or laboratory demonstration of muscle involvement. All five muscle enzymes should be checked (aspartate transaminase, alanine aminotransferase, lactate dehydrogenase, aldolase, and creatine kinase) to increase sensitivity. Magnetic resonance imaging,

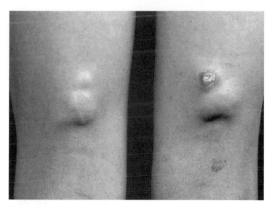

Figure 12-10: Dermatomyositis. Calcinosis cutis on the legs

usually of the hip and thigh musculature, has largely replaced painful electromyography and muscle biopsy as the definitive test for muscle involvement. ANA is frequently elevated but more specific serologies such as anti-Jo-1 are usually not.

The scalp and elbow rash of JDM is easily mistaken for psoriasis or seborrheic dermatitis. The facial rash can look like the eruption of SLE. Dermatitis, pityriasis rubra pilaris, sunburn, or other sun-induced eruption enter into the differential diagnosis. Skin biopsy will help rule out other skin diseases but is not usually necessary.

Pathogenesis

The pathophysiology of JDM probably relates to an immune-mediated vasculopathy leading to endothelial injury of the capillaries, venules, and small arteries of muscle, skin, and gastrointestinal tract. Narrowing of the vessel lumen leads to ischemic injury of the tissues.

Treatment

High-dose systemic corticosteroids are the mainstay of therapy for JDM. There is some evidence that monthly pulses of intravenous steroids (30 mg/kg per pulse of methylprednisolone) are more effective in preventing long-term sequelae such as calcinosis. Depending on the severity of the disease and the response to steroids, steroid-sparing agents such as methotrexate, cyclophosphamide, cyclosporine, azathioprine, and mycophenolate mofetil should be considered. Intravenous immunoglobulin and inhibitors of tumor necrosis factor (TNF)-α are other possible treatments.

The skin disease responds sluggishly to topical corticosteroids. Sun avoidance is very important as UV light exacerbates skin and muscle disease. Hydroxychloroquine, 5 mg/kg per day, is useful for recalcitrant cases.

Skin Signs of Inflammatory Bowel Disease

Key Points

- Mucocutaneous lesions can predate gastrointestinal disease
- Association with pyoderma gangrenosum (PG), erythema nodosum (EN), Sweet syndrome and aphthous ulcerations
- Oral lesions of cobblestoning, nodules, angular cheilitis, diffuse lip swelling, gingival hyperplasia, and pyostomatitis vegetans
- Contiguous or metastatic dusky, red nodules that form ulcers, fistulae, and sinus tracts
- Biopsy shows granulomatous inflammation

Clinical presentation

Inflammatory bowel disease (IBD) involves chronic inflammation of the gastrointestinal tract in the absence of an infectious cause. Varieties include Crohn's disease (CD), ulcerative colitis (UC), and indeterminate types. All forms are more common in adults but about one-third of cases begin before 20 years of age. The annual incidence is about 3–6 cases per 100 000, with CD being more common than UC and with a slight predominance of boys.

Mucocutaneous involvement with IBD may be related to direct or metastatic extension of the underlying disease (particularly CD), a manifestation of associated nutritional disorder, or a nonspecific inflammatory reaction pattern, usually PG or EN (discussed below), but also Sweet syndrome and aphthous ulcerations (Chapter 6). Vesiculopustular eruptions, seen in both CD and UC, may represent a variant of PG. Clubbing of the digits has been observed in IBD, most commonly with CD.

Pyostomatitis vegetans is seen in both forms of IBD and consists of oral erythema, edema, pustules, ulcerations, and vegetating papilloma-like projections. It is a highly specific marker for IBD. CD may have other oral manifestations, including cobblestoning, nodules, angular cheilitis, diffuse lip swelling, and gingival hyperplasia.

Cutaneous CD is a rare occurrence and is a challenging dilemma in the 20% of patients whose skin manifestations precede the diagnosis of their bowel disease. Perianal and perineal lesions are most common and usually appear in the setting of colorectal CD. Erythema, swelling, and a dusky cyanotic discoloration (Figure 12-11) herald the more advanced lesions, consisting of infiltrative plaques, erosions, ulcers, draining sinuses, fistulae, and scarring (Figure 12-12). Edematous, polypoid, tag-like projections are characteristic of perianal CD (Figure 12-13) and may be mistaken for a skin tag, condyloma acuminatum, or condyloma latum.

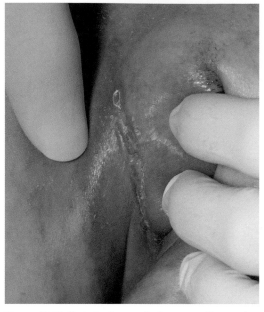

Figure 12-11 Crohn's disease. Erythema, swelling, and a dusky cyanotic discoloration in early cutaneous disease

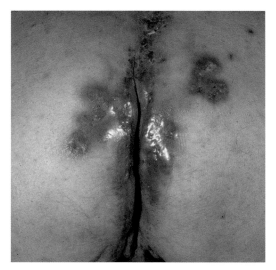

Figure 12-12 Crohn's disease. Infiltrative plaques, erosions, ulcers, draining sinuses, fistulae, and scarring of more advanced disease

Metastatic CD is the term used for cutaneous lesions that are not directly contiguous with the bowel disease. The abdomen and lower extremities are the most common locations. Lesions are dusky, red papules and nodules that ulcerate (Figure 12-14).

Diagnosis

A skin biopsy showing a granulomatous infiltrate, corroborated with appropriate bowel work-up, will confirm the diagnosis of IBD. The differential diagnosis of perianal disease includes warts,

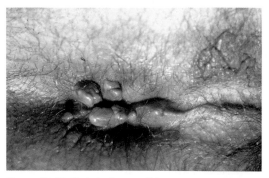

Figure 12-13 Crohn's disease. Edematous, polypoid, tag-like projections

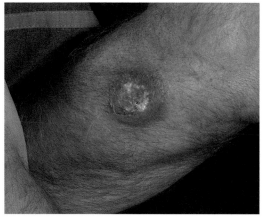

Figure 12-14 Crohn's disease. Metastatic lesion consisting of a dusky, red nodule on the arm

skin tags, perianal pyramidal protrusion, erosive diaper dermatitis, Langerhans cell histiocytosis, Behçet disease, hidradenitis suppurativa, peri-orificial dermatitis, child abuse, and infections such as perianal streptococcal disease. Cheilitis granulomatosa (Melkersson–Rosenthal syndrome when accompanied by facial swelling and furrowed tongue) is characterized by lip edema that looks just like CD.

Pathogenesis

It is believed that IBD is an autoimmune phenomenon with a genetic predisposition. Some environmental trigger, possibly pathogenic or commensal bacteria or other antigenic stimulus, may kindle an aberrant inflammatory response.

Treatment

Oral sulfasalazine or 5-aminosalicylic acid medications (mesalamine, olsalazine, and balsalazide) form the first-line agents for mild IBD. More severe disease may warrant intravenous corticosteroids and parenteral nutrition. Immunosuppressive therapy with 6-mercaptopurine or azathioprine may be needed for severe, unresponsive disease. The newer biologic agents that block the effect of TNF-α have been very effective.

Mucocutaneous disease might respond to systemic treatment of the bowel disease, but topical and intralesional steroids, topical tacrolimus, and oral metronidazole can be used for resistant lesions.

Pyoderma Gangrenosum

Key Points

- Purulent, boggy ulcers with undermined inflammatory margins
- IBD, arthritis, and leukemia lead a long list of possible causes
- Treat with prednisone and other immunosuppressive medications

Clinical presentation

PG begins as a small papule or pustule (Figure 12-15) that evolves into an enlarging necrotic ulcer with a yellow-white, purulent, boggy, soupy base and irregular, dusky, violaceous, undermined borders (Figure 12-16). Ulcers typically appear on the legs, but children also tend to have facial, groin, and mucous membrane involvement. The painful ulcers may be preceded by trauma, the phenomenon known as pathergy, so debridement should be avoided. Bullous, pustular, vegetative, ulcerative, and vesiculopustular varieties have been described. Healing occurs with cribriform scarring.

PG occurs in the setting of a number of underlying conditions (Box 12-2). IBD, inflammatory arthritis, and leukemia stand out in the pediatric age group. Many cases are idiopathic.

Diagnosis

The clinical appearance is usually enough to make an accurate diagnosis. Biopsy may be considered to rule out other entities in the differential diagnosis, PG being a diagnosis of exclusion. In particular, tissue biopsy for cultures of bacteria, deep fungi, and atypical mycobacteria is important, especially in immunosuppressed children. The differential diagnosis includes spider bite, vasculitis, and factitial disease.

A thorough review of systems, physical exam, laboratory work-up and, possibly, specialty referral are needed to identify primary causes of PG. A minimum of a CBC, peripheral smear, sedimentation rate, and ANA should be checked with other tests determined by history or physical exam findings.

Pathogenesis

PG is a neutrophilic, reactive inflammatory process of unknown cause.

Treatment

Treatment is geared toward correcting any identifiable underlying cause. Systemic therapy with corticosteroids, dapsone, minocycline, cyclosporine, or other immunosuppressive agents is usually needed to control PG. Intralesional steroids are effective for small or localized lesions. Topical tacrolimus might be partially effective in some but topical therapy is not usually very helpful. Biologic agents that block TNF have been effective in some patients, especially those with IBD. Minimizing trauma, wound manipulation, or debridement is important.

Erythema Nodosum

Key Points

- Tender, ill-defined nodules on the pretibial area
- Many causes but β-hemolytic streptococcus is most common
- Treat with rest, nonsteroidal anti-inflammatory drugs (NSAIDs) and saturated solution of potassium iodide (SSKI)

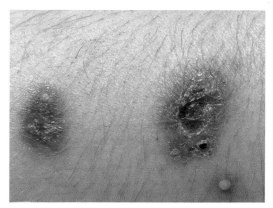

Figure 12-15 Pyoderma gangrenosum. Early evolving nodules and pustules

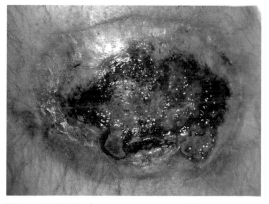

Figure 12-16 Pyoderma gangrenosum. Fully evolved ulcer with necrotic base and inflamed, undermined borders

BOX 12-2

Diseases associated with pyoderma gangrenosum

Inflammatory bowel disease

Hematologic disease

Leukemia

Lymphoma

Gammopathies

Polycythemia vera

Autoinflammatory conditions

Hidradenitis suppurativa

Acne conglobata

SAPHO (synovitis, acne, pustulosis, hyperostosis, osteitis)

PFAPA (periodic fever, adenitis, pharyngitis, aphthous ulcers)

Collagen vascular disease

Juvenile idiopathic arthritis

Lupus erythematosus

Takayasu's arteritis

Wegener's granulomatosis

Immunodeficiency

Sarcoidosis

Behçet's disease

Diabetes mellitus

Internal malignancy

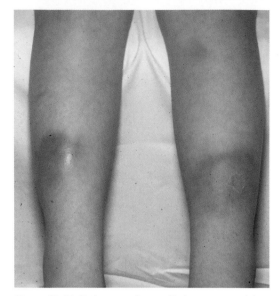

Figure 12-17 Erythema nodosum. Erythematous nodules with ill-defined, irregular borders on the pretibial region

Clinical presentation

EN presents with painful, bruise-like, erythematous, 1–6-cm nodules with ill-defined, irregular borders found most commonly on the legs, particularly the pretibial area (Figure 12-17). It can be seen in any age but is more common in teenagers and is rarely seen prior to 2 years of age. Female predominance occurs only in adolescence and adulthood. The legs are the classic location but thighs, trunk, and upper extremities may be involved. The course tends to be self-limited with most cases resolving in about 2 weeks, but chronicity tends to parallel the underlying cause.

Diagnosis

Most cases of classic EN can be diagnosed clinically. Biopsy is diagnostic but since EN is a panniculitis (an inflammatory condition of the fat), a good piece of subcutaneous fat is needed to confirm the diagnosis. A 4-mm punch biopsy may be adequate if it is pushed to the hub and pointed scissors are used in such a way to ensure that fat is obtained with the plug. A drill-like power punch or excisional specimen will yield a more generous degree of fat but is also more invasive. Pathology shows a septal panniculitis.

The differential diagnosis of EN includes trauma (battered child), vasculitis (Henoch–Schönlein purpura, polyarteritis nodosa), cellulitis, subcutaneous granuloma annulare, and other forms of panniculitis such as lupus. Recurrent palmoplantar hidradenitis is characterized by deep, painful nodules of the soles and, less frequently, the palms. It has been labeled as EN but is probably a distinct entity with a primarily neutrophilic abscess-like infiltrate centered on eccrine glands. Streptococcal and pseudomonal infections (*Pseudomonas* hot-foot syndrome) have been reported in some cases of palmoplantar hidradenitis.

In some respects, EN is like urticaria in that it represents an inflammatory response to some stimulus (Box 12-3). The challenge is finding the underlying cause so the review of systems, examination, and work-up are directed towards diagnosing these entities. Streptococcal disease, especially pharyngitis, is the most common cause and may account for nearly 50% of childhood cases. An ASO titer and/or streptococcus culture should be done. Other tests can be directed by symptoms, but a chest X-ray, stool culture, sedimentation rate, purified protein derivative, and mycoplasma titers could be considered in almost everyone.

Entities that may cause erythema nodosum

Infections

β-Hemolytic streptococcus (most common cause)

Mycoplasma pneumoniae

Viral upper respiratory infections

Coccidiomycosis

Histoplasmosis

Yersinia enterocolitica

Leptospira

Pseudomonas species

Mycobacterium tuberculosis

Others rarely reported

Malignancy

Hodgkin disease

Sarcoidosis

Inflammatory bowel disease

Behçet disease

Pregnancy

Medications

Oral contraceptives

Sulfonamides

Idiopathic (25–50%) of cases

Pathogenesis

EN is a reactive panniculitis with various underlying causes.

Treatment

The first line of treatment of EN is bedrest and limitation of vigorous activity. Medical treatment is geared toward the causative agent, particularly treating underlying streptococcal infections. Painful EN can usually be managed with NSAIDs until the lesions self-resolve. SSKI is a safe, albeit unpleasant, treatment for more severe or chronic cases. Dosing is 5 drops t.i.d., slowly increasing to 10 drops t.i.d. Intralesional or systemic steroids work well but are not generally needed.

Kawasaki Disease

* High fevers not responding to antipyretics
* Cervical adenopathy

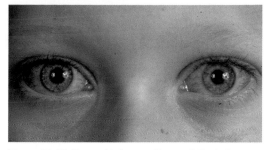

Figure 12-18 Kawasaki disease. Nonexudative bulbar conjunctival injection with a rim of sparing immediately around the iris

* Oral involvement, conjunctival injection, polymorphous cutaneous eruption, edematous, red hands and feet
* Coronary artery aneurysms
* Treat with intravenous immunoglobulin and aspirin

Clinical presentation

Kawasaki disease (KD) is a vasculitic syndrome of young children that may result in coronary artery aneurysms and/or occlusion, myocardial infarction, and death. Peak incidence is in children 2 years of age or younger, with almost all cases being younger than 5 years. Boys outnumber girls, and it is most common in Japan and among those of Japanese heritage.

KD begins with the abrupt onset of fever, usually greater than 39°C, which does not respond to antipyretic agents and lasts at least 1–2 weeks. Children tend to be irritable out of proportion to the severity of the fever.

Bilateral, nonexudative bulbar conjunctival injection (Figure 12-18) follows the fever and is one of the more characteristic features of KD. There may be a rim of sparing immediately around the iris, which can be a helpful sign. Oral mucous membrane involvement is characterized by red, cracked lips (Figure 12-19), strawberry tongue, and injected, red pharynx. Cervical lymphadenopathy of at least 1.5 cm in size may be seen but is the least common of the major diagnostic criteria. Generalized lymphadenopathy is not seen.

The rash of KD is polymorphous and nonspecific, variably described as scarlatiniform, erythema multiforme-like, urticarial, morbilliform, or erythrodermic. An interesting and important aspect of the KD rash is that perineal or diaper-area erythema (Figure 12-20) and desquamation can be an early and frequent finding, occurring in up to 60–70% of affected children. Nonpitting edema of the hands and feet with bright red palms and soles is later replaced by a fine desquamation beginning in the periungual area (Figure 12-21). Peripheral gangrene is a rare complication of KD. Vesicles, suggestive of

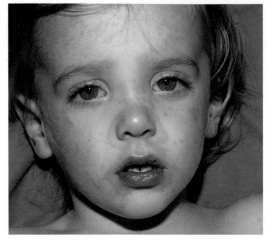

Figure 12-19 Kawasaki disease. Red, cracked lips and conjunctival injection

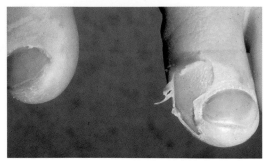

Figure 12-21 Kawasaki disease. Fine desquamation beginning in the periungual area is a late finding

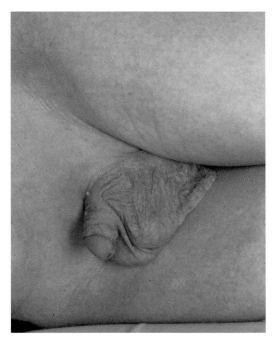

Figure 12-20 Kawasaki disease. Erythema in the "diaper region," a characteristic and helpful diagnostic sign

a viral illness or autoimmune blistering disease, and purpura, suggestive of a leukocytoclastic vasculitis, are not seen in the skin.

The most dreaded complication of KD is involvement of the coronary arteries with resultant aneurysms in about 15% of cases. Generally these regress with time but thrombosis can lead to myocardial infarction and death. Myocarditis, arrhythmias, and valvular dysfunction can occur. Other systemic complications include hydrops of the gallbladder, hepatic dysfunction, gastrointestinal problems, arthritis, sterile pyuria, and aseptic meningitis.

Diagnosis

There are no specific tests for KD so clinical criteria have been established to aid in diagnosis (Box 12-4). Fever of at least 5 days' duration must be accompanied by four of the five clinical signs of conjunctival injection, cervical adenopathy, rash, oral mucous membrane findings, and changes in the extremities. Not all children with KD fulfill these criteria and are labeled as incomplete or atypical KD. Diagnosis in these cases requires a great deal of clinical judgment and having adequately ruled out other entities in the differential diagnosis. Nonspecific but supporting laboratory studies include elevated C-reactive protein, sterile pyuria, thrombocytosis, hypoalbuminemia, and elevated transaminases. Skin biopsy is not helpful unless to rule out other skin disorders.

The differential diagnosis of KD includes inflammatory diseases such as Stevens–Johnson syndrome, toxic epidermal necrolysis, juvenile rheumatoid arthritis, and polyarteritis nodosa, and infectious processes such as scarlet fever, toxic shock syndrome, Rocky Mountain spotted fever, meningococcemia, hand, foot, and mouth disease, Epstein–Barr virus infection, fifth disease, and measles.

Pathogenesis

The pathogenesis of KD is unknown. Several factors point to an infectious etiology, including the scarcity of patients under 3 months of age or older than 5 years of age suggesting immunity to some agent, the clustering of cases in winter and early spring, and local epidemic outbreaks. There may be a genetic susceptibility since there is an increased risk in siblings of patients with KD and it is more common in Japanese children. The leading theory implicates a superantigen immune response to some – as yet unidentified – infectious agent.

Treatment

Children with KD should be hospitalized and cared for in an experienced pediatric unit. Intravenous immunoglobulin therapy given as

Diagnostic criteria of Kawasaki disease

Fever for 5 or more days, usually greater than 39°C

At least four of these five clinical features:

Bilateral, nonpurulent, bulbar conjunctival injection

Unilateral, cervical, nonfluctuant adenopathy greater than 1.5 cm in size

Polymorphous rash, particularly perineal

Oral mucous membrane changes – red, fissured lips, strawberry tongue, red pharynx

Hand and feet changes – erythema and swelling acutely, periungual desquamation 14–21 days

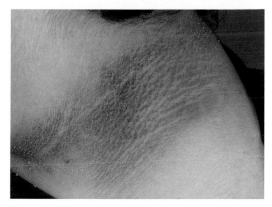

Figure 12-22 Acanthosis nigricans

a single 2 mg/kg dose should be started as soon as the diagnosis is established. Aspirin therapy is started at 80–100 mg/kg per day for 14 days and is decreased to 3–5 mg/kg per day thereafter. The use of pulse steroids is controversial and is not routinely advocated. There may be some role for inhibitors of TNF-α.

Acanthosis Nigricans

Key Points

- Velvety hyperpigmentation of the axillae and lateral neck folds
- Associated with hyperinsulinism
- No effective treatment exists

Clinical presentation

Velvety thickening and hyperpigmentation of the skin folds of the axillae and lateral neck characterize AN (Figure 12-22). Skin tag-like papules may be present. The brachial fossae, elbows, dorsal hands (Figure 12-23), knuckles, and inframammary regions may also be involved. African and Native American children have a particularly high incidence, although all races are represented. Most affected children are obese. Insulin resistance and a genetic tendency toward type 2 diabetes mellitus are the norm.

Other endocrinologic disorders such as hypothyroidism and genetic syndromes such as Crouzon syndrome have been reported to have AN but these associations make up a very small fraction of children with this condition. Underlying malignancy, particularly gastric carcinoma, has been reported in adults with AN, but this is extremely rare in childhood.

Diagnosis

AN is an easy clinic diagnosis. Retained keratin and confluent and reticulated papillomatosis (Chapter 7) may pose a diagnostic challenge. Biopsy is seldom needed. Fasting glucose levels are normal but insulin levels will usually be high. Work-up for the very rare associations of AN is not routinely necessary.

Pathogenesis

Obesity and insulin resistance are strongly correlated with AN, although the exact mechanism for the skin manifestation is not known. It is theorized that insulin acts as an epidermal growth factor.

Treatment

There is no effective treatment for AN. Weight loss is the optimal intervention but this is seldom achieved. Children should be counseled regarding their risk for adult-onset diabetes and consultation with a nutritionist may be helpful. Keratolytic agents such as 12% ammonium lactate cream offer modest help. Alcohol on a cotton ball may remove keratin debris that accumulates in the thickened grooves of the skin, lightening some of the dark color.

Hyperhidrosis

Key Points

- Almost always idiopathic but may rarely be from a secondary medical condition
- Treat with aluminum salts, iontophoresis, anticholinergic agents, botulinum toxin, or surgical interventions

Clinical presentation

Hyperhidrosis refers to localized or generalized sweating that exceeds the need to maintain thermal regulation. About 2–3% of the population suffers from this condition. The vast majority of pediatric patients with hyperhidrosis are otherwise completely well and may simply represent the far spectrum of normal. A number of medical conditions and/or medications may be the underlying cause of hyperhidrosis (Box 12-5), so the clinician must be aware that sweating can

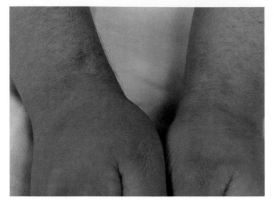

Figure 12-23 Acanthosis nigricans

be a manifestation of internal disease in a very small subset of patients.

Most cases of hyperhidrosis begin in childhood and adolescence, and sweating can range from a focal nuisance to extreme debility. The chief complaint may involve the social stigma of clammy hands or saturated armpits, but work and school may be hampered by inability to write or hold tools. It may worsen with stress and heat but these are not required to produce excessive sweating. Examination reveals moist skin, sometimes with noticeable faucet-like dripping. Socks and shirts may be damp.

An interesting variant of hyperhidrosis is *Frey syndrome*. This consists of an erythematous flush of the cheek with focal hyperhidrosis after gustatory or olfactory stimulation. It may result from a congenital cross-wiring of the seventh and eighth cranial nerves or from nerve damage after trauma or surgery. It is easily mistaken for food allergy.

Diagnosis

Starch iodine testing nicely demonstrates areas of focal hyperhidrosis but is not readily available in most clinics and is seldom necessary. A quick inspection of palms, soles, axillae, and face is all that is needed to confirm the diagnosis. A thorough review of systems and drug history is necessary to rule out the entities listed in Box 12-5. Laboratory work-up or specialty referral is only needed if one of these conditions is suspected.

Pathogenesis

Three million eccrine sweat glands are distributed over the entire body and they are innervated by the cholinergic fibers of the sympathetic nervous system. No abnormalities of the sweat glands can be detected histologically and hyperhidrosis may result from a complex dysfunction of the autonomic nervous system. Genetics may play a role, as 30–50% of patients report a family history of hyperhidrosis.

BOX 12-5

Causes of hyperhidrosis

Endocrinologic disorders

Hyperthyroidism

Hyperpituitarism

Diabetes mellitus

Diabetes insipidus

Pregnancy

Pheochromocytoma

Carcinoid syndrome

Acromegaly

Neurologic disorders

Head trauma

Hydrocephalus

Spinal cord injury

Cerebrovascular accident

Malignancy

Myeloproliferative disorders

Hodgkin disease

Central nervous system tumors

Castleman disease

Chronic infections

Tuberculosis

Brucellosis

Medication

Tricyclic antidepressants

Selective serotonin reuptake inhibitors

Acyclovir

Opioid analgesics

Alcohol and drug abuse or withdrawal

Pesticides

Dermatologic conditions

Eccrine nevus

Eccrine angiomatous hamartoma

Blue rubber bleb nevus syndrome

Glomus tumor

Treatment

A treatment algorithm is given in Table 12-1. Most patients can be managed nicely with topical use of aluminum salts such as aluminum chloride. Commercial preparations come in various strengths (Drysol 20%, Maxim 15%, Certain

Table 12-1 Treatment algorithm for hyperhidrosis

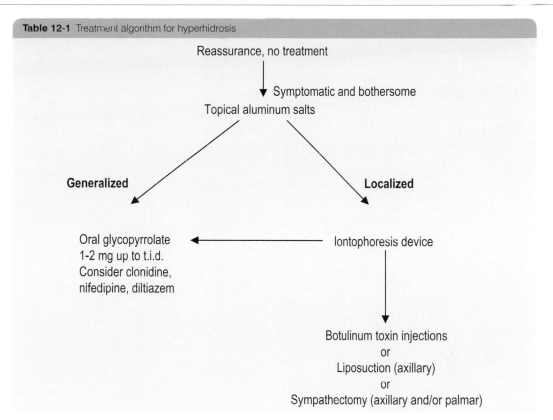

Dri 12.5%, Xerac AC 6.25%). A pharmacy can mix a 30% solution in water that might work better than the commercial products. Higher concentrations may cause irritation in the axillae. The solutions are applied daily until the desired level of dryness is achieved and then tapered until sweating recurs. Some patients can manage nicely with just weekly or twice-weekly application. Formaldehyde and glutaraldehyde may help with sweating but can cause contact sensitization and should be avoided.

Iontophoresis involves the use of an electrical current delivered through tap water. The ions that are generated are thought to cause a hyperkeratotic plug in the sweat gland pore, although the exact mechanism of action is not known. It is inconvenient but appears safe and reasonably effective. One device, the Drionic, can be purchased though www.drionic.com. A more sophisticated unit, the Fischer galvanic generator, may be beyond many patients' price range. The addition of glycopyrrolate to the solution may significantly increase the effectiveness of iontophoresis.

There is a jump in side-effects, price, and invasiveness once the first lines of treatment have failed. Oral anticholinergic treatment with glycopyrrolate (Robinul), 1–2 mg up to 3 times daily, is a good choice for generalized sweating or for significant focal sweating not controlled by the above treatments. Side-effects include dry mouth,

drowsiness, blurred vision, dizziness, constipation, nausea, loss of taste, headache, difficulty sleeping, and nervousness. Clonidine, nifedipine, and diltiazem have been used with some reported success but lower safety profile.

Injection of botulinum toxin has been highly successful when used in focal areas, particularly the axillae, for which it is approved by the Food and Drug Administration. Its use is limited by painful needle pokes and high expense. Remissions last for 9–12 months.

Surgical excision of focally bothersome axillae skin or liposuction of the axillary vault can be carried out with some success. Transthoracic, endoscopic sympathectomy is an invasive but effective means of curing debilitating palmar or axillary hyperhidrosis. It should be reserved for extreme cases. Most procedures are done without complication but compensatory hyperhidrosis elsewhere, especially the face, is a vexing sequela in some.

Further reading

Buka RL, Cunningham BB. Connective tissue disease in children. Pediatr Ann 2005;34:225–238.

Burns JC. Kawasaki disease. Adv Pediatr 2001; 48:157–177.

Crowson AN, Mihm MC, Magro C. Pyoderma gangrenosum: a review. J Cutan Pathol 2003; 30:97–107.

Eisenach JH, Atkinson JLD, Fealey RD. Hyperhidrosis: evolving therapies for a well-established phenomenon. Mayo Clin Proc 2005; 80:657–666.

Furukawa F, Hiroi A. Collagen diseases in children. Clin Dermatol 2000;18:725–733.

Gottlieb BS, Ilowite NT. Systemic lupus erythematosus in children and adolescents. Pediatr Rev 2006;27:323–329.

Haidir A, Solish N. Focal hyperhidrosis: diagnosis and management. CMAJ 2005;172:69–75.

Kakourou T, Drosatou P, Psychou F, et al. Erythema nodosum in children: a prospective study. J Am Acad Dermatol 2001;44:17–21.

Kethu SR. Extraintestinal manifestations of inflammatory bowel disease. J Clin Gastroenterol 2006;40:467–475.

Labbé L, Perel Y, Maleville J, et al. Erythema nodosum in children: a study of 27 patients. Pediatr Dermatol 1996;13:447–450.

Ploysangam T, Heubi JE, Eisen D, et al. Cutaneous Crohn's disease in children. J Am Acad Dermatol 1997;36:697–704.

Rennebohm R. Juvenile dermatomyositis. Pediatr Ann 2002;31:426–433.

Schwartz RA. Acanthosis nigricans. J Am Acad Dermatol 1994;31:1–19.